MediSin

The Causes & Solutions to Disease, Malnutrition And The Medical Sins That Are Killing the World

by Dr. Scott Whitaker, ND & José Fleming, CN, MH

Highly Recommended by Dick Gregory

This book is designed to provide accurate and authoritative information in regard to the subject matter covered. It is sold with the understanding that the publisher is not engaged in rendering medical or related professional services and that without personal consultantation the authors cannot and do not render judgement or advice about a particular patient or medical condition. If medical advice is required, the services of a competent professional should be sought. While every attempt has been made to provide accurate information, the author and publisher cannot be held responsible for any errors or omissions. There is no guarantee of disease prevention or survival.

Divine Protection Publications DPP
P.O. Box 36126 Hoover, AL 35236
1-888-MEDISIN
divineprotectionpublications@hotmail.com

2nd printing, July 2005
3rd printing, January 2006
4rd printing, July 2006
5th printing, October 2006
Revision, February 2007
2nd Revision, June 2010

Printed in the United States of America

Library of Congress Number 2005901519

ISBN 0972035222
Divine Protection Publications DPP

TABLE OF CONTENTS

FOREWORD

"MediSin", a book long overdue! I found it extremely informative & thought provoking. This book consists of over ten years of careful investigative research. Guaranteed to present every reader with a well-balanced understanding of natural medicine & allopathic medicine. The two writers use medical evidence as a basis to boldly testify before the American public, the criminal assault being inflicted on the masses in the name of health care.

Do you really know the effects of the chemicals in the foods that you're eating? Did you know that your lack of awareness about the connection between the pharmaceutical industry and those who govern Agribusiness are at the core of most common illnesses? Yes, this book uncovers the conspiracy of the Medical Industry, while at the same time guiding its readers back to a pathway of sound health.

Not only after reviewing the text of this writing, I have known these two men and about their works across the country for the last ten years. For 2 1⁄2 years I worked personally with Master Herbalist Jose Fleming, first hand. You taught me well, thank you! Doctor Scott Whitaker's work speaks for itself, his travels to Southeast Asia & the Orient for the gain of enlightenment in the arena of natural medicine has benefited thousands who are blessed to come into contact with him.

To the best of my knowledge, never before have two individuals of this magnitude collaborated non-selfishly on this subject. Far too long has the public suffered from the tragic side effects of western conventional MediSin, due to the fact that the general public has not been aware of the rarely revealed truth that lies within the pages of this book. With well regards, and wishes of enlightenment to these two dynamic gentlemen; keep up the good work.

Alvin Morrow, Author of Breaking the Curse of Willie Lynch, and inventor of "The Original Green Tea Tonic"

IN THE BEGINNING...

In the beginning, God populated the earth with broccoli, cauliflower, spinach, green, yellow and red vegetables of all kinds, so Man and Woman would live long and healthy lives.

Then using God's great gifts, Satan created commercial dairy and doughnuts... And Satan said, "You want chocolate with that?" And Man said "Yea." And Woman said, "add another one with sprinkles." And they gained 10 pounds.

And God created healthful yogurt that Woman might keep the figure that Man found so fair. And Satan brought forth white flour from wheat, and sugar from the cane, and combined them. And Woman went from size 2 to size 16.

So God said, "Try my fresh green salad" and Satan presented thousand-island dressing and garlic toast on the side. And Man and Woman unfastened their belts following the repast.

God then said, "I have sent you heart healthy vegetables and olive oil in which to cook them." And Satan brought forth deep fried fish and chicken-fried steak so big it needed its own platter. And man gained more weight and his cholesterol went through the roof.

God then brought running shoes so that his children might lose those extra pounds. And Satan gave cable TV with a remote control so Man would not have to toil changing the channels. And Man and Woman laughed and cried before the flickering light and gained pounds.

Then God brought forth the potato, naturally low in fat and brimming with nutrition. And Satan peeled off the healthful skin and sliced the starch center into chips and deep-fried them. And man gained pounds.

God then gave lean beef so that Man might consume fewer calories and still satisfy his appetite. And Satan created fast food and its 99-cent double cheeseburger. Then he said, "You want fries with that?' And Man replied, "Yea! And super size 'em."

And Satan said, "It is good."

And Man went into cardiac arrest.

...and Satan created HMOs

ACKNOWLEDGEMENTS & DEDICATIONS

Jose' Fleming

I have to acknowledge the Supreme Being who allowed this book to manifest. It was a great pleasure working with someone as tenacious as Dr. Scott Whitaker, without you this project would not be successful. And, thank you, Mr. Kevin Bryant of Inkosi Designs for your magnificent artwork and patience.

First, I would like to thank my mother Lillie Mae Fleming and father Nathaniel Fleming who saw to it that I was raised and influenced to grow into a man of integrity, compassion, tenacity, intellect and perseverance. I would also like to thank two loving grandparents Mrs. Mary and Mr. George Woodberry for having a great influence on my life. It was my grandmother who gave me the first two books that would be the foundation of my path, "Cooking with Mother Nature" by Dick Gregory and "Back to Eden" by Jethro Kloss.

Since the age of 14, I was always inspired by the courage and tenacity of Dick Gregory. Because of him I developed the will to represent some sort of change in this society. It is an honor to have known one of the greatest men in American history. Another individual that has been by my side in the time of struggle and guidance is Dr. R. Gregory, Ph.D. who is one of the most charismatic, caring and wisest men I know. Thank you, Dr. R. "Knees" Gregory and his loving wife, Ms. Joanne.

Much gratitude goes out to my wife Joyce, for giving me moral and financial support while I pursued my endeavors as an entrepreneur. I would like to acknowledge my Aunt Liz, and my cousin Rick, for sharing that brotherly love. A special appreciation goes out to Sterling Moody who has strongly influenced my entrepreneurial spirit. During my time of stress I would like to give thanks to Munir Ahmad and Bishop Melvin Dunn who have always given me fatherly advice and support.

A special note of thanks goes to my first mentor and family friend Dr. George Love, Jr., one of the greatest physician's of

Asian medicine, and Anahitta Jafari (the queen of whole food healing.) If it had not been for their intriguing medical background and compassion for teaching me most of what I know, I probably would not have the confidence to write this book. Thank you, George and Anahitta for your love and education on wellness and life. A very special thanks goes out to Eternity Deli, the Hebrew Israelite community, the Christian and Islamic communities for their inspiration and education. Thanks Mr. Shapiro and Ms. Rosenthal for your moral support.

I definitely can't forget my extended family and friends: Marilyn Mack, Shirley Spencer, Mr. Ernest Stringfellow, George Buckner, Andre Logan, Tony Moore, Nafi Rafat, Hakim Rashad, Hafiz and Shakira, Ishmael Thoth, Brother Ron, Randy O'Jay, Mr. Shegoog and "The Institution", Mr. Eli of our former health talk show, "It's About U", Chris Hughes, Carolyn and Moses Cid, Terry Poiyant, James Clark, Etefia Umana, TJ, Brother Anu, Brother Malik, Shirley Fields, Debra and Beverly Moore and Mr. Joe Palm, MPH of the "Mens Health Cartel"; thanks for believing in me and for all your support.

Finally, I would like to dedicate this book to the individuals that have fallen to the fate of ill-health. First, my childhood and life time best friend, Fernandars "Scoop" Gillespie, a great pro-football player, who helped find the path and purpose in which I am to follow. He is no longer with us but his wisdom and compassion will remain with me forever. I will never forget Sister Rasheeda Saeed, a very kind woman who was like a mother to me, who lost the battle to cancer. Finally, this book also goes out to the following people who lost the battle with ill-health; Mr. Dave, Lula, John Moore, Charles Davis, Cynthia Clemens, Larry Ali, Mr. Gore, Matthew Sutherland, Edward Fleming, Kay Fleming, Sister Shakura, Mrs. Munir Ahmad, Lula McKinley, both my grandmothers and those that I have failed to mention.

Dr. Scott Whitaker

I would like to first and foremost thank the Creator of the heavens and the earth, The Master of the Day of Judgment who allowed me to learn a little about his creation. I send peace and blessings upon all the Prophets from Adam to Noah to Abraham to Ishmael to Isaac to Solomon to David to Jesus and to the completion of that Prophethood with Muhammad Ibn Abdullah who lived over 1400 years ago in the Arabian Peninsula. Their spiritual leadership and understanding of science is unmatched in the world today. To all the scholars, teachers, and freedom fighters who taught me the values of hard work and sacrifice, both directly and indirectly: Al-Hajj Malik El-Shabazz (Malcolm X), Dick Gregory, Imam Abdul-Halim Musa, Fred Hampton Sr., Muhammad Ali, Emmett Till, Nat Turner, Huey P. Newton, Sister Patricia Barbara, Mrs. Marchante, and Mrs. Broussard. To family and friends who have impacted me through encouragement or positive energy: Mattie Whitaker (mother) who taught me the value of education, Charles Whitaker (father) who was my first teacher of nutritional health, Gloria Truitt (sister) who set the academic standards prior to me being born, Eric Grant (thanks for taking me the Museum of Science & Industry), Jill Copeland (first to introduce me to herbal teas), Hashim Ali (thanks for introducing me to Islam), Erik Williams (thanks for being there when I made my transition), Tamara Green, Amir Rashad (always positive), Suleiman Robinson (morally strong) , Rashad Badqir, Dr. Nathan Rabb Jr., Aunt Juliet & Uncle Henry (always giving great advice), Uncle Norman Golliday, Aunt Marie Shack, Aunt Mildred Farmer, Aunt Betty, Aunt Doris, Faruq Salaam, Maryum Ali (inspired me to write the book), Munygia Lumumba (strong soldier), Yusuf & Nadirah Muhammad & family , Marotha Pasha, Muhammad Abdullah, Sheik Humza, Tony Galway, Gerard Mayo, Jose Fleming, Mr. & Mrs. Dan Palley, Abdul-Malik Ali, Ahmad Adisa, Calvin Andrews, Jamila El-Amin, Chris Barr, Mahmoud Abdul-Rauf (always grateful for your generosity), Troy Henry, Marcia Logan, Erik Knox, Mrs. Charlotte Williams & family, The Watkins Family, Renee Smith, Public Enemy, KRS-One, X-Clan, Intelligent Hoodlum, all my cousins, and last but not least, Bridgett Whitaker.

This book is also dedicated to family & friends who were victims of MediSin: Joe Golliday (grandfather), Dora Golliday (grandmother), Aunt Lizzie, Aunt Versey, Clarence Whitaker (uncle), Brother Najeeb, Sherrie Taylor, Marie Russo, Uncle James Huntley, Inga Woodfork, Aunt Ruby, Uncle HC, and Agnes Schlef, may they all rest in peace.

A special thanks goes to Kevin Bryant of Inkosi Design Studio for his graphic art brilliance.

A special thanks goes to Chayah Yisrael & Sister Gayle for their editing expertise.

INTRODUCTION

"Dark, dark will be her nights; not even a lamp in a window will ever be seen again. No more joyous wedding bells and happy voices of the bridegrooms and the brides. Her businessmen were known around the world and she deceived all nations with ***sorceries****." Revelation 18:23*

Since the beginning of mortal existence, the deceivers of arrogance have always attempted to lead the masses astray from the divine path of knowledge and holy submission. It is the very nature of these unholy beings or entities to bamboozle the minds and capture spirits of all mortal beings by institutionalizing various degrees of trickery and falsehood. Various sciences of politics, religion, education, entertainment and commercialization are used to intentionally lead the masses astray by the protocols of evil. Men and women of the dark circle of intrigue and power have advocated this blueprint of deception through generations of devilment. In order to execute this master plan of worldly deception, laws, rules and regulations had to be implemented. There also has to be an authority or institution that will enforce these laws, rules and regulations in order to give what is wrong, precedence over what is right.

The verse in Revelations 18:23 states "...her businessmen were known around the world and she deceived all nations with sorceries." The word "sorceries" translated from Greek is "pharmakeia", which means:

1. The use or the administering of drugs.
2. Poisoning.

This word is from the Greek word pharmakon (a drug, i.e. spell-giving potion). It is this Greek word where we get our present day word "**Pharmacy**."

Like the works of an unholy sorcerer, doctors are taught how to market the illusions of trickery. The physician understands the system of vulnerability and submission. When you attempt to summarize your symptoms and health concerns, you have opened the door of opportunity for your doctor. Your laymen level of understanding becomes no match for the medical professional's oratory talent. Eventually, your mind is delivered to a state of submission having no alternative to your health concern, except the prescribed medications which could both be a worthless and lifetime application.

There are occasions when the physician changes the course of the game. For example, when the deadly adverse effects of Vioxx and Aleve finally made national news, doctors were already prepared to switch to another drug, with a sophisticated explanation as to why there was such an adverse effect from a drug that made over $3 billion in sales. So, in order to maintain control over the patient there has to be an "ace in the hole" available to prevent any doubts in the next prescription. Remember, as long as they remain the authority you are not to question their judgment.

Patients easily find themselves being a guinea pig by allowing a doctor to label their condition. For example, a patient goes to the doctor constantly complaining of a headache or pain, and then shares with him/her that they are contemplating quitting their job or separating from their spouse. They've just opened an opportunity for a prescription of Vioxx, Naproxen or Prozac. So, now they have a prescription for pain, discomfort and depression, which could put them at risk for a heart attack, kidney failure or violent behavior. These are common side effects from the prescriptions of MediSins.

MediSin is a newly coined word that describes the chemical poisons, pollutions, and other forms of anti-life and demonic technology that plague humanity. MediSin is any food, liquid, or substance that alters the state of the body's natural chemistry. For example, white refined sugar is a MediSin, because it causes tooth decay, constipation, acidic pH levels, and neurological imbalance, to name a few. Therefore, anything that contains white sugar is a MediSin. Sodium laurel sulfate, a popular body care and hygiene ingredient, is a MediSin, because it is a chemical that accumulates in the kidneys, eyes and liver causing severe damage to these and other organs. Therefore, any product (i.e. shampoo, toothpaste, etc.) that contains sodium laurel sulfate is a MediSin.

Processed foods are MediSins because of the chemicals that are used in the manufacturing process, which includes food dyes, benzoate, Splenda, hydrogenated oils, aspartame and other chemical by-products. White bread that has a shelf life of 21 days without molding is manufactured with preserving MediSins. Frozen foods, which contain carcinogens, like acryl amide (plastic), formaldehyde and aflatoxins (fungus) are MediSins that will destroy your liver and drain your life force.

The United States and the people of the world are at a serious crossroads with the continuing sickness on this planet. America, having used its military and economic might across the globe has turned into the monster of midway. Not only is America threatened by so-called "terrorists", but also from within. Disease, corrupt politics, religion and business are destroying the moral fabric of the nation. From an outsider looking in, America appears to be headed for the annuals of history along with Communism. She has been so deceived by sorcery (pharmaceuticals) that her sickness will eventually bring economic and social collapse.

Millions of people worldwide are waking up to the fact that the pharmaceutical (Greek word for sorcerer) industry is an investment industry based on the continuation of disease. The survival of the pharmaceutical investment industry is threatened by four main factors:

1) **Unsolvable business conflict**: The nature of the pharmaceutical investment industry is the business of disease. Its basis is the patentability of new synthetic drugs (MediSins) that merely target symptoms but do not eliminate the root cause of disease. The continued existence of disease and their expansion is a precondition for further growth of this industry. Prevention and eradication of disease undermines the economic basis of this business.

2) **Unsolvable legal conflicts:** A wave of patient litigation against the deadly side effects of pharmaceutical drugs threatens to cripple this industry. Since drug side effects are the fourth leading cause of death in the industrialized world, an end to this litigation is not in sight. (Journal of the American Medical Association, April 15, 1998).

3) **Unsolvable ethical conflicts:** The pharmaceutical industry faces an intrinsic conflict between maintaining profits from patent fees and meeting the health needs of people. In developing countries, the profitability of drugs has been a major factor contributing to the spread of AIDS and other degenerative diseases.

4) **Unsolvable scientific conflicts:** Advances in vitamin research, cellular medicine and natural health can eliminate today's most common diseases. These safe, effective and affordable natural therapies focus on the prevention and eradication of disease-not only the alleviation of symptoms. This fact, and the profitability of these non-patentable natural approaches, threatens the economic base of the pharmaceutical investment business.

The only solution for America and the rest of the world is to return to the Creator's natural food laws. By applying the principals of fasting, eating of wholesome foods, meditation, charity, exercise, and good hygiene, to name a few, would put America and the rest of the world back on the straight and narrow.

MEDICAL SINS I

1. MEDICAL SINS OF THE HEALTHCARE INDUSTRY

"According to the National Center for health statistic there are probably over 600 million doctor visits annually and probably less than 10% is ever introduced to natural food or medicine."

The primary motive for today's medical profession is derailed by greed, prestige and power of the industry. One percent of the population owns more than seventy percent of the nation's wealth and ten percent owns all of it. In the medical arena, power and wealth cannot co-exist with integrity and humanitarianism. They are totally two different natures. One is the nature of divine guidance, which will submit to truth and deliver to the masses what is needed: the right to health and prosperity. The other is the nature of the beast, which cannot exercise compassion and integrity because of its arrogance and desire to only control.

America has made outstanding accomplishments in modern medicine with life saving drugs and trauma medicine. There are some great doctors of medicine who due to their excellent training and wisdom have saved lives from the result of accidents, gunshot wounds, and poisons. A well-trained staff with competent surgeons in the emergency room is not the area of medicine that is the problem. Instead, it is the area of prescription drugs, treating chronic disease and the application of a food pyramid that is irrational and unnatural. The problem is that the Medical-Industrial-Complex (MIC) controls the rationale and the "live or die" decision of the physician at hand simply because they control the revenue and govern the administrative policies of what the patient is allowed to receive, regardless of whether it be right or wrong. This is why today's American medical system is also guilty of fraud, trickery, suppression and murder! For example: if you are ever diagnosed with cancer, you need to know that your MD or Oncologist is legally forbidden to use a natural cancer treatment that could possibly cure you. Regardless of what they know about a cure or how they feel about the treatment, their hands are tied by the American Medical Association (AMA) and Food & Drug Administration (FDA). You may have options such as going to Mexico or Germany for natural protocols, but if you cannot afford the expenses you will be at the mercy of the butcher committee or the radiation corporation. They have the power to pass legislation that forbids any licensed MD from treating cancer with anything other than chemotherapy, radiation or surgery. This avenue has only left a trail of dead hope!

The crazy thing about allopathic medicine is that it has used many forms of trickery to convince the masses that there is no other application but allopathic medicine. Dr. Hebert L. Ley, former Commissioner of the FDA quoted, "The thing that bugs me is that people think the Food and Drug Administration is protecting them – it isn't. What the FDA is doing and what the public thinks its doing are as different as night and day."

Another idea to ponder is that the average life span of an American is 68 years, and the average life span of a MD is only 58 years! Now somebody please redo the math on that! Is it that the doctors put so much energy into saving lives that they exhaust their own life force or is it because of Karma (Universal Law): "you reap what you sow?" Since MD's are prescribing poisons and playing God, maybe this is the price for practicing without divine guidance. Or maybe the medical doctor needs to humble themselves and ask the Creator what are they doing wrong and submit, for the seeker of true knowledge has a great reward.

Any natural treatment that you can obtain and self-administer threatens to remove your doctor from the medical treatment program. Although your doctor may not object to this, the AMA is vehemently opposed to any application other than cut, burn, or drug. This is the reason that this demonic organization advocates legislation to prevent the public from ever being educated on holistic approaches. Sounds like a conspiracy, maybe? The term "conspiracy" has become the cornerstone of "Political Correctness," persecuting anyone who represents change, speaks out or acts against the system. In others words they are considered paranoid schizophrenic or a "fruitcake." This is why we have a docile mainstream society whose only contact with information is through controlled media outlets.

In a corporation, a Board of Directors meeting is a conspiracy, a private club is a conspiracy, and a secret organization is a conspiracy! Once you begin to seek knowledge and allow yourself to become enlightened, you will know that Big Pharma has Congress practically in the palm of their hands. For decades, Congress has been for sale, hell, this country is for sale, just ask your Chief Executive. While the "Sleeping Giant" (you the citizen) is asleep, the agent provocateurs and conspires enact laws like the Patriot Act I & II. So as you continue to read MediSin, you will see that the legislation is actually governed and implemented by the Corporations. Welcome to the age of wicked capitalism and greed.

Western medicine has obtained three words that created a medical monopoly of a trillion dollar a year industry: Diagnose, Prescribe, and Treat. Though these three words are the determining factor of life or death to a patient under the administration of allopathic medicine, the purpose of practice is not to favor the patient but to benefit the profit share of the corporation. It is not about the personal lives that are saved; it is about how many lives can be treated with patented drugs. Let's pay close attention to the function of these words:

"Diagnose" or sometimes, "examine" is when a MD or other licensed professional examines a patient and determines the recognized medical term for the "disease" or "condition." Now the physician does not look at lifestyle, your diet, your blood type, your constitution or other signs of your malady.

"Prescribing" is when a licensed professional under the auspices of the FDA and the Big Wigs of the pharmaceutical industry authorizes specific medications or treatment, in writing. The patient then takes the prescription to the "drug store" to receive their medicine or MediSin to address the symptoms of their disease.

"Treat" is the process of providing drug materials or other recognized medical treatments for the diagnosed "disease" or "condition." Most medical treatments such as hysterectomies, thyroid or gallbladder removal, not only leaves the patient minus an important organ or gland, but the removal of a body function that will never be normal again.

"Cure" is when the observed symptoms from which the licensed professional deduced a "diagnosis" are no longer detectable and the patient is said to have been "cured" by the authorized "treatment," even if the patient dies several years later. For example, a patient is treated for a certain type of cancer with the application of chemotherapy, radiation or surgery. The patient falls into a remission state for a couple of years, and then the cancer returns in another area of the body, but at an alarming rate. The patient's immune system is compromised even more as they succumb to death.

The Medical-Industrial-Complex is a pyramid of power that controls every corporate entity of the pharmaceutical, health care and commercial food chain industries. The provocateurs of this corporate pyramid have managed to place their representatives or agents into influencing positions throughout the boards of all major food and drug corporations which includes: American Tobacco, AT&T, General Electric, General Foods, General Mills, Kraft Foods, Sara Lee, Kellogg's, Hewlett-Packard, IBM, Monsanto, ADM, Minute Maid, Sears, Shell Oil, BP Amoco (British Petroleum Amoco), Time Life Publications, Pfizer, Aventis, Tyco Chemicals, and Pillsbury-just to name a few!

When the masses allow one group such as the FDA or AMA to monopolize the health care industry, you will always have a medical system like the one existing today. The problem is not only medicine and the Government; it is the docile mind set of the masses. It is not the lack of laws or a faulty constitution, nor do we need more schools. The problem lies squarely on the fact that we have allowed ourselves to be brainwashed, run amuck, and led astray from the righteous and sovereign path of freedom and health. For example, take pregnancy. What could be more normal? Our ancestors were having babies that were just as healthy and as normal as ours, and in even larger numbers, without ever visiting a doctor. However, in the name of medical science, the mother becomes a pawn on the chessboard of the medical system. The baby is set into parameters that have to meet all the statistical norms. Then if mother's weight should happen to increase, the doctor reprimands and scares her. From now on she is worried. That worry carries into the developing fetus causing emotional damage. But it gets worse if any one parameter does not fit the norm or is in doubt. If the baby is not following its pre-determined schedule, birth is induced, or a caesarean is ordered. For so-called normal births, it is routine to have an episiotomy. That is to say, a large deep cut in the vagina so as to prevent lacerations. Every normal stage in a woman's life is treated as an illness. This is true of menstruation, PMS and menopause. As for mammograms to prevent breast cancer, this is not prevention. It is only a detection device to treat it earlier. The tests are often wrong, but the treatment continues all the same.

It is not only women, however. Children who do not fit the accepted pattern are also subjected to medication. A child who is rebellious or doesn't fit into the standardized statistical norm is considered to be "hyperactive" and is made to take medication for a fictitious illness. The pharmaceutical companies conveniently forget to tell us that their advertising and promotional budget is two to three times greater than their research budget. They are also not the ones who will tell us that medication is the CAUSE of many illnesses, a third of the cost of hospitalizations, and of many deaths. All of this is the **"medicalization"** of society which is a medical sin!

People are going hungry in America, not just for food, but truth, in education, truth in politics and truth in health. America's population has soared 13.2% (281 million) in the last decade, and people are not living longer; they are getting sicker. Ill health practically has no bias, as we have witnessed Bill Clinton's need for bypass surgery, the loss of Florence Griffith-Joyner, Robert Palmer, Gregory Hines and a host of many others of both wealth and poverty. Knowledge of divine health has no price and certainly does not care who is rich or poor. Whatever is sown in the early stages of life will surely be reaped before the end because you will become a victim of MediSin. These people of divine creation didn't just parish from a disease but an absence of holistic wisdom on the behalf of western and allopathic practice.

CODEX: THE KING OF TYRANNY AND ANTICHRIST OF HEALTH!

"Because the interests of the Pharma-Cartel are against the health interest of entire mankind, the battle will be fierce; therefore, the Cartel tries to force other industries behind its unethical plans by means of laws."
- Matthias Rath, MD, famous Germ physician, outspoken critic of Codex Alimentarius

The Birth of CODEX

There is an international crisis that could destroy health freedom worldwide as we know it. As of 2005, the implementation of a program called CODEX will severely restrict the limits of nutritional consumption in all so-called "free" countries of the world like Germany, Norway, Australia and America. CODEX claims that it is a set of standards for food and nutrition created by the United Nations (UN) and backed by the World Trade Organization (WTO). Its primary mission is to control how and what type of foods people can grow, sell, eat, and dictate what type of dietary supplements can be manufactured, sold and the amount that can be bought. Though this might have been the initial motive behind the Codex Alimentarius of 1963, the Codex Alimentarius of 2005 has nothing to do with good intentions according to health freedom activist.

CODEX states that its purpose is to protect the health of the consumer and regulating fair trade. However, like "9/11" and all the other political scams and cover up's by the elite, it is a public relations ploy to convince you that they care about you, when they don't give a damn about you! The Codex Alimentarius of 2005 is manipulated and controlled by massive multi-national corporations and provocateurs that seat on the boards of companies that hold interest in pharmaceuticals, synthetic food manufacturing, chemicals, pesticides, bio-technology and industrial agriculture.

These are the most powerful, most toxic industries, the most heavily subsidized in the world and they control the biggest "sellouts" and "bootlicker's" (lobbyist) in the political world.

Why?

Natural health products like whole food vitamin, mineral, herbs, amino acids, essential fatty acids, green foods, and super immune formulas are a direct threat to the profits of pharmaceutical icons. Why spend $8-$10.00 for a good B-complex formula or $7-9.00 for a good magnesium product or $12-$18.00 for 5-HTP to help reduce stress when they can just get you hooked on Zoloft or Prozac and make hundreds of thousands of dollars on your perpetuating prescription! In essence, the more natural applications that are used to resolve the common problems of health, the less pharmaceutical drugs are consumed which lowers their profit margins. Natural or holistic medicine is aimed to treat the underlying cause of the condition not just the symptoms without the toxic adverse effects of prescriptions drugs. Drugs are only design to suppress the symptoms, not cure the disease.

Codex Alimentarius is Unscientific

CODEX is comprised of many so-called "guidelines." One of these is the "Vitamin and Mineral Guideline." It claims to protect consumer health against dangerous levels of vitamins, mineral and amino acids. But in reality it's not about the well being of the common man, women or child, in fact it is reported that CODEX declares nutrients as a "sort of toxin." This is executed by distorting real science into a senseless, pseudo-scientific ideology hoping that you would be docile enough to fall for this sham! CODEX intends to restrict the amount of vitamin C you can purchase, for example instead of you having the freedom to purchase a 1000 mg of vitamin C, the CODEX law can reduce the product to 200mg.

The American public and congressional bodies are being bombarded and overwhelmed with the propaganda concerning CODEX in order to prevent the real nature of this beast from being exposed, which simply stated CODEX is about economical profits causing consumer hazard and population control. It is very important that people who strive for optimum health start focusing on being a sovereign people again instead of being so caught up in the Super Bowl, The Pennant, Boule' Conferences, Pretenders, American Idol, Dance Halls, Revlon Products or who's getting paid, certainly not you or I. Congress is the gatekeeper of your rights on the American front, that's why you need to exercise the little power you have by communicating with your congressman/woman regarding the truth about CODEX and your freedom of health. So become a member of the Health Freedom USA Campaign before it's too late!

Why Health Freedom is Vital to health and Longevity

What is the Freedom of Health? The freedom of health is the liberty to make a comfortable decision about the type of health care you want for you and your family, the right to choose mineral and vitamin therapy over blood pressure, diabetic and pain medication. Health freedom is being free to choose your own health treatment protocol and nutritional supplements such as minerals, amino acids, herbs, homeopathic remedies, wholesome edible foods that are right for you and your family without being persecuted by state, government or corporate entities. Health freedom is the right to purchase fruits, vegetables, meats, and other foods for human and animal consumption that has not been irradiated or manipulated by some sort of genetic engineering. Any finally, no man or women, government or multi-national entity is above the divine law governed by our Creator because natural health is crucial to the attainment and the essentials of optimal health and longevity.

2. THE PROVOCATEURS of THE AMA

Rockefeller once said "competition is a sin" and in order to avoid the competition two propositions in the early days of the establishment were created. One proposition was that all doctors should have a "suitable education" implemented only by the "medical circle of intrigue", and the second was to uniform and elevate a standard of requirements for the degree of M.D. This could only be achieved by meeting the prerequisites and exercising the philosophy of western medicine via American medical schools. These high profile medical professions must follow the protocols of western medical philosophy without deviating, otherwise the privileges of medical practice would be state and law restricted. For example, a doctor who decided to incorporate a detoxification, nutritional, metabolic or herbal therapy would be considered an outcast and would be sanctioned for having such a practice.

At the turn of the 20th century, the integrity of modern allopathic medicine began to neutralize the foundation of health care with a direction towards capitalism and gluttony. Names like Flexner, Farben, Fishbein and other distinguished names of the financial elite decided to mold and form a new ideology and theory about medicine and health care. The financial elite invested millions of dollars in medical institutions and hospitals that would eventually lock the door on natural medical applications like Homeopathy, Naturopathy and Chiropractic treatment for decades possibly centuries to come. The pharmaceutical corporations created "Business with Disease" and made a point to destroy the mind-set of natural health care. Homeopathy, the most formidable competitor of the allopathic medical profession during the 19th century gradually dropped in status. The direct competition that homeopathy posed to allopathic physicians led to campaigns excluding them from medical societies and hospital privileges.

The Massachusetts Medical Society began excluding homeopaths in 1860, and by the 1870's the AMA launched an attack on homeopathy and other treatments that posed a threat to the cornerstone of modern medicine. Physicians were forbidden to violate the code of ethics if they consulted with Eclectic physicians (herbal healers), females or African-American doctors. In the 1870's, the restrictions against female physicians was rescinded due to pressure from the growing women's rights movement, and the exclusions of African-American doctors continued with institutional racist practices.

The AMA was founded in 1847 merely as a social and scientific organization. Initially it was a private clique for practitioners to get together, trade knowledge and to have some fun. The AMA was taken over by Dr. Morris Fishbein who originally studied to be a clown, but saw the opportunity to make more money as a doctor. He entered medical school (where he failed anatomy), and then barely graduated. Fishbein never treated a patient in his entire career. He became the head of the AMA where he enriched himself while attempting to undermine legitimate natural therapies, completely. He was solely interested in money and control, which speaks for all the provocateurs of the modern medical industry.

For 25 years (1924-1949), Fishbein decided which drugs could be sold to the public based only on how much media money he could extort from drug manufacturers. He would require drug companies to place expensive ads in the Journal of American Medical Association (JAMA). There were no drug trials or testing, every approval was based on Fishbein's decision regardless of the adverse effects to the host. This man was not only an endorser of MediSin, but also a provocateur of greed and deception. Yet today there is a Morris Fishbein Center for the History of Science and Medicine at the University of Chicago.

Fishbein's orchestration of the AMA is responsible for national and international bribery, corruption, and fraud in the testing of drugs. Technically, the pharmaceutical industry has a worse record of law breaking than any other industry. In 1978, there were 1.5 million Americans hospitalized because of medication side effects alone. In 1991, 72,000 Americans were killed due to iatrogenic (doctor caused) compared to 24,073 fatalities from gunshots wounds, **which make doctors nearly three times more lethal than guns!**

The industry of health care and drugs has perfected this form of trickery by programming the mind-set of the masses to think that disease is largely an inevitable part of life. Most people actually believe that you are destined to die from some form of disease, which is really a sick frame of mind to begin with. This is part of that divine connection we have lost due to the MediSins that we are ingesting. It is unfortunate that young allopathic doctors are repeatedly brainwashed throughout their medical careers that natural medicines are fraudulent and quackish. They are told that there is no scientific evidence to support any claims of Iridology, Pulse Diagnosis, or Chelation Therapy. Modern medicine, as we know it today, is as much a dogmatic cult as Satanism. The basis of its doctrine is a germ theory based on irrational and unscientific proof.

For nearly 150 years the icons of the medical industry continues to have a monopoly on the entire health care system and generate billions of dollars through a innovative system of pharmaceutical medicine at the cost of many lives. The Pharmaceutical and Medical elite had the perfect game plan from the beginning. For example, when you control the educational system you control the curriculum, when you control the curriculum then the end result is in your favor.

These institutions produce the Medical Doctor and you worship them as the medical deities, "Mortal Gods" in white coats. Tell your MD you want to use the herb Feverfew or fish oil for a migraine headache instead of aspirin or acetaminophen (Tylenol) or Magnesium & Docosahexaenoic acid (DHA) for ADD instead of Ritalin or Dimethyl Sulfoxide (DMSO) or bananas for a peptic ulcer instead of Prevacid or Nexium, your physician may not only fire you but report you to the authorities. Just ask the parents who decline vaccine shots for their children, they'll tell you they had a hell of a time keeping their children in school. This is the crisis you and your future are faced with when you don't demand a choice of healthcare, instead you allow yourself and your children to be inoculated like sheep.

Mass Media: The Greatest Tool of Mind and Dietary Control

"The sole purpose of propaganda is to make the mindset of the masses so naïve, so complacent and so comfortable that even the aware are not aware that they are unaware, in essence, make the rabbit hole so deep that even when they see light, they will forever wonder blindly. "

Jose' Fleming
Co-Author of Medisin

The masses of America for the most part think that they are in control, they think that they are normal when it fact they are being controlled, manipulated, influenced and not actually normal. For many years scientist of the psych have explored the many facets of mass mind manipulation. Everyday psychological and influential tactics are exercised daily by the advertising industry for the sole purpose of complete consumerism. Mind control through advertising connects with the emotional and the belief foundation of the mind and guides the masses into a like minded thinking. This has been shown to have a magnetic influence on the way Americans think about health and why they have become so submissive to the American doctors recommendation of pharmaceutical medisins.

Since the turn of the 20th century, emotions and mental sovereignty have been continually challenged and manipulated by governments, political structures, corporations and television programming. For example, Orson Wells "War of the Worlds," became the essence of how media programming captures the human mind when people actually thought that the world was actually under attack by an alien force. Not to say that can't happen now because there are other life forms in other galaxies maybe even ours, but from innovative media programming anything is believable. P.T. Barnum once said "there is a sucker born every minute" which is why the pharmaceutical and medical industry have so much control of the masses. Regardless of the millions of people that have died from adverse effects and medical blunders, people still give conventional drugs precedence over the greatest gift the Creator has blessed human kind with, the ability to use judgment and common sense.

The material presented through television programming is designed to keep you so amused and entertained that you will become docile and lose that creative thought process you once had. One of the principle tools used in programming the human mind is the television (tel-LIE-vision), this device infiltrates ocular components and proceeds on to the human hard drive where the universe of electrical impulses and neurotransmitter activity function. Television, Satan's greatest tool of mass temptation and brainwashing, maintains, stabilizes and reinforces ideas, attitudes, behavior and actions.

Television programming influences your ideology, your choice of lifestyle, and it consumes your mind into the world of make believe. Though it is not regulated on how much truth and falsehood is allowed to be used in news media and commercial programming, the fact of the matter is that what is projected through food, pharmaceutical, and health care commercials are a mixture misnomers, untruths, and straight-out lies. For example, Wonder bread claims that it's enriched, refined, and adulterated white bread product can build your body twelve ways which is misleading consumer information. First and foremost white bread was used in the early 1900s to stop diarrhea because it is very constipating. It has no nutrition value whatsoever, you should "Wonder" how you're still alive after eating it!

It is time for you to realize that people who program television entertainment and news serve but one purpose: to lead you like sheep into the surgery room or drug you to death. They give false hope that the medical establishment is just a little closer to issues like solving the cancer mystery. Since 1971, Nixon's "War on Cancer" has been one big joke! Remember, in the book of Hosea 6:4 "My people are destroyed for lack for knowledge." Or take the so called political concern regarding children's education the "leave no child behind" program. Since when does a politician or a member of the "minority elite" become so concern about the children of the future, other than making them a more submissive and robotic. The real meaning of "leave no child behind" is "leave no child unrecruited" the military will have a direct route to your children's records so that they can give you their sales pitch to send your child across the waters to go and fight for Zionist Israel & Oil Men! In other words, if they are not an asset or a slave of the corporate or political system that controls the world, then they are a dependant, expendable and a causality of war.

What Corporations really want is revenue at the physical and social expense of the masses. As far as Big Pharma and Commercial food corporations are concerned every child could grow up on Ritalin, Zoloft and other psychotropic drugs and make a stronger pharmaceutical transition when they reach adulthood. The innovative advertising continues to feed you entertainment to create that impulse of buying. Let's take the famous comedian "Bruce Bruce" now here is a guy who is obviously over weight and should be advocating a health food commercial to challenge obesity. Instead he has allowed the fast food chicken icon "Popeye's" to convince him to convince you (the consumer) that it's alright to consume fried chicken with fries and other food items that contribute to heart disease, diabetes and obesity. The same thing goes for malt liquor commercials that market toward the African -American community: "if you want to have a good time then drink malt liquor." The advertisement department recruits or hires some bootlicking entertainer that is really a whore for money to mislead the community into drowning themselves with an alcoholic product that has been proven to change the mindset of a human being converting man into beast.

3. THE "FLEXNER REPORT"

One of the names that created the cornerstone of medical education was a scholar technician by the name of Abraham Flexner. Most of you, including the scholarly medical student and doctor are probably unfamiliar with this individual. Abraham Flexner was an able fund raiser, an experienced educator, and an organizer who decided that he was the solution to both the supposed failure of American education, and the General Education Board.

Flexner, a John Hopkins and University of Berlin Graduate became a researcher at the Carnegie Foundation for the Advancement of Teaching in New York City. Flexner's expertise was retrieving large amounts of information and making it palatable to others. Flexner's first impact on America was in the form of "Germanizing" the American medical education. While Flexner held a position at the Carnegie foundation, he was invited to conduct a major study among medical schools in America and Canada. Within eighteen months, he investigated 155 medical institutions and issued his "Flexner Report." Flexner soon became the lens that brought the Rockefellers and Carnegie fortunes into focus on the unsuspecting and vulnerable medical profession.

The Flexner Report, as it was called, was published in 1910. The report correctly pointed out the inadequacies of medical education at that time. It also proposed a wide range of sweeping changes, most of which were entirely sound. The alert observer, however, would note that the recommendations included strengthening courses in pharmacology and the addition of research departments at all "qualified" medical schools. Please note that at this time, there were twice as many practitioners of alternative medicine than there were of allopathic medicine. Taken at face value, the Flexner Report was above reproach and, undoubtedly, it performed a service that was much needed. It is what followed in the wake of the report that reveals its true purpose in the larger plan. Rockefeller and Carnegie began immediately to shower millions of dollars on those medical schools that were susceptible to CONTROL. Those that did not conform were denied the funds and eventually were forced out of business by their well-funded competitors.

Prior to 1910, the practice of medicine was relatively cheap. Medical degrees could be obtained via mail or marginal training at understaffed and inadequate medical schools. The profession was suffering from bad public reputation, and reform was in a desperate position. In 1905, there were 168 schools that were in operation, by 1927 the number had dropped to 80. Most of these schools that did not make the roster of legitimacy had been sub-standard, but educational excellence was not the primary criterion for determining which institution received Rockefeller funding. The determining test was integrity, the willingness of the school's administration and faculty to accept a curricula supporting DRUG research. This is how the profiteering began in the medical industry; historian Joseph Goulden describes the process this way:

"Flexner had the ideas, Rockefeller and Carnegie had the money, and their marriage was spectacular. The Rockefeller Institute for Medical Research and the General Education Board showered money on tolerably respectable schools and on professors who expressed an interest in research."

Since 1910, the foundations have invested over a billion dollars into the medical schools of America to promote chemically oriented MediSin in America. Naturopathic, homeopathy, and chiropractic medicine was denied funding because its foundation was not based upon chemical drugs. That's why medical doctors know NOTHING about nutrition after spending four years in these Rockefeller approved schools, because its not part of the curriculum and its not profitable.

4. EXPLODING THE GERM THEORY OF DISEASE

For the past seventy-five years, investigation and promulgation of the germ theory of disease has progressed by organized medical researchers and practitioners with mixed results. The present situation of this theory is that organized medicine has now produced such mass propaganda, for years, to the public to accept this theory that most uniformed people have now accepted it as a fact. At this writing, our Chief Executive is advocating mass immunization against disease by inoculation of the entire public, based upon the theory that by killing germs we can get rid of disease through anti-toxins injected into the blood stream.

The germ theory is the doctrine that disease can be communicated to the human system by minute animal organisms generally described as bacteria, found in great abundance in both air and water. Bacillus, spirilla, micrococcus, streptococcus, diplococcic, etc., are of the same origin and have been respectively named according to their varying forms or modes of growth.

When one thoroughly investigates the germ theory, there is no longer any doubt that bacteriologists have raised a superstructure on a false premise, which can be disproved by history, by logic and by laboratory demonstration. Both the laboratory and the clinic abound with evidence that shows conclusively that bacteria are no more related, primarily, to the cause of disease symptoms in which they are found than a dam is related to the cause of the waterfall that pours over it. There needs to be a universal demand that both the germ theory and the mass inoculation practice be given a full scale investigation as to its truth and merits in the cause of alleviating a suffering humanity. Those who profess to believe in this theory should be required to demonstrate their claims, both in the laboratory and clinically, under test conditions from which all tendency to misinterpret the findings have been removed. They should be required to openly discuss these findings with natural scientists that hold to the concept that it is the filth that is present in every type of disease symptom, rather than the bacteria that grows therein, that furnishes the REAL cause of disease-that the germs are merely incidental to this clinical picture instead of the cause of it.

If it were true that germs cause disease, without consideration of the internal environment, then the populations of the world would have been wiped out many thousands of years ago. The germ theory is not based upon logical facts. It is based upon the alteration of facts to fit the theory. However, in spite of all attempts at alteration and rationalization, the germ theory fails to answer many important questions.

A few examples of these are:

1) It is common to find pathogenic bacteria in a healthy person with no disease present, such as diphtheria and tuberculosis. Why can we find pathogenic germs in our body and still not have a disease?

2) It is not uncommon to find the disease without the bacteria. If the germ is the cause, how can we have the disease without the presence of the germ?

3) It often happens that when a disease organism is injected into an animal, the animal acquires a disease bearing no clinical resemblance to the original organism. Why? Because it's internal environment completely changed the original microbe.

4) After exposure, one person has a disease and another person doesn't. Why? It may be suggested that one person has a stronger immune system. Well, that is exactly one of our points. The only reason some of us have a stronger immune system than others is because of what we have done to ourselves. This explains why only a percentage of a group of people, all exposed to the exact same pathogens-perhaps in a school room will acquire the disease. The germ theory

can't explain why a person in a close relationship with another person who has a serious disease such as AIDS, does not acquire the disease. Disease is never acquired. It is always earned. Disease is not a question of exposure. It's an internal development, which can lead to exposure susceptibility. In other words, germ survival depends entirely upon its environment. A clean, healthy host destroys the germ.

The scientific world sets various postulates as guidelines to prevent alteration of facts to fit personal goals. In other words, a postulate is a rigid foundation based upon universal truths. Anything factual that does not fit that outline is not in fact pertaining to the postulate. There have been many scientists and authors who are quite willing to modify these rigid rules to suit their personnel interpretation of the facts. This is exactly what has happened to the germ theory. The facts have been modified and do not fit the scientific postulates.

There is a postulate for pathogenic microorganisms; it is called "Koch's Postulate." Any pathogenic microorganism must fit into this postulate. To establish whether a microorganism is pathogenic or not, it must be:

1) Found in each and every case of disease
2) Not found with any other disease
3) Isolated in pure culture
4) Able to produce the disease again

This is the original postulate. It is one thing to modify facts to the postulate, but what modern science has done, was to modify the postulate to fit their goals. Modern science has removed the second element to this postulate, because it nullifies or complicates the germ theory. This is their loophole to allow acceptance.

During the late 1800's, Antoine Be' champ (1816-1908) was the first to announce the pleomorphic cycle of bacteria creation. He found that there is a certain living organism, which he called microzyma that are responsible for this pleomorphic cycle. He found that the somatids (microzymas) could not be killed by heat, cold, chemicals, drugs, or anything else. They are virtually indestructible. They are found in the blood and in the cells of our bodies. The somatic is so small that we cannot see it under a good medical microscope. However, as they evolve, they enlarge into spores, which we can see through the microscope. They then advance into double spores, then into bacteria, fungus, and on into higher levels of pathogenic pleomorphic bodies.

Be' champ and Pasteur held completely different views about the cause of disease. Be' champ believed that disease evolved from within the body, and Pasteur believed that diseases were caused by bacteria, which invaded the body from the outside. Be' champ believed that living entities change or mutate into various other forms due to putrefaction, fermentation, and acid/ alkaline environment. Pasteur believed that nothing changed or mutated and it did not matter what condition the body's internal environment was in. Later, Pasteur admitted that he was wrong. When he was dying, Pasteur said (in terms of the germ theory) that he was mistaken and that Be' champ was the one who was correct. His actual words were: "The microbe is nothing; the terrain (environment) is everything." It is interesting that Pasteur often plagiarized Be' champ's work, claiming that he (Pasteur) was responsible for certain important scientific discoveries. Discoveries that have been incorrectly credited to Pasteur which were discovered by Be 'champ: 1. Discovered that urea was formed through oxidation of albuminoids (proteins). 2. Isolated series of soluble ferments secreted by living organisms. 3. Explained the process of digestion and fermentation.

There are two reasons why the germ theory is so devastating. **First:** It encourages harmful habits by suggesting that it doesn't matter what we do or eat, because diseases are usually caused by germs attacking us, and there is nothing we can do to avoid them except by having vaccines. The theory perpetuates an extremely harmful and unnatural dietary lifestyle, which floods our bodies with toxic acids, mucus, and many other poisonous substances. These acids and toxins activate a disease cycle, which is a pleomorphic (multiform) process that causes mutation of normal life forms within our bodies. From this gradual mutation process, disease develops, and if the cause is not abated, various diseases are allowed to advance into chronic and degenerative states. This explains why medical schools do no teach nutrition. They purposely believe that it doesn't matter what we eat that eating has nothing to do with health or disease yet even most children know better than that! It has only been in the last few years that the trend has begun to change. More and more medical doctors are realizing that their college professors did not have all the answers, and there is a great need for doctors to think for themselves.

Second: The germ theory encourages medical doctors to use costly, ineffective, often harmful, and sometimes deadly methods of treatments-treatments that cause serious futuristic diseases. Medical practices, with the blessings of the FDA, bombard our bodies with even more contaminants by using treatments (drugs and radiation), which seldom produce the desired affect and much too often contribute towards even more weakness and more disease. Drugs often poison healthy cells and suppress the body's elimination processes, driving disease deeper into the tissues, which may cause temporary relief, but only postpones the body from ridding itself from of the potential deadly condition that caused the disease in the first place.

So what did medical science decide to do? They accepted Pasteur's original concepts that disease was caused by outside entities, which attack our bodies hence, the birth of the "Germ Theory." Here was the beginning of the downfall of the healthiest nation in the world. It is because of the Germ Theory, that even today, most medical doctors do not believe that it matters what we eat. They seem to believe that all the filthy, slimy, moving garbage we see in a sick person's blood is sterile. They want to give us all sorts of vaccines, shots, tests, radiation, drugs, operations, etc., because they want us to believe that we need to attack and kill these entities, which have invaded our bodies, rather than clean the environment that makes their propagation possible. So why medical doctors are taught this? How much money will drug companies or doctors make if they send their patients home and tell them to change their diet, cleanse their bodies using herbs, fasting, and enemas, or simply use natural means to help improve the body's elimination? What will be their future profits if disease is eradicated?

The problem is that the disease industry (allopathic medicine) does NOT WANT us to believe that we create our own disease within our bodies. Why? There is no money in it! If people understood that we are responsible for our health and that our health is based upon how we conduct our lives, there is the possibility that we might actually change our lifestyles and if we did, we could end disease within a few years. The disease industry makes about 17% of America's gross national product, and that 17% is just the medical part of it. Consider the meat and dairy industries, all the supermarkets, restaurants, fast food, processed food companies, chemical companies, etc. All of these businesses make up the DISEASE INDUSTRY. Whether knowingly or ignorantly, they still support, encourage, and promote disease. Take all that away and America would go bankrupt.

We can see that neither the President nor the Congress of the U.S. is about to kick the medical industry and the money mongers in the rear and say "Start telling the truth and let's clean up America." It's just not going to happen from the manipulative end; there is too much to lose. If this is going to change, we, the people, will have to make it happen. If we don't, we can expect giant epidemics in the near future. People in power do not have the wisdom to guide a nation into health. People in power have gone money mad and power hungry. They are willing to kill their own grandchildren, millions of people and the earth itself, as long as they can enjoy their temporary power and their temporary, money today.

5. CHEMICALS IN MY FOOD: THE BUREAU OF CHEMISTRY

"15 out of 21 deaths in the United States are related to nutrition."
Dr. Evert Koop, Surgeon General

The regulatory era may have started with industries manipulating the government in their own best interest but regulatory legislation has also been initiated through public pressure for the government to curtail harmful industrial practices, set safety guidelines which protect our natural resources. When WE THE PEOPLE demand it, surely, those regulatory agencies serve the public's best interest. Don't count on it.

In 1907, after 25 years of public agitation over harmful food adulteration and misbranding, the Bureau of Chemistry, precursor of the Food and Drug Administration (FDA), was officially put in charge of policing the food supply. Bureau Chief Harvey W. Wiley, the Ralph Nader of his day, took on the food processing industry with a vengeance. Once established in his post at the USDA, Wiley successfully helped Congress in answering their questions about the safety of food chemical preservatives. Back in 1902, Wiley was granted $5,000 to actually study the health effects in humans when chemical preservatives, food coloring and other substances were put into foods. A true champion of the people's interest, Wiley enlisted the services of young, healthy volunteers, mostly employees of the Department of Agriculture. They agreed to follow a strict regime of natural foods, provided by the department, so that over a period of a month, a particular additive could be added to the food for testing. The idea was that if healthy young adult men had even the slightest adverse reactions, then unhealthy people, the young and the elderly would be even more vulnerable.

The criteria for these human tests were meticulous. Feces and urine were measured daily, and various other measurements were made along with noting if any physical or behavioral changes occurred such as fatigue, headaches, lack of appetite, indigestion and the like, at which time the subject would be put back on a pure diet. The participants in the tests were named "the Poison Squad" and became the subject of national news stories as the public became more and more interested in how adulterations in food might affect their health. During this same period of time, interest in finally passing a pure food law came to fruition thanks to the vigorous work of Wiley, who wanted to see that the federal government had the authority to force removal of all manner of chemical preservatives and other additives from America's food supply.

When the ***Pure*** Food and Drug Act of 1906, (please note the emphasis on the word "pure") this new law gave Wiley the authority he sought to start cleaning up the food supply. His Poison Squad studies, some of which had been published by the government printing office, had shown that many health problems were caused by the presence of an array of chemical additives in food. The Coca-Cola corporation was at the top of his hit list. But any hopes that enforcement could become reality were quickly put to rest. Political influence worked its magic and Coca-Cola flourished with impunity. One such additive on the ropes was the artificial sweetener, saccharin and herein lays the incredible tale of how the ***Pure*** Food and Drug Act was sidetracked from its original purpose by none other than the great "populist" president, Teddy Roosevelt. As the story goes, some years earlier, two chemists, Constantine Fahlberg and Ira Remsen, had accidentally discovered saccharin during other chemical research. Fahlberg later patented the substance, then, later still, John Queeny founded a company he named after his wife's family, Monsanto (which means Mono=One, Santo= Satan: One Satan), to manufacture the product.

It was well known that Wiley was opposed to allowing saccharin to remain in the food supply. Going over Wiley's head, immediately after the Pure Food and Drug Act was passed, future Vice President of the United States, James S. Sherman, then of the Sherman Brothers food manufacturing firm, met with President Roosevelt to discuss the fact that his firm had saved $4,000 the previous year using saccharin, rather than sugar in the company's canned corn. Wiley, who was present at the meeting, explained to Roosevelt that saccharin was made from coal tar, totally devoid of food value and injurious to health. Roosevelt, who was trying to control his weight and had been advised by his personal physician to use the sweetener chose to believe his doctor and challenged Wiley's explanation, to which Wiley replied, "Mr. President, he probably thinks you may be threatened with diabetes." Roosevelt angrily replied, "Anybody who says saccharin is injurious to health is an idiot."

The following day, Roosevelt undermined Wiley and appointed Ira Remsen (who discovered saccharin), President of Johns Hopkins University, to head up a Referee Board later to be known as the Remsen Board to protect the interests of the chemical industry. The Remsen board became very successful in blocking any authority Wiley had to remove adulterants from the food supply. Then, over the next several years, bit by bit, regardless of the law, the authority to police chemicals in food was transferred out of the Bureau of Chemistry.

Finally, thoroughly disgusted, Wiley quit. His departure was noted by the Rocky Mountain News, under the caption, "The Borgias of Business."

"...For twenty years at least, the food poisoners of the country have waged warfare on Dr. Harvey W. Wiley, and since the passage of the Pure Food Act in 1906 they have trebled efforts to have him discharged. These Borgias of business have won, for the circumstances attending Dr. Wiley's recent resignation makes it, in practical effect, a dismissal..."

Fortunately, Wiley's saga didn't end there. While giving up on any hope of honest oversight of food from government agencies, in the true never-say-die tradition of real health freedom fighters, Wiley set up the Good Housekeeping Bureau of Foods, Sanitation and Health, where voluntary evaluations of consumer products were to be conducted. Even today their findings are published in Good Housekeeping magazine. In addition, in 1929, Wiley wrote a detailed account of the destruction of the purpose of the Pure Food and Drug Act in a book he entitled, *THE HISTORY OF A CRIME AGAINST THE FOOD LAW - The Amazing Story of the National Food and Drugs Law Intended to Protect the Health of the People Perverted to Protect Adulteration of Food and Drugs*.

Some years later the modern FDA was created to oversee regulation of all foods and drugs and by 1970, a fresh-out-of-law-school lawyer by the name of James S. Turner became the next gladiator in the fight in an attempt to protect the public from unsafe food additives. Turner, one of Ralph Nader's original "Nader's Raiders", a cadre of young lawyers out to make government work right, eventually published a book on the failings of the FDA called, "The Chemical Feast: the Nader Report on the Food and Drug Administration". A short time later, Turner, largely at his own expense, made every effort to keep aspartame off the market. And what a fight it was.

As Turner described it, G.D. Searle, a drug company whose scientists had discovered aspartame quite by accident and a company with little experience in food regulation, made the motions of complying with the law, but screwed up royally. Early tests showed aspartame produced microscopic holes and tumors in the brains of experimental mice and epileptic seizures in monkeys. Animal tests also showed that aspartame was converted to dangerous substances such as formaldehyde. (See Chapter 28 about Aspartame). A documentary called "Sweet Misery" documents this entire affair and is available to the public for sale.

During much of the time the aspartame scandal was in high gear, a little known natural sweetener, stevia, was making its way into American markets. According to the American Herbal Products Association in an affirmation petition submitted to the FDA in 1992, "Stevia leaf is a natural product that has been used for at least 400 years as a food product, principally as a sweetener or other flavoring agent. None of this common usage in foods has indicated any evidence of safety problem. There are no reports of any government agency in any of the above countries indicating any public health concern whatsoever in connection with the use of stevia in foods." The Thomas J. Lipton Company, in a petition to the FDA, cited over 120 articles about stevia written before 1958 and over 900 articles as of 1995. The Ambassador to Paraguay where stevia is grown, in a letter to the FDA (1993), pointed out that stevia is a completely safe health promoting herb and in its refined form, in Japan, it held 41% of the sweetener market. (Aspartame is banned in Japan.)

Yet, despite glowing reports on stevia, products have been confiscated from stevia manufacturers; thousands of stevia cookbooks have been burned by order of the FDA; and the industry is unable to have stevia approved as a safe food additive. In the convoluted logic of FDA officials only Washington insiders can understand, stevia is currently allowed to be sold as a standalone "dietary supplement" or an herb, if properly labeled as such, but not as a sweetener. In FDA parlance, "If Stevia is used in a dietary supplement for a technical effect, such as use as a sweetener or flavoring agent, and is labeled as such; it is considered an UNSAFE FOOD ADDITIVE."

Millions of Americans in the health freedom movement are grateful we can get our hands on stevia, and use it as a sweetener. However, the stevia story reinforces our skepticism of the longtime behavior of FDA officials in their job to protect the public from unsafe food. Based on decades of this same anti-natural products regulatory doublespeak and harsh enforcement activity, we look at every bill introduced in Congress to ratchet up the FDA's authority to "regulate" nutritional supplements as yet another potential threat to our health.

The Purpose of Preservatives and Additives

The purpose of technology today is not just to make life better but to challenge the divine laws of the Creator in every facet of creation, especially when it comes to our food. Dr. Harvey Wiley, Dr. Weston Price and a few other humanitarians who saw this monstrous idea of synthetic food manufacturing and where it was going.

The Twinkie is probably the most fascinating creation of synthetic delicacy.

The ingredient list reads more like a formula for an automobile or jet fuel than for human consumption. Even though, the Twinkie's "synergy of chemicals" passed the test of palatable food consumption it has became a taste-bud delight, their bright plastic husks are found in landfills all over the planet!

In America we live like no other generation has anywhere on the planet, in America we eat like no other human being on the planet, in America we consume pharmaceuticals and over the counter drugs like no other people on the planet. In America, we are the victims of stockholders investments, a giant experiment of toxic ingestion and the Devils Protocol! In the game we call economics and free enterprise, the stakes are always high and the average American consumer is on the tip of it as it pokes a hole in our very lives. American's consider their standard diet normal but in reality you're only a few hundred years away from total genetic mutation from all the over consumption of corporate junk they call a standard diet.

Your human structure consists of billions of living cells that cannot be recognized by human eyes but is comprised of practically everything that makes this universe whole. The only reason why some people have eaten the Standard American Diet (SAD) without serious harm for the first few decades of their lives is due their body's DNA, physical constitution and divine resistance. But rest assure, the cellular breakdown is coming! Though your genetic weakness is hidden by youth and vitality, the repetitive accumulation of toxins will take effect and eventually manifest into degenerative diseases, i.e. diabetes, heart disease, kidney failure, cancer and ultimately premature death. This is due to the fact that cellular resistance to disease diminishes as the abuse of high fructose corn syrup, chemical meats, homogenized dairy, white sugar, and white flour continues. So, the next time you visit a friend or relative in the hospital or someone drops dead after dinner, remember the biochemistry of the human body will tolerate toxicity only to a point.

Chronic diseases such as arthritis, IBS, cancer and an array of psychological and psychiatric disorders are only a manifestation from the accumulation of chemicals you've consumed since birth. These chemicals become imbedded in every cell within the body. These chemical are capable of producing mutations through chromosome damage called mutagens which cause disruptions of your genetic code. This genetic process will cause a monstrous consequence among our offspring and their offspring. For example, pregnant mothers who constantly consume refined foods eliminate vital nutrients like chromium, zinc and vanadium from the body which lead to diabetes. The pharmaceutical shareholders take advantage of this created disorder caused by the 'food' made in their laboratories by developing a diabetic vaccine, because they know that the children could be born with onset diabetes.

The chemical engineers of the food industry can practically make anything taste like anything without providing any nutritional value. Lemon juice adds flavor and zest to many meals, but unfortunately the industry can now replace the wholesome juice from the lemon with 2-methyly-3-(pisopropylphenyl)-propionaldehyde, a name not of this universe among thousands of other chemical additives humans consume every single day.

The corporate food manufactures provide an array of products like sulfur dioxide (a known carcinogen) to preserve dried fruits. Formaldehyde which is used to delay the decomposition of human remains has been used as a common disinfect in frozen vegetables. If you look closely at commercialized luncheon meats you will notice a glitter which is sodium nitrate which coverts into a nitrous acid causing stomach cancer. Would you believe that all commercial chicken feed contains arsenic to stimulate growth, increase egg production and give chickens a yellowed skin? Looks like chickens with jaundice!

Here are some other ways the industry increases profits while preserving our food but increasing toxicity within our bodies:

1) Aluminum destroys our dietary lifestyle because the compounds are added to our baking powder, margarine, aspirins, antacids, beer, table salt and antiperspirants. The soft metal also leaches into our food and water through cookware and commercial can beverages. It is a scientific and clinical fact that aluminum concentrates in the human brain leading Alzheimer's disease.

2) For all you commercial cream lovers, be mindful of the brand of choice because you could be consuming propylene glycol, the same chemical used in the production of anti-freeze and paint removal. Also, a stabilizer called Carbonmethycellulose used as a stabilizer in not only ice cream but salad dressings, cheese spreads and everybody's favorite chocolate milk! This "very important" additive has produced cancerous tumors in at least 80% of the rats injected; even though the FDA denies this, because it does not cause cancer in rats that consume it orally. Would you as the consumer be just a little concerned?

3) For over 50 years brominated oils have been used in bottles of fruit juice to maintain an appeal of freshness, but the effects of thyroid enlargement, kidney damage, liver malfunction and potential shrunken testicles have caused Canada, Holland and Germany to ban this chemical from their bottled drinks. However, your FDA allows it in the great USA!

4) Take the chemical cyclamate (cyclohexylamine), even though this toxic chemical was banned it was once used to sweeten children's favorite domestic drink "Kool-Aid." It was found to cause chromosome damage in animals, increase the chances of still-born children and birth defects. Lipton the manufacture of the sweetener donated this artificial additive to mental hospitals and prisons in Ohio. Great job Lipton!!!

Food coloring (causes hyperactivity) is another complicated health influence. Many food colors that were introduced to the food chain have been banned after 20 years of damage on the market. These chemicals were removed after it was discover to have caused cancer. Today, "certified food colors" in a class called polycyclic aromatic hydrocarbons are still considered carcinogenic. In spite the toxic potential, the FDA continues to claim that food coloring is safe for human consumption, because it only causes cancer when it is injected into lab rats! The industry knows that children respond to bright colors i.e. skittles, popsicles, Hi-C, Fruit Loops and Now & Later candy, which all contain food coloring and a lot of refined sugar.

We have all been victims of acidifiers, modifiers, dyes, bleaches, preservatives, chemical flavors, buffers, emulsifiers, thickeners, stabilizers, pesticides, fungicides, insecticides, herbicides, anticaking, anti-foaming, hydrolyzed oils, soy fillers, wheat by products, hormones, antibiotics, steroids and genetically modified ingredients. Believe it or not most of us consume one of these chemicals daily, while they begin to corrupt every cell within our body, disrupting the natural biochemistry of the body and setting the stage for disease.

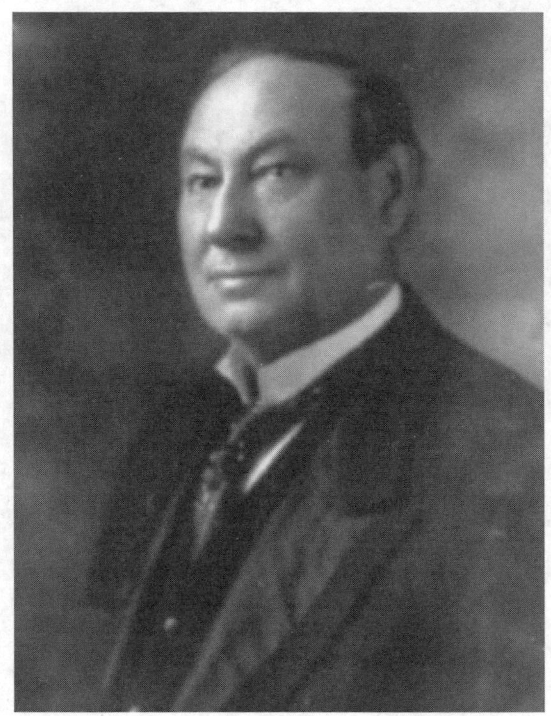

Dr. Harvey Wiley
Director of the Bureau of Chemistry

6. MILESTONES IN U.S. FOOD AND DRUG LAW HISTORY

FDA Backgrounder
May 3, 1999
Updated August 5, 2002

Milestones in U.S. Food and Drug Law History

From the beginning of civilization, people have been concerned about the quality and safety of foods and medicines. In 1202, King John of England proclaimed the first English food law, the Assize of Bread, which prohibited adulteration of bread with such ingredients as ground peas or beans. Regulation of food in the United States dates from early colonial times. Federal controls over the drug supply began with inspection of imported drugs in 1848. The following chronology describes some of the milestones in the history of food and drug regulation in the United States.

1820

Eleven physicians meet in Washington, D.C., to establish the **U.S. PHARMACOPEIA**, the first compendium of standard drugs for the United States.

1848

DRUG IMPORTATION ACT passed by Congress requires U.S. Customs Service inspection to stop entry of adulterated drugs from overseas.

1862

PRESIDENT LINCOLN appoints a chemist, Charles M. Wetherill, to serve in the new Department of Agriculture. This was the beginning of the Bureau of Chemistry, the predecessor of the Food and Drug Administration.

1880

PETER COLLIER, chief chemist, U.S. Department of Agriculture, recommends passage of a national food and drug law, following his own food adulteration investigations. The bill was defeated, but during the next 25 years more than 100 food and drug bills were introduced in Congress.

1883

DR. HARVEY W. WILEY becomes chief chemist, expanding the Bureau of Chemistry's food adulteration studies. Campaigning for a federal law, Dr. Wiley is called the "Crusading Chemist" and "Father of the Pure Food and Drugs Act." He retired from government service in 1912 and died in 1930.

1897

TEA IMPORTATION ACT passed, providing for Customs inspection of all tea entering U.S. ports, at the expense of the importers.

1898

Association of Official Agricultural Chemists (now AOAC International) establishes a **COMMITTEE ON FOOD STANDARDS** headed by Dr. Wiley. States begin incorporating these standards into their food statutes.

1902

The **BIOLOGICS CONTROL ACT** is passed to ensure purity and safety of serums, vaccines, and similar products used to prevent or treat diseases in humans.

Congress appropriates $5,000 to the Bureau of Chemistry to study **CHEMICAL PRESERVATIVES AND COLORS** and their effects on digestion and health. Dr. Wiley's studies draw widespread attention to the problem of food adulteration. Public support for passage of a federal food and drug law grows.

1906

The original **FOOD AND DRUGS ACT** is passed by Congress on June 30 and signed by President Theodore Roosevelt. It prohibits interstate commerce in misbranded and adulterated foods, drinks and drugs.

The **MEAT INSPECTION ACT** is passed the same day.

Shocking disclosures of unsanitary conditions in meat-packing plants, the use of poisonous preservatives and dyes in foods, and cure-all claims for worthless and dangerous patent medicines were the major problems leading to the enactment of these laws.

1907

First **CERTIFIED COLOR REGULATIONS**, requested by manufacturers and users, list seven colors found suitable for use in foods.

1911

In **U.S. v. JOHNSON**, the Supreme Court rules that the 1906 Food and Drugs Act does not prohibit false therapeutic claims but only false and misleading statements about the ingredients or identity of a drug.

1912

Congress enacts the **SHERLEY AMENDMENT** to overcome the ruling in U.S. v. Johnson. It prohibits labeling medicines with false therapeutic claims intended to defraud the purchaser, a standard difficult to prove.

1913

GOULD AMENDMENT requires that food package contents be "plainly and conspicuously marked on the outside of the package in terms of weight, measure, or numerical count."

1914

In **U.S. v. LEXINGTON MILL AND ELEVATOR COMPANY**, the Supreme Court issues its first ruling on food additives. It ruled that in order for bleached flour with nitrite residues to be banned from foods, the government must show a relationship between the chemical additive and the harm it allegedly caused in humans. The court also noted that the mere presence of such an ingredient was not sufficient to render the food illegal.

THE HARRISON NARCOTIC ACT requires prescriptions for products exceeding the allowable limit of narcotics and mandates increased record-keeping for physicians and pharmacists who dispense narcotics.

1924

In **U.S. v. 95 BARRELS ALLEGED APPLE CIDER VINEGAR**, the Supreme Court rules that the Food and Drugs Act condemns every statement, design, or device on a product's label that may mislead or deceive, even if technically true.

1927

The Bureau of Chemistry is reorganized into two separate entities. Regulatory functions are located in the **FOOD, DRUG, AND INSECTICIDE ADMINISTRATION**, and nonregulatory research is located in the **BUREAU OF CHEMISTRY AND SOILS**.

1930

McNARY-MAPES AMENDMENT authorizes FDA standards of quality and fill-of-container for canned food, excluding meat and milk products.

The name of the Food, Drug, and Insecticide Administration is shortened to **FOOD AND DRUG ADMINISTRATION (FDA)** under an agricultural appropriations act.

1933

FDA recommends a complete revision of the obsolete **1906 FOOD AND DRUGS ACT**. The first bill is introduced into the Senate, launching a five-year legislative battle.

1937

ELIXIR OF SULFANILAMIDE, containing the poisonous solvent diethylene glycol, kills 107 persons, many of whom are children, dramatizing the need to establish drug safety before marketing and to enact the pending food and drug law.

1938

THE FEDERAL FOOD, DRUG, AND COSMETIC (FDC) ACT of 1938 is passed by Congress, containing new provisions:

- Extending control to cosmetics and therapeutic devices.
- Requiring new drugs to be shown safe before marketing; starting a new system of drug regulation.
- Eliminating the Sherley Amendment requirement to prove intent to defraud in drug misbranding cases.
- Providing that safe tolerances be set for unavoidable poisonous substances.
- Authorizing standards of identity, quality, and fill-of-container for foods.
- Authorizing factory inspections.
- Adding the remedy of court injunctions to the previous penalties of seizures and prosecutions.

Under the **WHEELER-LEA ACT,** the Federal Trade Commission is charged with overseeing advertising associated with products otherwise regulated by FDA, with the exception of prescription drugs.

1939

FIRST FOOD STANDARDS issued (canned tomatoes, tomato purée, and tomato paste).

1940

FDA TRANSFERRED from the Department of Agriculture to the Federal Security Agency, with Walter G. Campbell appointed as the first Commissioner of Food and Drugs.

1941

INSULIN AMENDMENT requires FDA to test and certify purity and potency of this lifesaving drug for diabetes.

1943

In **U.S. v. DOTTERWEICH**, the Supreme Court rules that the responsible officials of a corporation, as well as the corporation itself, may be prosecuted for violations. It need not be proven that the officials intended, or even knew of, the violations.

1944

PUBLIC HEALTH SERVICE ACT is passed, covering a broad spectrum of health concerns, including regulation of biological products and control of communicable diseases.

1945

PENICILLIN AMENDMENT requires FDA testing and certification of safety and effectiveness of all penicillin products. Later amendments extended this requirement to all antibiotics. In 1983 such control was found no longer needed and was abolished.

1948
MILLER AMENDMENT affirms that the Federal Food, Drug, and Cosmetic Act applies to goods regulated by the Agency that have been transported from one state to another and have reached the consumer.

1949
FDA publishes **GUIDANCE TO INDUSTRY** for the first time. This guidance, "Procedures for the Appraisal of the Toxicity of Chemicals in Food," came to be known as the "black book."

1950
In **ALBERTY FOOD PRODUCTS CO. v. U.S.** , a court of appeals rules that the directions for use on a drug label must include the purpose for which the drug is offered. Therefore, a worthless remedy cannot escape the law by not stating the condition it is supposed to treat.

OLEOMARGARINE ACT requires prominent labeling of colored oleomargarine, to distinguish it from butter.

DELANEY COMMITTEE starts congressional investigation of the safety of chemicals in foods and cosmetics, laying the foundation for the 1954 Miller Pesticide Amendment, the 1958 Food Additives Amendment, and the 1960 Color Additive Amendment.

1951
DURHAM-HUMPHREY AMENDMENT defines the kinds of drugs that cannot be safely used without medical supervision and restricts their sale to prescription by a licensed practitioner.

1952
In **U.S. v. CARDIFF**, the Supreme Court rules that the factory inspection provision of the 1938 FDC Act is too vague to be enforced as criminal law.

FDA CONSUMER CONSULTANTS are appointed in each field district to maintain communications with consumers and ensure that FDA considers their needs and problems.

1953
FEDERAL SECURITY AGENCY becomes the Department of Health, Education, and Welfare (HEW).

FACTORY INSPECTION AMENDMENT clarifies previous law and requires FDA to give manufacturers written reports of conditions observed during inspections and analyses of factory samples.

1954
MILLER PESTICIDE AMENDMENT spells out procedures for setting safety limits for pesticide residues on raw agricultural commodities.

First large-scale **RADIOLOGICAL EXAMINATION OF FOOD** carried out by FDA when it received reports that tuna suspected of being radioactive was being imported from Japan following atomic blasts in the Pacific. FDA begins monitoring around the clock to meet the emergency.

1955
HEW SECRETARY OVETA CULP HOBBY appoints a committee of 14 citizens to study the adequacy of FDA's facilities and programs. The committee recommends a substantial expansion of FDA staff and facilities, a new headquarters building, and more use of educational and informational programs.

The **DIVISION OF BIOLOGICS CONTROL** became an independent entity within the National Institutes of Health, after polio vaccine thought to have been inactivated is associated with about 260 cases of polio.

1958
FOOD ADDITIVES AMENDMENT enacted, requiring manufacturers of new food additives to establish safety. The Delaney proviso prohibits the approval of any food additive shown to induce cancer in humans or animals.

FDA publishes in the Federal Register the first list of **SUBSTANCES GENERALLY RECOGNIZED AS SAFE (GRAS)**. The list contains nearly 200 substances.

1959
U.S. CRANBERRY CROP recalled three weeks before Thanksgiving for FDA tests to check for aminotriazole, a weedkiller found to cause cancer in laboratory animals. Cleared berries were allowed a label stating that they had been tested and had passed FDA inspection, the only such endorsement ever allowed by FDA on a food product.

1960
COLOR ADDITIVE AMENDMENT enacted, requiring manufacturers to establish the safety of color additives in foods, drugs and cosmetics. The Delaney proviso prohibits the approval of any color additive shown to induce cancer in humans or animals.

FEDERAL HAZARDOUS SUBSTANCES LABELING ACT, enforced by FDA, requires prominent label warnings on hazardous household chemical products.

1962
THALIDOMIDE, a new sleeping pill, is found to have caused birth defects in thousands of babies born in western Europe. News reports on the role of Dr. Frances Kelsey, FDA medical officer, in keeping the drug off the U.S. market, arouse public support for stronger drug regulation.

KEFAUVER-HARRIS DRUG AMENDMENTS passed to ensure drug efficacy and greater drug safety. For the first time, drug manufacturers are required to prove to FDA the effectiveness of their products before marketing them. The new law also exempts from the Delaney proviso animal drugs and animal feed additives shown to induce cancer but which leave no detectable levels of residue in the human food supply.

CONSUMER BILL OF RIGHTS is proclaimed by President John F. Kennedy in a message to Congress. Included are the right to safety, the right to be informed, the right to choose, and the right to be heard.

1965

DRUG ABUSE CONTROL AMENDMENTS are enacted to deal with problems caused by abuse of depressants, stimulants and hallucinogens.

1966

FDA contracts with the National Academy of Sciences/National Research Council to evaluate the **EFFECTIVENESS OF 4,000 DRUGS** approved on the basis of safety alone between 1938 and 1962.

CHILD PROTECTION ACT enlarges the scope of the Federal Hazardous Substances Labeling Act to ban hazardous toys and other articles so hazardous that adequate label warnings could not be written.

FAIR PACKAGING AND LABELING ACT requires all consumer products in interstate commerce to be honestly and informatively labeled, with FDA enforcing provisions on foods, drugs, cosmetics, and medical devices.

1968

FDA BUREAU OF DRUG ABUSE CONTROL and Treasury Department Bureau of Narcotics are transferred to the Department of Justice to form the Bureau of Narcotics and Dangerous Drugs (BNDD), consolidating efforts to police traffic in abused drugs.

REORGANIZATION of federal health programs places FDA in the Public Health Service.

FDA forms the **DRUG EFFICACY STUDY IMPLEMENTATION (DESI)** to implement recommendations of the National Academy of Sciences investigation of effectiveness of drugs first marketed between 1938 and 1962.

ANIMAL DRUG AMENDMENTS place all regulation of new animal drugs under one section of the Food, Drug, and Cosmetic Act-Section 512, making approval of animal drugs and medicated feeds more efficient.

1969

FDA begins administering SANITATION PROGRAMS for milk, shellfish, food service, and interstate travel facilities, and for preventing poisoning and accidents. These responsibilities were transferred from other units of the Public Health Service.

The **WHITE HOUSE CONFERENCE ON FOOD, NUTRITION, AND HEALTH** recommends systematic review of GRAS substances in light of FDA's ban of the artificial sweetener cyclamate. President Nixon orders FDA to review its GRAS list.

1970
In **UPJOHN v. FINCH** the Court of Appeals upholds enforcement of the 1962 drug effectiveness amendments by ruling that commercial success alone does not constitute substantial evidence of drug safety and efficacy.

FDA requires the first **PATIENT PACKAGE INSERT**: oral contraceptives must contain information for the patient about specific risks and benefits.
The **COMPREHENSIVE DRUG ABUSE PREVENTION AND CONTROL ACT** replaces previous laws and categorizes drugs based on abuse and addiction potential compared to their therapeutic value.

ENVIRONMENTAL PROTECTION AGENCY established; takes over FDA program for setting pesticide tolerances.

1971
PHS BUREAU OF RADIOLOGICAL HEALTH transferred to FDA. Its mission: protection against unnecessary human exposure to radiation from electronic products in the home, industry, and the healing arts.

NATIONAL CENTER FOR TOXICOLOGICAL RESEARCH is established in the biological facilities of the Pine Bluff Arsenal in Arkansas. Its mission is to examine biological effects of chemicals in the environment, extrapolating data from experimental animals to human health.

Artificial sweetener **SACCHARIN**, included in FDA's original **GRAS** list, is removed from the list pending new scientific study.

1972
OVER-THE-COUNTER DRUG REVIEW begun to enhance the safety, effectiveness and appropriate labeling of drugs sold without prescription.

REGULATION OF BIOLOGICS-including serums, vaccines, and blood products, is transferred from NIH to FDA.

1973
THE U.S. SUPREME COURT upholds the 1962 drug effectiveness law and endorses FDA action to control entire classes of products by regulations rather than to rely only on time-consuming litigation.

LOW-ACID FOOD PROCESSING regulations issued, after botulism outbreaks from canned foods, to ensure that low-acid packaged foods have adequate heat treatment and are not hazardous.

CONSUMER PRODUCT SAFETY COMMISSION created by Congress; takes over programs pioneered by FDA under 1927 Caustic Poison Act, 1960 Federal Hazardous Substances Labeling Act, 1966 Child Protection Act, and PHS accident prevention activities for safety of toys, home appliances, etc.
1976
MEDICAL DEVICE AMENDMENTS passed to ensure safety and effectiveness of medical devices, including diagnostic products. The amendments require

manufacturers to register with FDA and follow quality control procedures. Some products must have pre-market approval by FDA; others must meet performance standards before marketing.

VITAMINS AND MINERALS AMENDMENTS ("Proxmire Amendments") stop FDA from establishing standards limiting potency of vitamins and minerals in food supplements or regulating them as drugs based solely on potency.

1977

SACCHARIN STUDY AND LABELING ACT passed by Congress to stop FDA from banning the chemical sweetener but requiring a label warning that it has been found to cause cancer in laboratory animals.

1980

INFANT FORMULA ACT establishes special FDA controls to ensure necessary nutritional content and safety.

1982

TAMPER-RESISTANT PACKAGING REGULATIONS issued by FDA to prevent poisonings such as deaths from cyanide placed in Tylenol capsules. The Federal Anti-Tampering Act passed in 1983 makes it a crime to tamper with packaged consumer products.

FDA publishes first **RED BOOK** (successor to 1949 "black book"), officially known as Toxicological Principles for the Safety Assessment of Direct Food Additives and Color Additives Used in Food.

1983

ORPHAN DRUG ACT passed, enabling FDA to promote research and marketing of drugs needed for treating rare diseases.

1984

FINES ENHANCEMENT LAWS of 1984 and 1987 amend the U.S. Code to greatly increase penalties for all federal offenses. The maximum fine for individuals is now $100,000 for each offense and $250,000 if the violation is a felony or causes death. For corporations, the amounts are doubled.

DRUG PRICE COMPETITION AND PATENT TERM RESTORATION ACT expedites the availability of less costly generic drugs by permitting FDA to approve applications to market generic versions of brand-name drugs without repeating the research done to prove them safe and effective. At the same time, the brand-name companies can apply for up to five years additional patent protection for the new medicines they developed to make up for time lost while their products were going through FDA's approval process.

1985

AIDS TEST FOR BLOOD approved by FDA in its first major action to protect patients from infected donors.

1986

CHILDHOOD VACCINE ACT requires patient information on vaccines, gives FDA authority to recall biologics, and authorizes civil penalties.

1987
INVESTIGATIONAL DRUG REGULATIONS REVISED to expand access to experimental drugs for patients with serious diseases with no alternative therapies.

1988
FOOD AND DRUG ADMINISTRATION ACT of 1988 officially establishes FDA as an agency of the Department of Health and Human Services with a Commissioner of Food and Drugs appointed by the President with the advice and consent of the Senate, and broadly spells out the responsibilities of the Secretary and the Commissioner for research, enforcement, education, and information.

THE PRESCRIPTION DRUG MARKETING ACT bans the diversion of prescription drugs from legitimate commercial channels. Congress finds that the resale of such drugs leads to the distribution of mislabeled, adulterated, subpotent, and counterfeit drugs to the public. The new law requires drug wholesalers to be licensed by the states; restricts reimportation from other countries; and bans sale, trade or purchase of drug samples, and traffic or counterfeiting of redeemable drug coupons.

GENERIC ANIMAL DRUG AND PATENT TERM RESTORATION ACT extends to veterinary products benefits given to human drugs under the 1984 Drug Price Competition and Patent Term Restoration Act. Companies can produce and sell generic versions of animal drugs approved after October 1962 without duplicating research done to prove them safe and effective. The act also authorizes extension of animal drug patents.

1989
FDA issued a nationwide recall of all over-the-counter dietary supplements providing 100 milligrams or more of **L-TRYPTOPHAN**. The recall was instituted because of a clear link between the consumption of L-tryptophan tablets and its association with a U.S. outbreak of Eosinophilia-Myalgia Syndrome (EMS) in 1989. Symptoms of EMS include fatigue, shortness of breath, rash, swelling of the extremities, and in some cases congestive heart failure. By 1990, The Centers for Disease Control and Prevention confirmed over 1,500 cases of EMS with 38 deaths. Officials estimate that there may have been 3,000-10,000 unreported cases. Numerous trace levels of impurities were identified in the L-tryptophan implicated in many of the EMS cases and the links between L-tryptophan and EMS are still being investigated in the laboratory. In 1990 FDA put an import alert in place prohibiting its importation.

1990
NUTRITION LABELING AND EDUCATION ACT requires all packaged foods to bear nutrition labeling and all health claims for foods to be consistent with terms defined by the Secretary of Health and Human Services. The law preempts state requirements about food standards, nutrition labeling, and health claims and, for the first time, authorizes some health claims for foods. The food ingredient panel, serving sizes, and terms such as "low fat" and "light" are standardized.

SAFE MEDICAL DEVICES ACT is passed, requiring nursing homes, hospitals, and other facilities that use medical devices to report to FDA incidents that suggest that a medical device probably caused or contributed to the death, serious illness, or serious injury of a patient. Manufacturers are required to conduct post-market surveillance on permanently implanted devices whose failure might cause serious harm or death, and to establish methods for tracing and locating patients depending on such devices. The act authorizes FDA to order device product recalls and other actions.

1991

Regulations published to **ACCELERATE THE REVIEW OF DRUGS** for life-threatening diseases.

1992

GENERIC DRUG ENFORCEMENT ACT imposes debarment and other penalties for illegal acts involving abbreviated drug applications.

PRESCRIPTION DRUG USER FEE ACT requires drug and biologics manufacturers to pay fees for product applications and supplements, and other services. The act also requires FDA to use these funds to hire more reviewers to assess applications.

MAMMOGRAPHY QUALITY STANDARDS ACT requires all mammography facilities in the United States to be accredited and federally certified as meeting quality standards effective Oct. 1, 1994. After initial certification, facilities must pass annual inspections by federal or state inspectors.

1994

DIETARY SUPPLEMENT HEALTH AND EDUCATION ACT establishes specific labeling requirements, provides a regulatory framework, and authorizes FDA to promulgate good manufacturing practice regulations for dietary supplements. This act defines "dietary supplements" and "dietary ingredients" and classifies them as food. The act also establishes a commission to recommend how to regulate claims.

FDA announces it could consider **REGULATING NICOTINE** in cigarettes as a drug, in response to a Citizen's Petition by the Coalition on Smoking OR Health.

URUGUAY ROUND AGREEMENTS ACT extends the patent terms of U.S. drugs from 17 to 20 years.

ANIMAL MEDICINAL DRUG USE CLARIFICATION ACT allows veterinarians to prescribe extra-label use of veterinary drugs for animals under specific circumstances. In addition, the legislation allows licensed veterinarians to prescribe human drugs for use in animals under certain conditions.

1995

FDA declares **CIGARETTES** to be "drug delivery devices." Restrictions are proposed on marketing and sales to reduce smoking by young people.

1996

FEDERAL TEA TASTERS REPEAL ACT repeals the Tea Importation Act of 1897 to eliminate the Board of Tea Experts and user fees for FDA's testing of all imported tea. Tea itself is still regulated by FDA.

SACCHARIN NOTICE REPEAL ACT repeals the saccharin notice requirements.

ANIMAL DRUG AVAILABILITY ACT adds flexibility to animal drug approval process, providing for flexible labeling and more direct communication between drug sponsors and FDA.

FOOD QUALITY PROTECTION ACT amends the Food, Drug, and Cosmetic Act, eliminating application of the Delaney proviso to pesticides.

1997

FOOD AND DRUG ADMINISTRATION MODERNIZATION ACT reauthorizes the Prescription Drug User Fee Act of 1992 and mandates the most wide-ranging reforms in agency practices since 1938. Provisions include measures to accelerate review of devices, regulate advertising of unapproved uses of approved drugs and devices, and regulate health claims for foods.

1998

MAMMOGRAPHY QUALITY STANDARDS REAUTHORIZATION ACT continues 1992 Act until 2002.

First phase to **CONSOLIDATE FDA LABORATORIES** nationwide from 19 facilities to 9 by 2014 includes dedication of the first of five new regional laboratories.

7. THE BARBER, THE FIRST INSTITUTIONALIZED SURGEON

One of the most respected professions today, the barber was once an institution of surgery that goes back to the year 1096. The era began when William, the Archbishop of Rouen, prohibited the wearing of a beard (to stop the spread of Islam). The word "Barber" comes from the Latin word "Barba," meaning beard. These men of this profession were also the practitioners of medicine and priesthood. They were even commissioned to perform acts of surgery.

The barber was responsible for drawing blood or performing surgery since there were no surgeons back at that time. Most diseases that are curable today were fatal during the dark ages of Europe. "Bloodletting" was the popular method of curing all forms of ill health (President George Washington died from this practice). The clergy who enlisted barbers as their assistant first performed this form of ignorant medicine. This was the first step in the progression of the barber profession. Barbers became the assistant to the physician/clergy until the 12th century.

The modern barber pole represented the bloodletting of the barber. The two spiral ribbons painted around the pole represented the two long bandages, one twisted around the arm before bleeding and the other used to bind afterward. Originally, when the pole was not in use it had a bandage around the outer surface and was used as a door sign. But later on, for the sake of convenience, instead of hanging out the original pole, another one was painted imitating the original so that it could become a permanent symbol outside the shop.

At the council of Tours in 1163, the clergy were forbidden to draw blood or perform any surgery because it was sacrilegious for the ministers of God to draw blood from the human body. This is when the barber-surgeon practice began. The connection between barber and surgeon continued for over six centuries. The barber was institutionalized as being a sound profession that even embraced dentistry. Barbers were allowed to perform surgery in dentistry for several centuries.

Up to the year 1416, the barbers were not interfered with by the practice of surgery and dentistry. However, the profession was beginning to go beyond their means of practice by performing procedures that became too complex for standard applications of surgery. People became sick instead of well; soon the barber-surgeons resorted to quackery in order to cover up their medical ignorance. Soon the complaints reached the Council of London in 1446 where an ordinance was passed forbidding barbers from practicing surgery.

In 1450, the Guild of Surgeons was incorporated with the Barbers Company act of parliament. Barbers were restricted to blood-letting, tooth drawing, cauterization and tonsorial operations. However, the board of governors, regulating the operations of the surgeon and barber-surgeons, consisted of two surgeons and two barbers. When a surgeon was presented with a diploma ordaining him to practice his profession, the diploma had to be signed by two barbers as well as two surgeons. The surgeons were opposed to this, but since the barbers were very much favored by the monarchs, this ordination preserved their privileges until the middle of the 18th century.

Even though the barber uses a totally differently application on the public today, he/she is still respected as a practitioner of health and one of the most important institutions in society. The barber shop is a refuge where people can relieve their social stress while being recreated from a shampoo, hair cut or shave. The barber shop helps turn boys into young men by elevating their minds with everything from history to current affairs. Let us not forget the women's beauty salon, which is an institution within itself. If it were not for this community cornerstone, the immaculate beauty of a woman would be hard to achieve.

MEDICAL SINS II

8. DIETARY NEGLECT: THE CAUSE OF DISEASE

In today's society, disease is accepted as a common part of life, "you were born to die from something" ideology. We all have relatives, friends and colleagues who have passed on from one some sort of degenerative or chronic disease. There is an underlying reason that causes disease to manifest in the first place. We can assume that blood sugar imbalance, lupus, cancer, diabetic coma, heart attack or even Alzheimer's disease is the underlying cause of death. However, the real cause of our ultimate demise is the disharmony with the universe and the Creator, i.e. spiritual imbalance, nutritional imbalance, physical and mental imbalance. These entities are the tools that fast food restaurants, drug corporations, processed food manufacturers, doctors and politician's use to lead us astray from the divine law that keeps us balanced. This is why America leads the world in degenerative diseases like arthritis, heart disease, cancer, diabetes, autoimmune disease and psychological illnesses. Practically everything we consume from processed foods to medications has altered our state of mind and health. Diseases like dental decay, kidney failure, multiple sclerosis, hyper or hypothyroidism, and irritable bowel syndrome are manifested through dietary neglect.

Human disease increases when the vital and essential nutrients in the human body decrease. After 20 to 30 years of consuming white bread products, white sugar, tap water, hydrogenated oils, and now irradiated food, your life has technically been sucked out of you! The majority of the people who have eaten processed Frankenstein foods for the last ten years are really creating within themselves genetic bodies without any life. Vital nutrients are non-existent, because the foods and drugs that are consumed tax the body of vitamins, minerals, enzymes and essential cofactors. Soon the production of immune enhancing cells like the T-lymphocytes, Beta cells, valuable hormones and neurotransmitters become so limited that the human body cannot defend itself from various forms of ill health. Your arterial walls become damaged, the liver becomes clogged, the kidneys fail to perform and the gastrointestinal area becomes a dump site for mucoid plaque. The final result is a compromised immune system where free radicals take over your body, and diseases like, cancer, diabetes, arthritis, lupus, MS, and various other degenerative diseases run rampant.

Let's examine some real statistics on America's ill health:

250 million people visit the emergency room each year.
250 billion cups of soda are consumed each year
13 billion barbiturates and amphetamines are taken
80 million people suffer from allergies
64% of the American population is overweight
60 million people are addicted to tobacco
50 million people are chronic alcoholics
Cancer is the number #1 death among children
30 million people have systemic arthritis
32 million people suffer from mental illness
Over 29 million suffer from high blood pressure
Over 13 million people have diabetes
(This is increasing at an alarming rate)
31 million people have no teeth
16 million suffer from ulcers
8 million children are mentally retarded
10 million suffer from psoriasis
50% of Americans die from heart disease (WOW!)
25 million submit to a surgeon's knife each year
Over 33% of America will have cancer and 80% will die within five years, with or without allopathic treatment
Over 50% of Americans have chronic digestive disorders.
Over 215 million people are still addicted to sugar
Over 36, 000 tons of aspirin are consumed
Over 86% of American children cannot pass a physical fitness test.
The elderly comprise 12% of the population of which 25% commit suicide

So what is disease and where does it begin? Disease is a breakdown of harmonious, cellular, biological and physiological activity within a living body. A disease is a manifestation of a foreign activity and disharmony within the body of life. Here are several underlying causes of disease:

Dietary neglect
Genetic engineering
Toxicity
Cloning
Unsanitary conditions
Stress
Chemical influence
Spiritual death

Before one is actually sick or diseased, there are a number of symptoms or warning signs that something within the body is wrong: tumors, cysts, colds, constipation, high/low blood sugar levels, smelly urine, etc. When a person's body begins to show the symptoms of diabetes or the onset of heart disease, the body gives you signals like uncontrolled sweating, fatigue, dehydration, heart palpitations, or bad body odor. Some people would respond by seeking help of their HMO practitioner, some people would not do anything and let the condition progress to its final stage. Once the disease continues to go untreated by detoxification, vitamin therapy, herbal medicine or conventional treatment, it eventually will cause cellular damage. Tissues, glands, nerve cells, and organ activity become altered and start to break down.

Most Americans have no idea that the food we eat, water we drink, and the over-the-counter drugs we take are the building blocks of premature aging and disease. Through chemical manipulation, the fast food industry and grocery outlets have caused the consumer to develop a great taste for toxicity. This is why the corporations depend upon the creative brainwashing through advertisement and the docile attitude of American behavior. They can continue to get away with synthetic manufacturing that contributes to profits and population control, because the masses have been lulled to sleep.

Another reason that disease begins in our bodies is due to an acidic internal environment. The body must maintain an alkaline pH of 7.2-7.4 in order to maintain a healthy chemical balance. If our body's pH level drops below that point it becomes acidic and disease begins to manifest. For example, if you develop a pH level of 5.0 you have become very acidic or if you develop a pH level of 9.0 you have become extremely alkaline. pH is referred to as potential for Hydrogen. We need oxygen to maintain an alkaline environment. The refined foods like white sugar, excessive commercial meats, added caffeine and all drugs develop an acidic environment that initially creates a potential for disease. When we lack oxygen fungus, bacteria, and germs all thrive within our bodies. Candida or yeast infections thrive in both men and women because of an acidic environment due to not only a lack of oxygen but to the over-consumption of dead foods, canned goods, soda pop, candy, fast foods and antibiotics. Your body loses that positive charge and oxygen, and this is where you experience the first symptoms of illness. To get a better understanding of this activity, please see the movie "Osmosis Jones." This movie gives a great example of how various immune functions work in the body on a cellular level.

9. SOIL TOXICITY: THE FOUNDATION TO MALNUTRITION

When crop growth begins to decrease, the modern day corporate farmer abandons the land instead of trying to figure out how to regenerate it. They migrate to virgin areas and exercise this same form of MediSin and move on. The modern farmer has been persuaded to use monoculture, artificial fertilization, pesticides, herbicides and mechanization in order to prevent ruinous taxation, inflation and the increasing cost of production. The end result of our domestic food needs has been "quantity" rather than "quality," and the gradual destruction of precious soil that has been preserved by the natives for thousands of years is almost extinct (Read Senate Document 264, 1936).

The MediSin behind "mono-cropping" is that chemical fertilizers are now used to replace the nutrients lost in the growth process. Pesticides have increased tenfold while crop losses due to insects have doubled. So who's really killing whom? Most pests have developed a resistance to the chemicals used against them, so farmers still have to purchase more deadly pesticides! A National Cancer Institute study found that farmers exposed to pesticides and herbicides had 6 times more risk of contracting cancer than the average person. An estimated 27,000 to 300,000 people are poisoned annually by these pest control chemicals.

The optimum of our physical and mental constitution solely depends upon the mineral and protein preserves in the soil. The grocery store is plentiful with attractive, and shiny but tasteless and nutritionally worthless fruits and vegetables. They are worthless in true value because of the chemical manipulation and depleted nutrition. The human body can thrive on fruits and vegetables that are grown on vital rich soil, which provide the body with enzymes, co-factors, antioxidants, and trace minerals. Companies that serve the "under-served" like Monsanto, Dow Chemical, ADM, DuPont and AgrEvo have no intention of maintaining the ecological balance of our earth. Monsanto's so-called weed killer Round Up became the third leading cause of farm worker illness with several fatalities from ingesting traces of Round Up. Now, this lethal chemical is distributed worldwide and is somewhere in our food chain.

People complain about the price of organic foods, but fail to realize the hidden cost of commercial farming, billion dollar subsidies, pesticide regulations & testing, hazardous waste clean up, adverse health effects, and deaths. There are tens of thousands of pesticides approved by the EPA long before research links them to cancer. Now the EPA considers 60% of all herbicides, 90% of fungicides, and 30% of insecticides carcinogenic (cancer causing agent). There are over 4.5 million known toxic chemicals and 375, 000 new chemicals produced annually.

Due to the provocateurs of the agricultural industry, the standard American food chain has been an ever-changing process. It leaves the American people more exposed to toxins, mineral depletion, and genetic foods. The human cell is constantly struggling between a normal and mutated state. If you look at the small print on your commercial snack label it would read more like a rocket fuel formula with unpronounceable test tube names than a food item for human consumption. For instance, the Twinkie (chemical cake) has been a successful experiment in taste-bud delight, containing the bright plastic husk found in dumpsites all over the planet. However, to the gullible American, it looks like a "snack delight" rather than "chemical fright."

The masses, not only in America but in the entire world, have become so docile and so programmed that they have no clue that they are consuming products that are harmful. Americans consume foods that contain more than five thousand chemical additives, which they enjoy at breakfast, lunch and dinner. About one-third is considered to be harmless another third is described by the FDA (Food and Drug Administration) as "GRAS" and acronym for "generally recognized as safe," and the other third, more than 2,000 chemicals are cell damaging and mutating. These chemicals are randomly selected as food additives and are never tested for possible harmful results, just as the prescription drugs are marketed for experimental purposes only.

10. UNDERSTANDING TOXEMIA AND THE STAGES OF DISEASE

Toxemia is a polluted condition of the body's own biological terrain, due to impurities in the bloodstream derived from adulterated foods and environmental toxins. These bodily pollutants are becoming more ingested creating a wide spread of allergies, ear infections, skin diseases, slow growth, neurological and mental retardation. One of the contributors to toxemia is the overworked digestive system. This starts from consuming foods from your fast food restaurant **(McKillers, Murder King, Jack n' the Casket, Hell Taco, Krispy Grease, Crack in the Box and KFC (Kidney Failure and Cancer)** with their drive-thru of death menus. Always remember, these food chains could care less about your health, its all about profits!

<u>The Progressive Development of Disease</u>

1st Stage: General Fatigue: A depletion of physical and mental energy. This condition is normally accompanied by muscular tension, hardening of the arteries, frequent urination, sweating, constipation, brain fog, and short periods of feeling cold or hot. Mentally, we start to lose our clarity, active perception and accurate response.

To recover from this stage: it usually takes a short time, from a few hours to a few days. Once adequate rest is obtained and the consumption of whole foods, herbal teas, tonics, quality water and exercise are incorporated then equilibrium and health once again begins to manifest.

2nd Stage: Aches and Pains: When feelings of general fatigue prevail, we begin to experience occasional pains and aches. Headaches, cramps and other various pain symptoms appear from time to time. Temporary shortness of breath, irregular heartbeat, fever and chills also begin to appear. Mentally, we may experience occasional depression, worry, and insecurity.

3rd Stage: Blood Stagnation: If the dietary lifestyle is continued through adolescence on to adulthood, along with environmental pollution, our quality of blood, including red blood cells, white blood cells and blood plasma, become unsuitable for maintaining harmony with our natural surroundings. The quality of our blood determines the quality of our body's cells and tissues, organs and systems. Blood disorders create various abnormal conditions in our body from which symptoms of sickness arise. Acidosis, high and low blood pressure, anemia, and other diseases occur during this stage including leukemia, epilepsy, asthma and skin disease.

4th Stage: Emotional Disorder: If an improper quality of blood is not in circulation for a prolonged period of time, various emotional disorders begin to surface. Short temper, excitement, anger, frustration and a general feeling of despair are frequent in daily life. Physical movement becomes more rigid and we gradually lose flexibility in both body and mind.

5th Stage: Organ Disease: This stage produces gradual changes in the quality and function of our organs and glands. This is where the symptoms of atherosclerosis, diabetes, gall/kidney stone formation appear and where the beginning stage of some organ cancers, multiple sclerosis and other auto-immune diseases begin to manifest.

6th Stage: Nervous Disorder: This is the stage where physical paralysis and mental illnesses like schizophrenia and paranoia begin. Physical and mental coordination of various functions gradually diminishes. A negative view of life and the alternative begins to dominate the mind, even suicidal tendencies may be discussed.

7th Stage: Arrogance: This is the most developed form of sickness, along with denial which is the foundation of humanity's fall altogether. Selfishness, egocentricity, vanity, self-pride, and self-justification becomes the core of hopelessness.

Every physical, mental and spiritual illness belongs to one of the seven stages listed. All diseases are inter-dependent and inter-connected with one another; they are symptoms stemming from the same root cause; diet, spirit and lifestyle toxicity. As life begins, we are only a natural and divine manifestation that is only familiar with the zest for life. We accept the idea that we will pass on from some type of illness, like heart disease, cancer, diabetes, or some other degenerative disease because our parents or grandparents did. This ignorant universal belief by modern society is certainly contrary to the divine law of nature and human life. As long as we continue to live away from the infinite laws of divine wisdom happiness, health and longevity, we will become only a fantasy as we proceed slowly down the road of self-blame and negative energy.

11. DEATH BY MEDICAL SINS

The Lazarou Study was based on statistical analysis of 33 million American hospital admissions in 1994 where hospitals that prescribed medications were analyzed. Two million people were injured from prescription drugs; 2.1% of the patients experienced a serious adverse drug reaction; 4.7% of all hospital admissions were due to adverse drug reactions; fatal adverse drug reactions occurred in .019% of the patients and 0.13% of admissions. Researchers concluded that a projected 106,000 deaths occur annually due to adverse drug reactions.

In the year 2000, a study in which the increase in hospitalization cost per patient suffering an adverse drug reaction was $5,483. Therefore, the cost for the Lazarou study's 2.2 million patients with serious adverse effects costing about $12 billion. Adverse effects commonly emerge after FDA approval of most drugs. The quality of the drug cannot be measured until it has been massively administered across the country or globe for several years.

THE BEDSORES OF THE HEALH CARE INDUSTRY

The complications of bedsores also known as Decubitic Ulcer or Hospital Gangrene are one of the many health concerns that are commonly overlooked during a hospital stay. It has been recorded that there are over one million patients in American hospitals who suffer from bedsores annually. It's not only a serious health concern for the family, but it generates excruciating pain for the patient. Unfortunately, 50% of those affected with bedsores are patients over the age of 70. The mortality rate from bedsores ranges from 23% to 37% due to infection. Bedsores are caused by poor circulation, unsanitary conditions, no fresh air, artificial lighting (no sun exposure) and no physical movement. This condition could be easily eliminated by getting exercise, sun exposure, skin brushing to increase circulation, and good hygiene. The resulting financial burden runs to a tune of $55 billion.

This is an unnecessary MediSin and is certainly avoidable if nurses and doctors were not so concerned about their nightlife rendezvous and entertainment agendas. Obviously, the hospital is not a place where compassion has precedence over chitchat, soap operas and sexual gossip. The hospital, which really means a place to die, has really become more of a cattle stall for the "sheeple" (brain dead people). Obviously, to protect the integrity of the institution the "bootlicking" critics would say that the cause of death would be from the patient's ill health or old age, as opposed to the seriously ulcerated skin condition.

The General Accounting Office (GAO), a special investigative department of Congress has cited 20% of the nation's 17,000 nursing facilities for violations between July 2000 and January 2002. The Coalition for Nursing Home reform states that at least 1/3 of the America's 1.6 million nursing home residents may suffer from malnutrition and dehydration, which eventually causes death. The need for adequate nursing staff is paramount, because most of the patients aren't able to manage the completion of a meal due to their limited mobility. The Coalition Report states that malnourished nursing home patients had a five-fold increase in mortality from the time they are admitted to a hospital. So, take 1/3 of the 1.6 million nursing home residents who are malnourished and multiply that by a mortality rate of 20%, and there would be 108,800 unnecessary deaths due to undernourished patients in nursing homes.

THE MEDISINS OF SURGERY

Another MediSin that plagues the ill-care industry is the thousands of unnecessary surgeries performed each year. Health concerns such as fibroid tumors, tonsillitis, and thyroid imbalance have given doctors an opportunity to capitalize on unnecessary surgical procedures. The majority of the surgeries are avoidable if the medical industry truly understood the cellular energies within the human body and the divine laws of health. Most controversial surgeries of "organ dysfunction" involve mineral, enzyme, and vitamin deficiency through consuming the wrong foods. In 1974, 2.4 million unnecessary surgeries were performed annually resulting in 11, 900 deaths at an annual cost of $3.9 billion. What a shame! In 2001, 7.5 million unnecessary surgical procedures resulted in 37,136 deaths at a cost of $122 billion (using 1974 dollars). Ridiculous! These controversial surgeries were for obesity, breast implants, and breast removal. Media-driven surgery such as gastric bypass for obesity "modeled" by Hollywood and media personalities like Mr. Al Roker of Good Morning America, entices the mind of the unconscious and uneducated American. Instead of setting an example of dietary leadership and lifestyle changes which includes detoxification, fasting and exercise, media personalities are paid to convince you to take the detour to grandma's house where you'll only find a wolf in doctors' clothing.

By 1994, there was an increase of 38% for a total of 7,929,000 cases for the top ten surgical procedures. In 1983, surgical cases totaled 5,731,000. In 1994, cataract surgery was number one with over two million operations, and the second was cesarean section (858,000 procedures), inguinal hernia operations placed third (689,000 procedures), and the surgeons of arthroscopy flock like vultures on the cases of knee surgery, especially in the athletic arena. This is the seventh most common surgery, which has grown to 153% (632,000 procedures).

It is important to know that the mortality rate associated with medical and surgical procedures is a very serious issue. When one signs a release form before undergoing any procedure, the mind is still in denial regarding the true risk involved. Do you really believe that surgery is the absolute remedy for your ill health? If you were to take the time and reflect on your diet, lifestyle, spiritual balance, and mental state you would never see the surgery line (exception: serious accidents). Besides why pay for your doctor's next yacht, let him/her go take out a loan like the rest of us.

THE FIRST IATROGENIC STUDY

One of the most important studies on modern medical sins was done by Dr. Lucian L. Leape. He opened "Pandora's box" in his 1994 JAMA paper, "Error in Medicine". He began the paper by reminiscing about Florence Nightingale's maxim – "first do no harm." However, he discovered the opposite of this philosophy. He uncovered a report in 1964 that stated 20% of the hospital patients suffer iatrogenic (doctor caused) injury, with a 20 % fatality rate. In 1981 it was reported that 36% of hospitalized patients experienced an iatrogenic injury with a 25% fatality rate.

Medical doctors are actually taught that medical mistakes are acceptable. Denial is a very common mind set in professional medicine. The term "infallibility model" of medicine leads to intellectual dishonesty with a need to cover up mistakes rather than admit them or correct them. Leape had hoped that his paper would encourage medicine "to fundamentally change the mind set about medical errors and as to why they really occur." Although you can't buy love, you can buy "scientific results." The only safeguard in reporting these case studies is when journalists remain ethical and unbiased. Unfortunately, this type of behavior is slowly becoming a thing of the past.

In 1997, during a press conference, Dr. Leape released a nationwide poll on patient iatrogenic injuries that was conducted by the National Patient Safety Foundation (NPSF), which is sponsored by the American Medical Foundation. The survey found that more than 100 million Americans are victims of medical mistakes. Forty-two percent were directly affected and a total of 84% personally knew of someone who had incurred a medical mistake. We suspect these numbers are a lot higher, but since the AMA sponsored the survey, you know they had to be conservative.

Dr. Leape also updated his 1994 statistics saying that medical errors in inpatient hospital settings nationwide are as high as three million and could cost as much as $200 billion. Leape used a 14% fatality rate to determine a medical error death rate of 180,000 in 1994. In 1997, using Leape's base number of three million errors, the annual deaths would be as much as 420,000 for inpatients alone. This does not include nursing home deaths, or people in the outpatient community dying of the adverse effects from drugs like Vioxx, Ibuprofen, or suicidal-homicides from other drugs like Zoloft and Prozac. These people are all victims of MediSin.

The American system of "Disease Management" is obviously in need of a complete and total reform: from the curriculum in medical schools to protecting patients from excessive medical intervention. Realistically, nothing will change because of denial, arrogance and greed. Change would cause such an upheaval, that it would rival a social and economical Armageddon. This is how devastating the deception and falsehood of medicine actually is. We want you to be fully aware of the bridge that needs to be crossed and the toll that needs to be paid. There are powerful pharmaceutical, medical technology, and special interest groups with an enormous interest in the business of medicine. They are the ones who fund medical research, support medical schools and hospitals and pay for advertisement in medical journals. Because they walk with deep pockets they can entice scientists and academic administrators to support their efforts, and believe it or not, the "puppets" and "sellouts" of these institutions trade in their integrity every day for a tangible incentive.

Such funding can be the determining factor of opinion from professionals who caution the acceptance of a new therapy or drug. Next time you're in a medical institution, just look at the names of the board trustees and you will see the conflict of interest as clear as day. For example, a 2003 study found that nearly half of medical school faculty who serve on Institutional Review Boards (IRB) to overview the clinical trail research, also serve as consultants to the pharmaceutical industry. Do you think these people are concerned about your health?

A news release by Dr. Erik Campbell, a lead author, said "Our previous research with faculty has shown us that ties to the industry can affect scientific behavior, leading to such things like trade secrecy and public information. It seems that the price for integrity and humanity does not have the value of greed and power, the medical profession has allowed itself to be lured onto the reef of a new medieval dogmatism in medicine. A dogmatism that forces all practitioners into a compliance with holy pronouncements of scientific truth, a dogmatism that has closed the door on the greatest scientific advance of the twentieth century."

<u>The Nature of Big Pharma</u>

The un-divine purpose and driving force of the pharmaceutical industry is to increase sales of prescription drugs for on going diseases and to find new diseases to market drugs. The information that you are about to read not only demonstrates profitable revenue but the continued use of these drugs regardless of the adverse affects experienced by the consumer/patient. The application of these drugs/medisins proliferates other conditions that will require other forms of medications which will lead to more side affects and the need for more prescription drugs. The capital objective is to continue the cycle until you eventually become the ultimate victim of a medisin!

By its very nature, Big Pharma has no interest in curing disease, it is the nature of the beast. Greed knows no ethic, has no morals or compassion but only the desire for profit and control. The eradication of any disease inevitably destroys a multibillion dollar market of prescription drugs as a source of revenue. Therefore, prescription drugs are primarily developed to relieve symptoms without ever curing the ailment.

If eradication therapies for many health concerns are discovered and developed, Big Pharma will by its nature have an inherent interest to suppress, discredit and obstruct any natural breakthroughs in order to make sure that diseases continue as the very basis for a lucrative prescription drug market. The economic interest is the main reason why no medical breakthroughs have been made for the control of most common diseases such as cardiovascular disease, cancer, high blood pressure, congestive heart failure, diabetes, and other degenerative diseases.

At the same time Big Pharma corporations withhold public information about the effects and risks of prescription drugs and potential life threatening side effects are omitted and openly denied; isn't that the very nature of a "devils advocate," to lie and deceive. Remember Revelations 18:23: "by sorcery were all nations deceived." The corporations truly understand the psyche of the masses when they run pharmaceutical commercials. The ad grooms and manipulates the already programmed mind of the consumer with calming music, smiles and family warmth just to set you up for the kill. Then at the very end of the commercial it announces the contraindications and dangerous adverse effects that can occur after short or long term usage, but they know that the average person is too docile to register the side affects of the medisins. So the patient's primary care physician reels in another source of revenue for Big Pharma, the pharmaceutical sales representative and the primary care physician.

In order to assure the status quo of this deceptive scheme, a legion of pharmaceutical lobbyists are employed to influence legislation, control regulatory agencies (e.g. FDA), and manipulate medical research and education.

BILLION DOLLAR MEDISINS

MEDISINS	PURPOSE	REVENUE IN BILLIONS	SIDE EFFECTS
Lipitor	Cholesterol Blocker (LDL)	6.30	closing of throat, flu-symptoms, blurred vision

Zocor	Cholesterol (LDL)	5.10	constipation bloating,
gas			
Prevacid	Decreases stomach acid	4.40	heartburn, antacids, stomach ulcers
Procit	Man-made protein, builds RBC's, treats anemia	3.20	swelling lips, increase blood pressure, fatigue, rashes
Nexium	Treat ulcers	2.80	headaches GERD disease, nausea, dry mouth, acid reflux
Zyprexa	Treats psychotic	2.60	Increase blood conditions, bipolar sugar, severe disorder, muscle stiffness confusion, Irregular heart beat, weight gain
Celexa	Treats depression	1.40	low blood pressure, sev-ere headaches

MEDISINS	PURPOSE	REVENUE IN BILLIONS	SIDE EFFECTS
Premerin	Hormone Replacement	1.0	increased risk of replacement, endometrial hy-perplasia that may lead to cancer of the uterus, heart

			attack, breast cancer, blood clots
Paxil	Antidepressant	1.50	causes depression, panic, anxiety, obsessive behavior, low blood pressure, tremor, anxiety
Glucotrol	Helps to control blood sugar	.30	may increase the risk of death from cardiovascular disease
Avandia	Improve glycemic control in patients with type II diabetes	1.30	anemia, edema and cardiac failure.
Prilosec	Short-term treatment of duodenal ulcers	1.10	swelling of stomach, lips and tongue, liver disease
Advair	A steroid, prevents the release of substances in the body that cause inflammation. Muscle relaxant	1.20	edema, chest pain, shortness of breath and weight gain

MEDISINS	**PURPOSE**	**REVENUE IN BILLIONS**	**SIDE EFFECTS**
Zoloft	Treats depression, obsessive compulsive disorder, Post-Traumatic Disorder (PTD)	2.50	high blood pressure, difficult breathing, low blood pressure insomnia, impotence

MEDISIN	PURPOSE	REVENUE IN BILLIONS	SIDE EFFECTS
Celebrex	Arthritus, pain killer and Cox-2 inhibitor	2.50	swelling of lips, abdominal pain, bloody stools and congestive heart failure
Epogen	Used to treat anemia	2.50	increased blood pressure, flu-like symptoms, numbness, tingling and rash
Nuerontin	Treat seizures and some types pain	2.40	blurred vision poor coordination, tremors, and drowsiness
Plavix	Prevents platelets from clustering and treatment for heart attacks	2.20	swelling of throat, lips, and tongue, headaches confusion, and easy bruising
Norvasc	Treats blood pressure, angina and chest pain	2.10	severe dizzness, juandice, slow heart beat and abnormal dreams
Effexor	Antidepressant, treats anxiety	2.10	irregular heart beat, seizures, high blood pressure, insomnia, and abdominal pain

Pravochol	Treats cholesterol and triglycerides	1.90	flu-like symptoms, blurred vision and yellowing of skin

These are only an example of the thousands of medisins that are prescribed on a daily basis to helpless and unconscious consumers and patients. Practically every condition can be controlled with diet, exercise, and proper supplementation. Remember, no man-made drug takes precedence over God's divine laws of healing and his garden of natural resources. My people are destroyed for what? A lack of knowledge!

MEDICATION/MEDISIN	NUTRIENTS DEPLETED
ANTACIDS/LAXATIVES	
• Aluminum hydroxide (Amphojel, Riopan) • Aluminum hydroxide and magnesium hydroxide (Mylanta, Maalox) • Aluminum hydroxide and magnesium carbonate (Algicon, Gaviscon) • Magnesium hydroxide (Milk of Magnesia) • Magnesium oxide (Mag-Ox) • Magnesium sulfate (Epsom Salts) • Sodium Bicarbonate	Calcium and Phosphorus
ANTIBIOTICS	
• Penicillin's (Amoxicillin) • Cephalosporins • Macrolides (Macro, Ziththromax) • Aminoglycosides (Garamycin, Cleocin)	Biotin Inositol Lactobacillus acidophilus Vitamin B1, B2, B3, B6, B12, K
• Tetracyclines, Sulfonamides (Vibramycin, Minoci)	Calcium, Iron, Magnesium, Lactobacillus acidophilus Bifodobacteria bifidum (bifidus) Vitamins, B1, B2, B3, B6, B12, K
• Neomycin (Mycifradin)	Beta-carotene Iron Vitamin A Vitamin B-12

MEDICATION/MEDISIN	NUTRIENTS DEPLETED
• Co-Trimoxazole	Bifidobacteria bifidum (bifidus) Lactobacillus acidophilus
• Insoniazid (Nydrazid)	Vitamin B3 Vitamin B6 Vitamin B12
• Rifampin (Rifadin)	Vitamin D
• Ethambutol (Myambutol)	Copper, Zinc
ANTICONVULSANTS	
• Barbituates (Tuinal, Seconal)	Biotin, Calcium, Folic acid Vitamin D, K
• Phenytoin (Dilantin)	Calcium, Folic acid, Vitamin B1 Vitamin B12, Vitamin D, K
• Carbamazepine	Biotin, Folic acid, Vitamin D
• Valpronic Acid	Carnitine, Folic acid

MEDICATION/MEDISIN	NUTRIENTS DEPLETED
ANTIDIABETICS	
• Sulfonylureas: Acetohexamide (Dymelor) Glyburide (Micronase, Diabeta) Tolazamide (Tolinase)	Coenzyme Q10
Biguanides: Metformin (Glucophage)	Vitamin B12
ANTI-GOUT DRUGS	
• Colchicine	Beta-carotene Potassium Sodium Vitamin B12
ANTI-INFLAMMATORIES	
• **Salicylates:** Aspirin (Epirin, Ecotrin, Asperum) Choline magnesium trisalicylate Trilisate	Folic acid Iron Potassium Sodium Vitamin C
• Nonsteroidal anti-inflammatory agents Celecoxib (Celebrex) Diclofenac (Cataflam) Diflunisal (Dolobid) Etodolac (Ultradol)	Folic acid

Fenoprofen (Nalfon)	
Ibuprofen (Motrin, Advil)	
Ketoprofen (Orudis)	
Ketorolac (Toradol)	
Meclofenamate (Meclomen)	
Mefenamic acid (Ponstan)	
Nabumetone (Relafen)	
Naproxen (Nalfon)	
Piroxicam (Clinoril)	
Tolmetin (Tolectin)	
• Indomethacin (Indocin)	Folic acid
	Iron
• Corticosteroids:	Calcium
Beamethasone (Celestone)	Folic acid
Budesonide (Entocort)	Magnesium
Cortisone (Cortone)	Potassium
Dexamethasone (Decadron)	Selenium
Flunisolide (Aerobid)	Vitamin C

MEDICATION/MEDISIN	**NUTRIENTS DEPLETED**
Fluticasone (Salmeterol)	Vitamin D
Hydrocortisone (Cortef)	Zinc
Methylprednisolone (Medrol)	
Mometasone (Nasonex)	
Predisone (Deltasone, Orasone)	
Triamcinolone (Aristocort, Kenacort)	
ANTIVIRALS	
• **Reverse Transcriptase Inhibitors**	Carnitine
Didanosine (Videx)	Copper
Lamivudine (Epivir)	Vitamin B12
Stavudine (Zerit)	Zinc
Zalcitabine (ddC, HIVID)	
Zidovudine (Retrovir)	
BENZODIAZEPINES	
• Alprazolam (Xanax)	Melatonin
• Diazepam (Valium)	
BRONCHODILATORS	
• Theophylline (Slo-Bid, Theolair, Slo-Phylline, Theodur)	Vitamin B-6
CARDIOVASCULAR DRUGS	
• Vasodilators:	Coenzyme Q10
Hydralazine (Apresoline)	Vitamin B-6

Loop diuretics: Bumetanide (Bumex) Ethacrynic Acid (Edecrin) Furosemide (Lasix)	Calcium Magnesium Potassium Vitamin B-1 Vitamin B-6 Vitamin C Zinc
• Thiazide diuretics Hydrochlorothiazide (Esidrex, Hydrodiuril) Indapamide (Lozol) Cardiovascular drugs cont. Methyclothiazide (Enduron) Metolazone (Zaroxolyn)	Caclium Magnesium Potassium Zinc
Potassium-sparing diuretics: Triamterene (Dyazide)	Calcium Folic acid Zinc

MEDICATION/MEDISIN	NUTRIENTS DEPLETED
• ACE inhibitors: Captopril (Capoten) Enalopril (Vasotec)	Zinc
• Centrally-acting antihypertensives: Clonidine (Catapres) Methyldopa (Aldomet)	Coenzyme Q10
Chlorthalidone	Zinc
• Cardiac glycosides: Digoxin (Lanoxin)	Calcium Magnesium Phosphorus Vitamin B1
• Beta-Blockers: Acebutolol (Sectral) Atenolol (Tenormin) Beta-Blockers Betaxolol Kerlone) Bisoprolol (Cardicor) Carteolol Cartrol Carvedilol (Coreg) Esmolol (Brevibloc) Labetalol (Normodyne) Metprolol (Lopressor, Toprox XL) Nadolol (Corgard) Pindolol (Visken) Propranol (inderal) Sotalol (Betapace) Timolol (Blocadren)	Coenzyme Q10 Melatonin

CHOLESTEROL-LOWERING DRUGS

• **HMG-CoA Reductase Inhibitors:** Atorvastatin (Lipitor) Cerivastatin (Baycol) Fluvastatin (Lescol) Lovastatin (Mevacor) Pravastatin (Pravachol) Simvastatin (Zocor)	Coenzyme Q10
• **Bile Acid Sequenstrants:** Cholestyramine (Questran)	Beta-carotene Calcium Folic acid Iron Magnesium Phosphorus Vitamins A, B12, E, K and Zinc

MEDICATION/MEDISIN	NUTRIENTS DEPLETED
Bile-Acids Sequestrants cont.	
Colstipol (Colestid)	Beta-carotene Folic acid Iron Vitamin A Vitamin B12 Vitamin D Vitamin E
ELECTROLYTE REPLACEMENT	
• Potassium Chloride (Time Release)	Vitamin B12
FEMALE HORMONES	
• Oral contraceptives	Folic Acid Tyrosine Vitamin B2 Vitamin B6 Vitamin B12 Vitamin C Magnesium Zinc
Estrogen replacement (ERT) and hormone Replacement (HRT) therapies: Conjugated Estrogens (Premarin) Esterified Estrogens (Estratab, Menest) Estrogens (Estrace, Estinyl)	Magnesium Vitamin B6 Zinc

MEDICATION/MEDISIN	NUTRIENTS DEPLETED
Medroxyprogesterone (Provera)	
Raloxifene (Evista)	
LAXATIVES	
• Mineral Oil	Beta-carotene
Calcium	
Vitamin A	
Vitamin D	
Vitamin E	
Vitamin K	
Bisacodyl (Dulcolax)	Potassium
PSYCHOTHERAPEUTIC AGENTS	
• **Tricyclic antidepressants:**	Coenzyme Q10
Amitripyline (Elavil)	Vitamin B2
Despiramine (Norpramin)	
Doxepin (Sinequan)	
Nortiptyline (Aventyl)	
• **Phenothiazines:**	Coenzyme Q10
Chlorpromazine (Thorazine)	Vitamin B2
Thioriddazine (Mellaril0	
Fluphenazine (Prolixin)	
• **Butyrophenonones:**	Coenzyme Q10
Haloperidol (Haldol)	
• **H-2 receptor antagonists**:	**Calcium**
Cimetidine (Tagamet)	Folic acid
Famotide (Pepcid)	Iron
Nizatadine (Axid)	Vitamin B12
Ranitidine (Zantac)	Vitamin D
	Zinc
• **Proton pump inhibitors:**	Vitamin B12
Lansoprazole (Prevacid)	
Omeprazole (losec)	
OTHER DRUG APPLICATIONS OR MEDISINS	
• Methotrexate	Folic Acid, Copper
• Penicillamine (Cuprimine)	Magnesium, B6, Zinc
• Acetaminophen (Tylenol)	Glutathione

Since these medical prescriptions can deplete the body of important vitamins, minerals, co-factors, and enzymes, the best action to take in order to prevent a compromised immune system is to replace them. Seek a qualified specialist that may be able to direct you to the most appropriate source for supplements and lifestyle changes. Shopping at health foods stores would be a start, and then start attending more lectures on natural health. Remember, you only have one mortal life, live it well, by seeking knowledge.

12. HOSPITAL FOODS: WHO WROTE THE MENU?

"A hospital is like a war. You should try your best to stay out of it. And if you get into it you should take along as many allies as possible and get out as soon as you can....For the hospital is the Temple of the Church of Modern Medicine, and thus one of the most dangerous places on earth...Children, again, provide us with a message from their unclouded perception: kids are unabashedly afraid of going to the hospital. Just as their fear of doctors is something we could all cultivate to our advantage, so is their fear of hospitals." Dr. Mendelson, Confessions of a Medical Heretic, 1979.

The medical institutions claim that they are well trained and are committed to excellence. But how are they committed to excellence when the patients are abused and forced to eat refined, irradiated and synthetically manufactured foods. As a matter of fact, practically every conventional hospital in the U.S.A. serves more food that devitalizes the human body than foods that nourishes it. If one were to actually analyze the nutritional base of their hospital breakfast, lunch or supper, they would find the following; their commercial dairy milk is laced with growth hormones and antibiotics, their instant breakfast cereals possibly contain genetically engineered, irradiated and chemical treated grains, their Jell-O is pork based, their breads are mucous producing, their meals are canola and vegetable oil based, and their commercial sweeteners such as Splenda, Equal, Sweet n Low and white sugar are all life taxing drugs.

In order for the human body to have any chance of full recovery it first has to have a non-chemical, whole food base and organic diet. You cannot expect the body to rebuild itself on foods that are not grown on a fertile organic foundation or that is genetically altered. Notice that Genesis 8:22 doesn't say, "harvest and seed-time" because harvest never comes first.

Now let's look at the first law of seedtime and harvest: *You will always reap what you sow.* We can see when the Creator first set this law into motion on this planet:

"And God said let the earth put forth [tender] vegetation: plants yielding seed and fruit trees yielding fruit whose seed is in itself, EACH ACCORDING TO ITS KIND, upon the earth. And it was so." *Genesis 1:11*

The patient should be given only wholesome fresh produce, not produce that is laced with sulfur dioxide, pesticides, insecticides that contain cancer causing compounds. Grains should be wholesome not genetically modified and chemical treated, breads should be freshly baked not preserved to last months without molding. The juice should be organically fresh squeezed, not reconstituted from concentrate. Foods should contain trace elements, vitamins, and minerals, just like pet food; yes pet foods are actually healthier because they contain trace minerals and micro nutrients! Finally, a patient needs whole grain salt, not sodium chloride (table salt). As far as the completely "salt-free" diet goes, this advice can cause your kidneys to breakdown and your respiratory function to collapse. So when a physician tells you to refrain from consuming salt, ask him or her about whole salt or Celtic sea salt? If they give you that stupid look just tell them to re-educate themselves by reading Jacque de Langre, PhD book titled "Sea Salt's Hidden Powers," The Biological Action of All Ocean Minerals on Body and Mind. In the mean time become a smart consumer by conducting your own research!

All allopathic hospital food menus are developed by registered dieticians. Dieticians enter universities with good intentions, but unfortunately they are only shown the same old American Standard Diet (SAD) protocol. Malnutrition is one of the main reasons patients die in hospitals, especially the elderly. This is a crime, because so many patients are injured unknowingly through the foods served in hospitals. Just think about it, have you ever said, "I'm going to go to a hospital for dinner" or "I'm going to a hospital to relax, meditate, fast, or eat nutritious meals." Finally, hospital foods are more of an experimental food protocol just to see how long the human body can endure it, believe it or not the roaches and mice would want better.

13. VACCINES: THE LIE OF THE NEEDLE

"I've heard drug experts say they believe if penicillin were discovered today, the FDA wouldn't license it."- Ronald Reagan

FEAR (**F**alse **E**vidence **A**ppearing **R**eal) has captivated the American mind and the world to accept ideologies that may not have even been considered if the FEAR factor was not shoved down their throats. The Neo-cons in Washington and their counterparts have gotten the world fixated on "the war on terror" which is an euphemism for the "war on Islam." The real terrorist's are the International Corporations, which include Pharmaceutical, Defense Contractors, and Producers of Genetic Foods. FEAR plays its role by causing individuals to view a certain look or culture with a long arm and condemn them for not wanting to look or accept the "Western European Model" or "Democracy." Remember the saying' "they hate us because of our freedom!" How arrogant and unintelligent of a statement to make! When was the last time you had some democracy or freedom? Speaking of democracy, that word **does not** appear in the US Constitution, Bill of Rights, Declaration of Independence, or any State Constitution! How many gullible Americans can actually define what or who is a terrorist? Most of their convictions were given to them by the perfidious press who, by the way, are all owned/controlled by major corporations. If you think that America is the land of the free and home of the brave then you need to consider this:

1) Former & Current Administrations have sent the good-paying jobs out of the country to foreign sweatshops (see the movie "The Corporation")

2) There are bills in congress for a military draft in the near distant future.

3) There are bills in congress to vaccinate the entire country against a biological agent created in a US Military laboratory.

The tactics that are used to scare a populace about a tragic event are also used in regards to your own body. When it comes to MediSin and vaccines, it is important to free your mind from the overriding conditioning that has been imprinted onto our brains like circuit boards. What we will find in history takes us right into the present, into a nightmare of unprecedented proportions, into the face of darkness that the world has tasted and forgotten only to be hit again with a scale that encircles the globe. When it comes to MediSin we all look to the FDA, the CDC, the AMA and the APA for comfort, and trust that what we eat or take as medicine in the form of vaccines is safe. It is to these people and organizations that we give our blind faith. It has long been known, and is on official federal records and testimony that many of the people in these organizations shuffle back and forth or own stock in one or more of the major pharmaceutical firms who all share similar philosophies and practices. Many have been part of huge conglomerates that were broken up after WWII.

The people who bring you your Bayer Aspirin are the same folks who built and ran the Auschwitz Concentration Camp. Auschwitz was the largest mass extermination factory in human history. Few people know that Auschwitz was a 100% subsidiary of IG Farben which now lives on as Bayer Aspirin Company. On April 14, 1941, in Ludwigshafen, Germany, Otto Armbrust, the IG Farben board member responsible for the Auschwitz project, stated to his IG Farben board colleagues, "Our new friendship with America (Rockefeller) is a blessing. We have determined all measures integrating the concentration camps to benefit our company." The pharmaceutical departments of the IG Farben cartel used the victims of the concentration camps in their own way: thousands of them died during human experiments such as the testing of new vaccines.

The pharmaceutical and chemical giant, IG Farben, attempted to shake its abominable image through corporate restricting and renaming after World War II and they succeeded beyond their wildest imagination. So great has been their success that the public has no idea that many of the men who were responsible for these atrocities were given a plane ride to America under

Government protection called Operation Paperclip. The story of pharmaceutical terrorism is the story of such men, which are the same men who are most responsible for creating the modern medical paradigm that relies exclusively on drugs that are highly toxic and poisonous in nature. These men were in control of the large chemical and pharmaceutical companies well before Hitler reached puberty and were around well after his alleged death.

By accepted legal standards, the Bayer Company of today is in fact, the Bayer of World War II. In 1998, Bayer conducted pesticide experiments on humans in what was called the 'Inveresk Trials.' The Sunday Herald in England reported that subjects were given a single dose of a substance called azinphis-methyl (AM) and then were observed for seven days. Sounds like the same experiments done on the black men in the south called the Tuskegee Experiment. This is just the tip of the iceberg that shows the kind of attitudes that have always been a part of pharmaceutical companies like Eli Lilly which lied about the safety of thimerosal in the 1930's and then proceeded to put its mercury based compound, almost secretly, into vaccines and many other medical products for decades without interference from the FDA.

The tradition lives on, and many of the techniques are the same. All of this is important when looking for medical truth and sanity because it is exactly that which was abandoned by the pharmaceutical and chemical giants in the beginning of the 20th century. It is a historic fact that it was the Rockefeller-Farben industrial complexes that were instrumental in fostering chemical-based drug treatment as the basis for health care, and true to form they have been the dominant adversaries against safer non-drug treatments. When John D. Rockefeller interlocked his American-based international empire with that of I.G Farben in 1928, "it created the largest and most powerful cartel the world has ever known. Not only has that cartel survived through the years, it has grown and prospered. Today it plays a major role in both science and politics of cancer therapy," wrote G. Edward Griffin in a World without Cancer and The Politics of Cancer Therapy.

A major reason why health care is in such shambles is that the medical establishment has allowed itself to be bought off by the pharmaceutical industry, whose prime motive is PROFIT. Eustace Mullins described very well the roots of this nightmare and how John D. Rockefeller, with the help of the American Medical Association and government officials, gained control of America's "health" care industry in the early part of this century. "Educating" medical students was instrumental in their plan. Mullins writes: "Rockefeller's Education Board has spent more than $100 million to gain control of the nation's medical schools and turn our physicians to physicians of the allopathic school, dedicated to SURGERY, and the HEAVY USE OF DRUGS." Many people are unaware that many of the medical schools in the early part of the century taught herbal medicine, fasting, vitamin/mineral therapy, colon therapy, and used non-invasive techniques. Today you'll be lucky if an allopathic physician has more than three hours of class instruction in nutrition.

Many are the horror stories that have come from this insanity. Forty years ago, for example, the world was shocked by the thalidomide tragedy when regulatory agencies in many countries approved a drug that caused damage to the fetus in early pregnancy. About 8,000 mothers worldwide who used the drug as a sleeping pill or as a remedy for morning sickness during the late 1950s and early 1960s gave birth to children with flipper-like arms and legs, missing fingers and toes and/or organs in the wrong place. The drug was ultimately banned in 1962. This was a high profile situation that has been repeated time and time again in more subtle ways with many other drugs and vaccines which are sold to us as safe but hold hidden horrors that we just do not want to see. Just look at the latest MediSin Vioxx, which was approved for children only weeks before it was pulled from the market. Vioxx, the painkiller (killer of humans) drug was responsible for 30,000 to 100,000 cardiovascular–related health risks. When an N.B.A. trainer recently doled out a week long dose of Vioxx to an ailing player, the player shot him an incredible glance. *"I'm not taking these anymore, especially after what happened to Alonzo."* Then the player said according to the trainer, *"Give me something else."* Since Alonzo Mourning, the current Miami Heat All-Star center was found to have a kidney disorder more than a year ago (he eventually had a transplant), the same disorder that caused the San Antonio swingman, Sean Elliott, to undergo a kidney transplant and eventually forced him to retire has caused many athletes to take a second look at popping a pill for pain. These anti-inflammatory MediSins are causing kidney disease at an alarming rate. The authors alone know of at least

20 men who are not even athletes who have been diagnosed with Focal Segmental Sclerosis, the same diagnosis as Alonzo and Sean. One (1) in thirteen (13) blacks will be diagnosed with this disorder that is fatal without kidney dialysis or a transplant. This is why you see the majority of kidney dialysis centers in the African-American community, since they are 75%-80% of the users. Is this some form of genocide?

Modern psychology has completely failed the human race for it has excluded from its curriculum, the roles of the criminally insane. The psychological profiles of a group of men who control the chemical and pharmaceutical industries are men who take it as their duty and destiny to slowly torture and kill uncounted millions of other humans through slow and sometimes quick chemical poisoning. History will one day show that the people at the top, and probably in the middle of these organizations are the greatest criminals that humanity has ever known, for it will be recorded that they have been responsible for the deliberate poisoning and death of uncounted millions of people which unfortunately includes newborn infants. This might seem like the most fantastic of fantastic statements you have ever read but when you put together the whole picture we come to see that the principle organizations involved with medicine and public health subscribe to the same philosophies of the same people and organizations involved in the extermination of millions of people. The science and philosophy of the CDC (Center for Disease Creation) and the FDA are that poisons are safe and absolute for mass consumption and the AMA backs them up to the hilt. People are gullible and have a natural tendency to believe that government approved products are safe.

The pharmaceutical companies live very comfortably behind the high walls of self-images that have been deliberately created to deceive us. They portray themselves in the light of Louis Pasteur, Robert Koch, and other pioneers in medicine successfully hiding the truth of who they really are. They claim to be interested in the eradication of diseases in order to serve humanity when the truth is that they deliberately create disease to expand their markets and profits. "The pharmaceutical industry does not act in the tradition of the protector of humanity, but in the tradition of IG Farben, a group of organized criminals willing to sacrifice countless human lives in order to maintain their profits" says Dr. Mathias Rath who has filed a case against them at the world court at the Hague.

When we were children, we never could understand why The Creator would create a perfect body, but at the same time you had to get vaccinated to 'protect' yourself from some foreign invader. In our adult years, we have come to the realization that the Creator made our bodies perfect and that man (corporations) has suggested that we are not made perfect so we need to ingest their poisons. The human family is repeatedly told that vaccines are safe, vital to our wellbeing and necessary for the prevention of many diseases. Most of us take it for granted that not being vaccinated endangers our health and safety. In a worst-case scenario, we envision worldwide plagues and even extinction. Our faith in vaccinations is so strong that we think of them as panaceas, and look to science to develop new ones for every affliction known to man, from the common cold to AIDS. One of the major mistakes is that politicians, who are suckered by lobbyists from the drug companies are convinced without proper investigation into believing that vaccines are not only the best method of preventing disease but also the **only** way of preventing them. This encouraged and developed a whole monopoly of thought on this idea that has dominated allopathic medicine for this entire century.

The issue is one of philosophy; holistic health care is the science of individuals. It looks at how individuals are affected by an herb or an inoculation or whatever. MediSin is the science of statistics. Every study is done with random sampling, statistical controls. The conclusions are percentages and they always compare percentages. If your child could be injured in the line of public health (vaccinations), your government feels that it's just the risk you have to take in the service of the general public. Why does he/she have to get vaccinated to go to school if the other children are **already** vaccinated anyway? If vaccines are as safe and effective as medical science says, then why are allopathic doctors not lining up for the shots? After all, allopathic doctors are exposed to infected patients everyday. In fact, physicians belong to a high-risk category and are urged to accept vaccinations because of their continued exposure to infectious disease.

The whole concept of penetrating the skin with a needle to inject foreign substances is an unnatural act, because it is injected directly into the blood system. That is not the natural port of entry for that MediSin. In fact, the whole immune system in our body is geared to prevent that from happening. What we're doing is giving the virus or the bacteria carte blanche entry into our blood stream, which is the last place you want it to be. This increases the chance for disease because viral material from the vaccine stays in the cells, and is not completely defeated by the body's own defenses. The antibody response to a vaccine entering the blood occurs purely as an isolated technical feat, without any general inflammatory response (mechanism to rid the body of infection) or any noticeable improvement in overall health of the individual. When allopathic doctors and others quote studies on how effective is this or that vaccine, very often the study is done purely on antibody production in the blood (i.e. 'This vaccine was shown to be 95% effective based on seroconversion rates.'). If not relying on true-life experiences, these statistics artificially inflate vaccine efficacy. Such methods clearly cannot be relied upon for proper scientific evaluation.

In all fairness, let's take a look at what these MediSin's contain. There are three categories of ingredients. The first are cultured bacteria and viruses. All viruses, even attenuated (so-called killed) viruses contain RNA and DNA. RNA and DNA sheds, and this can be picked up by the cellular organisms in which they are immersed. This process of shedding genetic material by the cells of one species and its subsequent absorption into another species is known as "tran session." Cells in which viral RNA have integrated into the DNA of the animal cells can lie dormant in tissues throughout the body, and be activated at a later stage, triggering autoimmune phenomenon, such as cancer, multiple sclerosis, lupus, allergies, and rheumatoid arthritis. Tran session explains autoimmune phenomenon, why the immune system cannot distinguish between foreign invaders and its own tissues, and why it begins to destroy itself.

The second ingredient in vaccinations is the medium in which they are cultivated. This can include rabbit brain tissue, dog kidney tissue, monkey kidney tissue, chicken or duck egg protein, pig blood and cowpox pus. These foreign proteins are injected directly into the bloodstream. They are very toxic since they do not get filtered through the digestive process or pass through the liver. These proteins are foreign to the body, and are in a state of decomposition. They are composed of animal cells, and therefore contain animal genetic material. It is possible for the genes in these cells to be picked up by the live viruses in vaccines. These viruses then implant a foreign alien genetic material from animal tissue cultures into the human genetic system. Undigested proteins in the blood are one of the causes of allergies.

Finally, there are stabilizers, neutralizers, carrying agents and preservatives. Many people try to feed their children healthy foods. They would never think of giving their children formaldehyde, mercury, or aluminum phosphate to eat. However, they rush their children to the arms of the vaccine manufacturer's for an injection of toxins, and then cry out when their son or daughter has the unwanted side effect. What sane person would consider using a hazardous substance into the delicate body of an infant? What could formaldehyde or mercury have to do with preventing disease? Clearly, the pharmaceutical industry's treatment of vaccine health and safety issues leaves much to be desired. The finding of the Simian Virus (SV) 40 in Rhesus monkey kidney cells during the early 1960s may have contaminated millions of Americans through the polio vaccine. The contamination occurred because the kidney cells the vaccine virus was grown in came from monkeys infected with SV40. Health officials say the problem was eliminated after 1963. You're a fool if you believe that one!

Michele Carbone of Loyola University Medical center in Chicago has announced results that suggest the Soviet polio vaccine was contaminated with SV40 after 1963, possibly until the early 1980s. The vaccine was almost certainly used throughout the Soviet bloc and probably exported to China, Japan and several countries in Africa. That means hundreds of millions could have been exposed to SV40 after 1963. Could this be the reason for cancer's assault upon the American populace after the age of fifty? The consequences of exposure to the virus are rare forms of cancers.

The evil leaders of the world have recently taken a keen interest in the field of vaccines. They have established a special task force to oversee the administration of vaccines to children and adults throughout the world, called the Global Alliance for Vaccines and Immunizations (GAVI). The first meeting of this eerie and evil GAVI task force was held in Davos, Switzerland in 2000. Its members include Microsoft's Bill and Melinda Gates, the United Nations World Health Organization (WHO), the Rockefeller Foundation, and the World Bank. The national governments of Russia and U.S.A are also involved.

Gates, whose Microsoft is at the forefront of developing new nanotransistor technology, says he has $24 billion of his own money to give away. A lot of this money is going to go toward the development of new vaccines, which the United Nations World Health Organization (WHO) will administer to injections of the world's poor. Gates and his wife Melinda are also known to support Planned Parenthood (a Rockefeller creation) and other pro-abortion and global depopulation causes. With that type of support you can rest assured that the vaccines being developed by the United Nations (WHO) with Gates money secretly contain chemicals, which act to kill unborn babies inside the mother's womb. These people do not care and will never care for the suffering of children, women, and the elderly. Their only concern is profits and population control.

Save the Birds

The propaganda machine will be at work in the next few years to frighten you and the rest of the world about the so-called dangers from a flu virus. Always remember the bottom line behind these scares is money. Take in point the Avian or Bird flu. This whole saga is something straight from some tell-lie-vision mini series or fiction novel. Prior to 1997, the wild bird flu was a rare and relatively mild condition affecting only birds. The first case of bird flu affecting a human appeared in Asia in 1997. Apparently the wild virus had mysteriously changed to H5N1 strain, a variety that could very rarely affect humans when ingesting infected meat or in very close contact with birds. The "high path" H5N1 strain appeared suddenly and has been known to be located in many bio-hazard labs around the world.

When the Associated Press reported the death of a 60-year-old woman allegedly of bird flu, the US government halted "all chicken imports from China in a move to curb the spread of the virus." Shortly after, the first wave of slaughter began with 1.2 million Asian chickens. By 2003, 40 million birds had been slaughtered and Tyson foods, the Arkansas based largest meat producer and packer in the world has been making steady inroads into the previously closed Asian poultry market, filling the gap in production. Sounds like sabotage to us! Meanwhile, since May 2005, new outbreaks of high path H5N1 bird flu strain has cut a swathe across poultry in Russia, Greece, Holland, Kazakhstan, Turkey, Romania, Mongolia and Croatis, where massive poultry exterminations have begun. The poultry infection near Eastern Europe has caused widespread suspicion. A member of the Liberal Democratic faction of the Russian State Duma, Aleksei Mitrofanov, has said in a parliamentary speech that bird flu was invented by Americans who wanted to dominate the world's poultry markets. That basically sums it up!

Without signs of a human epidemic, On October 28, 2005 the US Senate passed an $8 billion emergency bill to fund research, drugs, and vaccines, based on no scientific evidence that bird flu constitutes a significant human threat and overwhelming evidence to the contrary. The administration is seeking an additional $6 billion to $10 billion from US taxpayers, according to a current Business Week report.

"President Bush this week asked the leaders of the world's top vaccine manufactures-Chiron, Sanofi-Aventis, Wyeth, GlaxoSmithKline and Merck-to come to the White House on Friday to discuss preparations for pandemic flu," reports the New York Times in October 2005

Billions of hard earned taxpayer money will flow into the coffers of selected pharmaceutical giants such as Roche, which holds the sole license to manufacture Tamiflu, an anti viral drug that is meant only for reducing the symptoms of the seasonal influenza and has never been tested for use for the bird flu. Thousands of brainwashed Americans are lining up for their dose when there has not been a single case of H5N1 bird flu in the US. Without a single human case of H5N1, Tamiflu is in such demand that a new US factory is being planned to ensure there is more of the drug available by the 2006 "flu season." This worthless drug cost $100 per dose. That comes to a staggering $2 billion. (Let it be known that a guy named Donald Rumsfeld holds stock in Tamiflu and was a former CEO of the company that produced it).

To add insult to injury, the drug companies have made a sweet arrangement with the U.S. government that they are not liable for any of the side effects from the drugs. President Bush's $7.1–billion pandemic flu plan seeks broad limits on lawsuits against producers of vaccines and antiviral drugs, but it is silent on how those injured or killed by adverse reactions might be compensated. The liability shield is contained in the Pandemic Flu Countermeasure Liability Protection Act of 2005. It would protect producers and distributors of emergency vaccines from injury suits except in cases of "willful misconduct." A term to be defined by the attorney general, and the secretary of Health and Human Services at a later date.

So, even if these drugs or vaccines wind up killing innocent children, these companies will not be held liable. But you don't have to worry; the FDA announced that Tamiflu is safe. Of course, this is the same agency that gave Vioxx its safety blessing before it killed more than 55,000 people. When Tamiflu kills U.S. children, Roche will plead that they had no idea it could do such a thing!

The main purpose of scaring the public into flu frenzy is to vaccinate the entire population and put those who refuse into concentration camps. The agents of evil have the technology to put into vaccine's microchips that monitor your every move. Pharaoh Bush is discussing the use of the military to enforce quarantine of suspected bird flu carriers. The US plans to install a new quarantine station at Logan International Airport to diagnose travelers. Preliminary discussions include plans to impose 10 year jail terms on people who breach orders to stay at home, in hospital or within their city during an influenza outbreak.

The Boston Globe reported on October 8, 2005: "On Tuesday, the president suggested that the United States should confront the risk of bird flu pandemic by giving him the power to use the US military to quarantine 'part[s] of the country' experiencing an 'outbreak'. So we have moved quickly in the past few months, at least metaphorically, from the global war on Islam (terror) to a proposed war on hurricanes, to a proposed war on the bird flu."

Special Note:

At the time of printing, Tamiflu had already been linked to neuropsychiatric incidents in children, including seizures, loss of consciousness, and delirium. In Japan the following reports have been documented:

1) A 14-year-old boy with the flu took a dose of Tamiflu and two hours later jumped from the ninth floor of his apartment building.
2) Another child, hours after taking a dose, jumped from the second floor of his house.

Dy (e) ing to be Noticed

"Respectable Greeks and Romans did not indulge in decorative tattooing, which they associated with barbarians. The Greeks, however, learned the technique from the Persians, and used it to label slaves and criminals so they could be identified if they tried to escape." (Gilbert, Steve, Tattoo History: A Source Book, p.15)

An example of the above quote in United States history was seen during the physical enslavement of Africans from 1600-1900. When war captives (Africans were not slaves upon their arrival in America-the slave was made in America) were brought to the plantation the slave master (former Presidents, Senators, etc.) tattooed their property so that when they escaped and if unfortunately caught the bounty hunter could identify the owner of the escaped property. Today, the physical chains of slavery have been lifted, but the mental chains of slavery are still present. People of today openly identify themselves with tattooing and have no clue to the dangers they present.

Underneath that harmless tattoo is a very serious risk of acquiring a deadly blood-borne disease such as Leukemia, Hepatitis

B, Hepatitis C, Tetanus, Syphilis, Tuberculosis and other blood-born diseases. An alarming research study recently published by Dr. Bob Haley and Dr. Paul Fischer at the University of Texas Southwestern Medical School in Dallas uncovered that the "innocent" commercial tattoo may be the number one distributor of hepatitis C. Dr. Haley concludes, "We found that commercially acquired tattoos accounted for more than twice as many hepatitis C infections as injection-drug use. This means it may have been the largest single contributor to the nationwide epidemic of this form of hepatitis."

Incredible! According to Dr. Haley's research you are twice as likely to be infected with hepatitis C from getting a tattoo from a tattoo shop, than shooting up dope! There is a documented case of a 22-year-old grocery store employee who simply received his $45 tattoo, and four weeks later-needed a LIVER TRANSPLANT! (Myrna L. Armstrong and Lynne Kelly, Tattooing, Body Piercing, and Branding Are on the Rise, The Journal of School Nursing, Feb. 2001, Vol 17 No.1, p.15)

The fact of tattoos spreading deadly diseases is nothing new. It's been known and documented for years. According to the Hepatitis Control Report, spring 2001, "Outside the United States, several studies have connected tattoos to hepatitis B and C transmission…"

"By the middle of the nineteenth century, it was becoming more and more apparent that the practice was not without its medical hazards. For instance, in 1853 the first case was reported of syphilis, transmitted not in the old fashioned way, but via the tattooist's needle." (Ronald Scott, Art, Sex, and Symbol, 1974, p.133)

In 1961 an outbreak of hepatitis B in New York City was linked to the tattoo. And the "ultra-liberal" New York City OUTLAWED the deadly tattoo from 1961until 1997! Did you know that the American Red Cross prohibits donors from donating blood for 12 months after getting tattooed?

Why are tattoos so vulnerable to disease?

There are four eliminating organs in the body: the colon, the kidneys, the lungs, and the skin. The skin is the body's largest eliminating organ. The four eliminating organs work together to keep the body clean and healthy. When any one of the four is not able to do its job, the other three must work harder.

As an eliminating organ, the skin excretes about a pint of poisons through the pores every 24 hours. The skin also:

Breathes and absorbs air, light, and water
Reacts to external stimuli and against pain
Evaporates heat for the body as the body maintains a constant temperature
Acts as a storehouse for fats and water
Secretes oil called sebum which keeps the skin flexible

Tattoos kill the skin. The skin cells that are under the tattoos are no longer functioning. The more tattoos covering the body, the fewer skin cells left alive to work as the body's eliminators. The colon, kidneys, and lungs must work harder to remove the waste that would ordinarily have been removed through that part of the skin.

Tattoos are made by injecting colored pigment into small deep holes made in the skin. As with most trauma, pain and bleeding are part of the process. Immediately after the tattooing process and during the healing process there is an acute inflammatory response which usually includes local swelling, redness, scab formation, and bleeding. Since a tattoo is an open would until it heals, infection of the wound is always a potential problem.

Problems can appear after the tattoo has healed. These include: lichenoids (small bumps of reactive tissue); granulomas (firm balls of reactive tissue that form around the material that the body perceives as foreign, in this case the tattoo ink); lymphocytoma (a skin reaction that mimics lymphoma of the skin); scaling, itching, sores, and keloids. Most tattoo dyes contain metal which accumulates in the body creating tumors, cysts, and blood cancers. For instance, the color Red has mercury and cadmium sulfide, Blue has radioactive cobalt, Brown has lead and White has titanium, zinc oxide and lead carbonate. These colors are suitable for automobile paint not human bodies!

Autopsies reveal that ink from tattoos wind up in the lymph node closest to the tattoo. Talk about immune deficiency! We spend all day, everyday trying to avoid chemicals, hormones, preservatives, drugs and other substances that we know harm the body. So why go and put something on your body that will weaken your immune system?

In his book, "The Rebirth of Gods," Dr. Paul Goss reminds us:

"You have to go to the store and buy beauty only when you do not understand yourself. True beauty is a healthy colon, liver, heart, appendix, tonsils, spleen, gallbladder, etc. Beauty comes from perfect health.

"When you allow others to be your understanding they can control how you perceive yourself. They will then use your insecurity against you and encourage you to destroy yourself. What you have been programmed to accept as beauty aids destroy your genes and organs."

Hot Market

One of the biggest booms in business has been in the dermatology industry. According to the American Society of Dermatological surgery, over 50% of everyone receiving a tattoo wants it removed. Tattoo removal by way of laser surgery is among the fastest growing areas. Depending on the size of the tattoo and colors used, the laser tattoo removal surgery can be very painful and very expensive. Tattoos performed by commercial tattoo parlors are much more difficult to remove because the tattoo is deeper, the ink more complex and thicker, It normally takes between 10 and 15 laser surgery sessions to remove the average tattoo, but 25-30 sessions are not uncommon, depending on the complexity of the tattoo. When you consider the average single session costs from $400-$800, the removal surgery can be very expensive, costing as much as $20,000. That $25 tattoo might cost $5000 to remove. Your HMO or PPO does not cover tattoo removals-this is strictly an out of the pocket expense.

If you have one or many tattoos, please consider removing this stigma from your body. Considering the dangers from the tattoos we recommend: Milk Thistle, Alpha-Lipoic Acid, Selenium, Cilantro, and Cod Liver oil to help the liver eliminate the heavy metals from the colors and repair your skin internally.

14. FLUORIDE: HOW AMERICA REALLY GOT BRAINWASHED

For the last sixty years gullible Americans have been told one big fat lie. This lie is called fluoridation. We know many of you will say, "My government would never lie to me or intentionally allow a poisonous product to be used by Americans." Well, hold on to your seats, because this form of MediSin has been going on since 1939.

In Pittsburgh, Pennsylvania, an unethical biochemist by the name of Gerald J. Cox, who worked for one of the largest aluminum companies in America (ALCOA) proposed the use of fluoridation for America's water supplies. ALCOA took a propriety interest in this issue, since fluoride is a MAJOR by-product of aluminum production. The company (Corporation) wanted to know how much fluoride exposure people could tolerate without getting mottled, discolored teeth. Or, more specifically, how much fluoride could ALCOA release into the nation's earth, water, and air without the public realizing that the Corporation was polluting the environment with a powerful toxin? (1) That same question was addressed by a stooge named H. Trendly Dean, former Dental Surgeon for the US Public Health Service. His mentor was Andrew Mellow, founder and major stockholder of ALCOA. Start to get the picture? Dean claimed that *"fluoride levels of up to 1 ppm (parts per million) in drinking water did not cause mottled enamel"* based on his own research. (2) Dean came up with the notion that fluoride added to the water supply at the magic dosage of 1 ppm would prevent tooth decay, while avoiding damage to bones and teeth. (3) Now back at Alcoa's Pittsburgh Industrial Research Lab, Mr. Cox took that news and ran with it. Cox fluoridated some lab rats in a study and concluded that fluoride reduced cavities and that: "The case should be regarded as proved." How arrogant! So, in the year 1939, Cox, an industry scientist working for a corporation threatened by fluoride damage claims and burdened by the odious expense of disposing of tons of toxic industrial waste, went touring the country pushing for fluoride usage. (4)

The first city to use fluoridation in America was Grand Rapids, Michigan. Guess who was picked to oversee the use of fluoridation among the people of Grand Rapids H. Trendly Dean. The truth is that Dean's great discovery (MediSin) was based on wishful thinking and some very shaky science. Dean's findings did not stand up to scientific scouting at all. Let's examine his reasoning; he quoted that teeth that become mottled or discolored were especially resistant to decay. That's like saying, "Let's all drink formaldehyde so our bodies won't decay." This guy was Dean of the US Public Service! An independent study of Dean's results revealed that he had engaged in "selective use of data", employing figures from 21 cities that confirmed his findings, and ignoring those from 272 other localities that did not. (5) In a 1955 court case challenging fluoridation, Dean admitted under oath that his published conclusions were wrong.(6) In hearings conducted by the AMA in 1957, he was forced to admit that dental fluorosis, the first sign of fluoride overdose, could be caused by water fluoridated at 1 ppm.(7) However, these admissions were never publicized and never acknowledged by the USPHS, the ADA, or the government bodies responsible for foisting fluoride on the public. This denial is genocide all the way from government to industry to local agencies.

Once the acceptance of fluoride was pushed on the public, the economic realities became apparent to all involved. Dentists, Government agencies, and Corporations were licking their chops like wolves on sheep. Chemical Week, a publication for the chemical industry, described the terror of the times: "All over the country, slide rules were getting warm as waterworks engines figured the cost of adding fluoride to their water supplies."(8) There was such overwhelming acceptance to proceed hastily, albeit irresponsibly. The Grand Rapids experiment was supposed to last 15 years, during which time health benefits and hazards were being studied. In 1946, however, just one year into the experiment, six more U.S. cities adopted the process. By 1947, 87 more communities were treated; popular demand was the official reason for this unscientific haste. Your U.S. Government put on a major public relations campaign spearheaded by Edward L. Bernays, a nephew of Sigmund Freud (we wonder whether he was a cocaine user also?). Bernays, a public relations pioneer who has been called the "original spin doctor",

(9) was a masterful PR specialist. As a result of his influence, Griffiths writes, "Almost overnight the popular image of fluoride which at the time was being widely SOLD as RAT & BUG poison became that of a beneficial ponder of gleaming smiles, absolutely safe, and good for children, bestowed by a benevolent paternal government. Its opponents were permanently engraved on the public mind as crackpots."(10) At that time, the only two disgruntled voices were the John Birch Society and the Ku Klux Klan (how ironic). They raved that fluoridation was a plot by the Soviet Union and/or communists in the government to poison America's brain cells. (11)

By 1950, fluoridation's image was a glamorous one, and there was not much science could do at this point. The PHS was fluoridation's main source of funding as well as its promoter, and therefore caught in a fundamental conflict of interest. Today, nearly 250 million people worldwide drink fluoridated water, including about 130 million Americans in 9,600 communities. Out of the 50 largest cities in the US, 41 have fluoridated water.

What is fluoride and why use it?

Fluoride is any combination of elements containing the fluorine ion. In its elemental form, fluorine is a pale yellow, highly toxic and corrosive gas. In nature, fluorine is found combined with minerals as fluorides. It is the most chemically active nonmetallic element of all the elements and also has the most reactive electro-negative ion. Because of this extreme reactivity, fluorine is never found in nature as an uncombined element. There was no US commercial production of fluoride before World War II. The need for fluoride was prompted by the manufacture of the atomic bomb. It's a common ingredient in rat and cockroach poisons, as well as one of the basic ingredients in both Prozac (Fluoxetene Hydrochloride) and Sarin Nerve Gas (Isoproply-Methyl-Phosphoryl Fluoride).

The first occurrence of fluoridated drinking water on earth was found in Germany's Nazi prison camps. The Nazi Warlords had little concern about fluoride's supposed effect on children's teeth, their alleged reason for mass-medicating water with Sodium Fluoride was to sterilize humans and force the people in their concentration camps into calm submission.(12) Repeated doses of infinitesimal amounts of fluoride will in time reduce an individual's power to resist domination, by slowly poisoning and narcotizing the left hemisphere of the brain, thus making him submissive to the will of those who WISH to govern him. **The real purpose behind water fluoridation is to reduce the resistance of the masses to domination and control and loss of liberty.** Contrary to the well-entrenched belief in fluoridation, there is no scientific evidence that ingesting fluoride reduces tooth decay.

Since 1945, the longest on-going fluoridation trial to date between fluoridated Newburgh, N.Y. and non-fluoridated Kingston, N.Y., shows virtually no difference between the tooth decay rates of either city. However, fluoridated Newburgh has about double the rate of dental fluorosis (fluoride poisoning), as does non-fluoridated Kingston. To quote Canada's leading fluoride EXPERT, Dr. Hardy Limeback from an interview in Arizona's Mesa Tribune (December 5, 1999): *"Here in Toronto we've been fluoridating for 36 years. Yet Vancouver, which has never fluoridated, has a cavity rate lower than Toronto's."* He continues: *"In Canada we are spending more money treating dental fluorosis than we do treating cavities. That includes my own practice."* Further he said: *"Your well-intentioned dentist is simply following 50 years of MISINFORMATION from public health and dental associations. Unfortunately we were WRONG."* Finally, Dr. Limeback stated that: *"Poisoning our children was the furthest thing from my mind."* We say this with all the earnestness and sincerity of holistic healers who have spent nearly 15 years of research into chemistry, biochemistry, and pathology of fluoride -any person who drinks fluoridated water for a period of one year or more will NEVER again be the same person mentally, physically, or spirituality.

This MediSin is hard to get away from because it's in your bath or shower water, your kitchen and anywhere that public water is used. At this point in time, virtually no restaurants or beverage processors use advanced water systems to remove fluoride when you purchase items. The toxic materials contained in fluoride will be there waiting for you...in your coffee, your tea, your beer, soft drinks, and reconstituted juices, your soup, rice, pasta, and anything else that contains or is made with public water. Since most of the U.S. (about 70%) is fluoridated, food and beverage products, which are produced across the country, that circulate through interstate commerce also contain fluoride.

For example, a chemical analysis of several common products reveal that, Gerber's Graduates Berry Punch contains 3.0 mg/l, Coca Cola Classic 0.98mg/l, Minute Maid Premium Orange Juice 0.98mg/l, Dole Pineapple Juice 0.78mg/l, Lucerne 2% Milk 0.72mg/l. Everyday foods that have been processed with fluoridated water contain fluoride. Kellogg's Fruit Loops cereal contains 2.1mg/l due to the processing with fluoridated Battle Creek, Michigan water. Gerber's white grape juice contains 2 mg/l. The drying of grapes to produce raisins concentrates fluoride even more. The highest daily dose of fluoride comes from using fluoride toothpaste. Do you ever wonder why Crest, Aim, Colgate, or any other toothpaste would carry warning labels for children less than 6 yrs of age on their packaging? Please start using non-fluoridated toothpastes or just start using plain old baking soda!

Moreover, fluorides are cumulative and build up steadily with ingestion of fluoride from all sources, which include not just water but the air we breathe and the food we eat. The body can only eliminate half of the total intake, which means that the older you are the more fluoride will have accumulated in your body. Inevitably this means the aging population is particularly targeted. And even worse for the very young, there is a major element of risk in baby formula made with fluoridated water. The extreme sensitivity of the very young to fluoride toxicity makes this unacceptable. Since there are so many sources of fluoride in our everyday living, it will prove impossible to maintain an average level of 1 ppm as is suggested by your government.

The results of these toxic effects are, first, the immune system. The distortion of protein structures causes the immune proteins to fail to recognize body proteins, and so instigates an attack on them, which is autoimmune disease. Autoimmune diseases constitute a body of disease processes troubling many thousands of people: Rheumatoid arthritis, systemic lupus, and asthma to name a few. However, the thyroid gland is seriously affected by fluoride. The thyroid gland produces hormones which control our metabolism - the rate at which we burn our fuel. Deficiency of thyroid hormones is relatively common, much more than is generally accepted by many medical authorities: a figure of 1:4 or 1:3 by mid life is more likely. The illness is insidious in its onset and progression. People become tired, cold, overweight, depressed, constipated; they suffer arthritis, hair loss, infertility, atherosclerosis and chronic illness. Sadly, it is poorly diagnosed and poorly managed by many doctors in this country. One further factor that causes deep anxiety is that fluoride displaces iodine in the body, which results in hypothyroidism (thyroid hormone cannot be manufactured without iodine).

Since fluoride is an enzyme (complex protein compounds that speed up biologically chemical reactions) poison it affects the muscle-skeletal system. Collagen tissue of which muscles, tendons, ligaments and bones are made is damaged. This toxic effect extends to the inner surface of the tooth making the enamel weak and brittle. Its visible appearance is dental fluorosis (fluoride poisoning). The enzyme poison effect to our genes is that DNA cannot repair itself, and chromosomes are damaged. Also affected is the inter-uterine growth and development of the fetus, especially the nervous system. Increased incidence of Down syndrome has been documented. Fluorides are mutagenic; which means they cause the uncontrolled proliferation of cells we call CANCER. This applies to cancer anywhere in the body, but bones are particularly targeted. A report in the New England Journal of Medicine showed a 400% increase in cancer of the thyroid in San Francisco during the period their water was fluoridated. On top of its other effects, fluoride calcifies the pineal gland. The pineal gland, spiritually, is the entrance point to the body for divine revelation (Crown Chakra). On a physical level it controls skin pigmentation, mental sanity, and it helps the pituitary gland to hold the potassium and sodium levels in the body. We feel that the warlike and unspiritual character of individuals in places of power resemble calcified pineal glands.

Fluorine was a large factor in the health problems in London due to the "London Fogs" that stemmed from the burning of fluoride from "Sea Coal." These emissions produced fogs so thick that they were called "Pea Soup" and people had to lead carriages around the streets in broad daylight with lanterns. It is this same area that spawned the problems connected to Jack the Ripper, who appeared to be looking at the health effects of prostitutes connected to these effects while at the same time being protected by Masons (see the movie "From Hell").

Fluoride taken into the stomach is converted by stomach acid to hydrofluoric acid (HF), which is highly absorbed into the body and highly retained. The stain resistant compound "Scotch Guard" is made from HF and was linked to Sudden Infant Death Syndrome. Infants tend to cough up stomach contents while sleeping and this mixes with the Scotch guard surface of baby mattresses. Here the stomach acid liberates the fluoride used in the stain resistant coating and makes HF, which causes Sudden Infant Death (SID) through suffocation. This MediSin has recently been discontinued in the same way Freon has been discontinued. However, to the parents of children who have died from fluoride poisoning this discontinuance of Scotch Guard is futile, at best.

The big question is, "Why do doctors and dentist swear by fluoridation if it's bad?" They swear by fluoridation because their industry taught them to swear by fluoridation. Doctors and dentists are students of their industry. The main point is that this faulty pseudo-science was passed off as proof positive that fluoridation worked, along with lobby support that influenced the AMA and the ADA to officially rubber stamp fluoridation as "safe and effective." Once they committed their reputations to fluoridation, the "sacred calf" was born. From that point on the blind followed the blind and fluoridation became ingrained in the policy and education of conventional doctors and dentists. At this point the blind have been following the blind for over half a century. What will happen to the reputation and credibility of the AMA and the ADA when eyes are opened? How large will the liability be? Right now their survival is sustained by denial and arrogance. Europe is about 90% non-fluoridated. Fluoridation is banned in Denmark, Germany, Holland, and Sweden. The truth is out and the time is coming when fluoridation will join DDT, lead, tobacco, aspartame, hydrogenated oils as a self-evident poison, doing serious damage to people, especially children.

15. MY MOUTH HURTS: DENTAL QUACKERY

"If you want to keep your teeth, then don't go to a dentist"
– Mrs. Nellie Whitaker *(grandmother of Dr. Whitaker)*

When an individual or organization tells a falsehood there is a need for more falsehoods to support the original untruth. The American Death Association (ADA) is currently in an untenable position because of lies they have told in the past. Now if they come clean about these issues they will be swallowed up in a flood of lawsuits they cannot win.

There are 5 issues that place the ADA in the liar's chair:

Falsehood #1: Fluoride is safe in our drinking water.
Dr. Cornelius Steelnik, Emeritus Professor of the Department of Chemistry at the University of Arizona in Tucson, AZ. studied fluoride exposure in 26,000 school children in 1992. The results showed that the more fluoride a child drank the more cavities the child experienced. The toxicity of fluoride was well established by a later study which compared 10 large US cities fluoridating their water with 10 similar sized cities that did not use fluoride. After a 20 year follow up the cities fluoridating their water were found to have 20% more cancer than the cities not using fluoride. These results prompted Dr. Dean Burk, the Chief Chemist Emeritus of the US National Cancer Institute to remark "fluoride (see Chapter 13) causes more human death, and causes it faster, than any other CHEMICAL."

Falsehood #2: Mercury amalgams are completely safe.
The ADA continues to fight for the alleged safety of mercury amalgams (tooth fillings), because to not do so would bury them in lawsuits they surely would loose. Many dentists have been persecuted and prosecuted for speaking out against mercury

amalgams. In 1984 a new policy was enacted by the ADA to remove the license of any dentist who mentioned that mercury "might" be dangerous. Dentist Mark Breiner had an ongoing battle with the ADA about his right to write articles in local Connecticut newspapers in which he called attention to the toxicity of mercury amalgams. He states "the ADA's rule of forcing silence on the part of dentists has been one of the greatest impediments to consumers learning the truth about amalgams or even learning that they are mainly mercury, and not silver. The majority of the dental boards are agents of the ADA.

Falsehood # 3: Gingival surgery is an effective way to heal gum disease.

The conventional dental approach to gum disease is antibiotic therapy and surgery. Periodontal disease (gum infections) affects approx. 80% of adults. Dr. Paul Cummings of Wilmington, North Carolina taught gingival (gum) disease at the University of North Carolina Dental School. He now recommends using hydrogen peroxide as a mouthwash and brushing with baking soda for diseased gums. He states that this method obtains a 99% success rate far better than he ever obtained with surgery or antibiotics. Cummings stated that "Not one clinical study has ever shown that periodontal surgery was necessary." This surgery only brings monetary reward to surgeons but does not eliminate receding gums, bleeding gums or nutritional deficits. People suffering from gum disease have a breakdown in the connective tissue supporting the gums which is directly related to a nutritional deficiency in Vitamin C.

Falsehood # 4: Root Canals are a safe operation.

Many chronic diseases, perhaps most, are a result of root canal surgery. Root canals trap anaerobic (cancer causing) bacteria in the tooth. Once in the tooth bacteria can eat through the enamel into the dentin and pulp and create festering pockets of microbes that can travel through the veins, cranial nerves, or lymph passages throughout the entire body. The results are head pain, neuritis, mental illness, depression, hyperactivity, and chronic fatigue syndrome. Ninety-five percent of root canal patients develop CANCER. Approximately 24 million root canal operations are performed annually in the United States. Nearly every dentist is oblivious to the serious health risks this operation produces.

Dr. Weston Price who traveled worldwide studying the teeth, diets and bones of native populations living without the benefit of "western modern food" learned that primitive tribes had perfect teeth without cavities or gum disease and had no bone diseases. Dr. Price learned after thousands of animal studies that a root canal tooth is always infected regardless of its appearance and lack of symptoms. When Dr. Price took a root canal tooth of a patient who had a chronic disease and placed this tooth in an animal, the patient became well and the animal developed the same illness the patient had previously suffered from. The patient whose root canal tooth was placed in an animal not only became well, they became well in 24 to 48 hours. This research completely changes the way allopathic physicians (MDs) need to think about disease causation.

Every root canal infection may have a different bacteria residing in it. Thus the individual who has three root canals could have three different infectious organisms continuously seeding the blood stream. This could result in three different degenerative diseases simultaneously affecting this person. Dr. Price learned that the most common bacteria infecting a root canal tooth was streptococcus. Staphylococci, spirochetes and fungi were also frequently identified. These bacteria caused many oral and dental illnesses as well as enormous degenerative diseases in other parts of the body.

Dentin (dense tissue formed under the enamel) makes up 95% of the structure of a tooth. It has the appearance of a solid stone like structure. The tissue of the dentin consists of very fine tubules. Undamaged dentin tubules contain a nutrient dense fluid that keeps the teeth alive and healthy. These nutrients reach the teeth by an artery which is accompanied by a nerve and vein in the root canal. When a tooth becomes decayed or injured conventional dentistry encourages the use mercury (poison) amalgams, which serves to protect the tooth from ongoing decay or injury. If the decay is neglected or not discovered until it has spread into the root canal the bacterial infection begins to rapidly engulf the nerve and blood vessels of that root canal. Once inside the root canal bacteria enter the dentin tubules which spread to the rest of the body. The bacteria, spirochetes and fungi have become established in a new home where they are free to multiply and grow without any impediments. Dr. Price found that not one of 100 disinfectants was able to penetrate and sterilize the dentin. Neither are any antibiotics capable of sterilizing root canals. Some dentists are convinced that the removal of pulp and packing the root canal cavity with a disinfecting substance blocks the supply of nutrients to the dentin tubules ensuring eradication of infection. This does not occur.

Once established in the root canal the bacteria become capable of mutating and changing their form. Price found out that established root canal bacterial organisms became more virulent and their toxins became more dangerous. A German oncologist named Josef Issel (1) was able to confirm these observations of Dr. Price. He learned that the toxins released from these root canal bacteria were closely related to the chemicals used by the Germans in World War I to create MUSTARD GAS.

This ability of bacteria to mutate and change in root canals is the same process occurring in bacteria after exposure to antibiotics. The changes bacteria are able to undergo permit them to become resistant to antibiotics (anti-life) that previously had no difficulty killing them. The ability to mutate relates to the genetic capabilities in the bacteria. On the other hand natural substances do not result in bacterial resistance because natural substances do not produce any genetic changes in the bacteria.

The desire of endodontics to pressure and save root canal teeth is commendable. However, far too often the tooth is saved but the patient dies. This happens because of false confidence in the ability of disinfectant substances used to sterilize the root canal tooth. Their myopic view of this problem is ignoring the presence of live bacteria in dentine tubules. Some intelligent open minded dentists have begun to try to solve the problem of universal infection in root canal teeth. These individuals are using colloidal silver, garlic, calcium oxide therapy from France, and prayer as solutions to this infectious problem.

Falsehood #5: Wisdom Teeth Removal.
If you're one of the rare individuals who still has all his/her wisdom teeth after the age of 40 then consider yourself blessed. It seems dentists in America feel that they have to suggest surgery to remove them when there is no sign of disease or discomfort.

The procedure generates lots of revenues for oral surgery (while causing considerable pain and suffering on the part of patients), but it has absolutely no rational justification, nor any real benefit, in most cases.

Today, in the UK, it is standard policy to avoid removing asymptomatic (show no sign disease or discomfort) wisdom teeth. But in the United States, it remains standard operating procedure to surgically remove even asymptomatic wisdom teeth, simply because they are there. It makes about as much sense as saying we should cut off everybody's fingers because they have so many! A dentist looks in your mouth, and in three seconds, determines that you need dental surgery? Hogwash! It's just a revenue generating procedure that's dishonestly pushed onto patients who gladly go along with anything their dentist says, even when it's utter nonsense.

However, it turns out, that the removal of wisdom teeth has been found to be an utterly worthless procedure to begin with. It "may do harm than good" says the British Medical Journal, after reviewing thousands of case studies. Folks, you need to start questioning your dentist. Don't believe everything they tell you. Often they're full of bunk, or they're trying to sell you on whatever procedure they get paid for performing. They're not all evil-many actually believe these procedures will help you, which is why they seem so sincere-but they are grossly misinformed. Their beliefs are based on medical dogma, not scientific fact. Their beliefs in these procedures are nothing more than a sort of medical pathology, where certain things are just considered "true" and never questioned even though the original basis for accepting them as truth has been proven entirely false.

In the vast majority of cases, you will be healthier and wiser by ignoring the advice of your conventional doctor or dentist and seeking out a naturopathic doctor and a natural health dentist. In fact, it's very important to avoid allowing a doctor or dentist to even hit you with a scare story or other manipulation tactic, because most people will just go right along with their advice even when it makes no sense. People don't question medical authorities as much as they should. And dentists know it. They know that most patients will go ahead and agree to practically anything they recommend (like sheep led to their slaughter).

The Immune System Factor

Creating a permanent abscess in the body with a root canal operation sets the patient up for serious degenerative diseases. Whether these diseases occur soon after root canal surgery or begin many years later depends on the patient's immune system. About 70% of the patients with impaired immune system function may become ill immediately after the root canal operation. The 25 to 30% of persons with a strong immune system may remain in perfect health for many years after root canal surgery. The strong immune systems of these persons engulf the living bacteria in the infected dentin of the root canals site preventing spread to distant sites. However, when these immune healthy individuals suffer a severe accident or trauma their immune system can become compromised that they proceed to develop a degenerative disease.

Every individual is responsible for their own health. You must remember that nearly all physicians as well as 99% of dentists know nothing about the danger of root canals. To make matters worse your MD does not inquire about root canals in taking a comprehensive medical history. This means that when you bring up the topic of your new arthritis, anemia, or low white blood cell that it may be related to that root canal you had ten years ago you most likely will be greeted by arrogance and ignorance from your physician. If you forget to remember the possible link between the new illness and the old root canal operation you will suffer. For the individual with a history of root canal surgery you have to face the truth that you for certain have a compromised immune system. If you intend to get rid of your chronic disease you must obtain competent dental care. You must seek a biologic trained dentist even if it means traveling a longer distance to get dental care.

Biologic Dentist

Biologic dentistry is worlds apart from conventional dentistry. These dentists have a consciousness of how treatment of the teeth and jaws affect the health of the individual. There is awareness that once a dental procedure has been done on a tooth (amalgam placement or gum surgery) it becomes more vulnerable to needing future dental care. Conventional dental cleaning removes a thin layer of enamel from the teeth with each trip to the dental office. Teeth cleaning with ultrasonic techniques do not remove enamel.

Metals placed in the mouth from dental procedures are regarded as toxic substances. Different metals in the mouth (mercury, gold, nickel, etc.) dissolve in the oral fluids. These dissolved metals produce electrical charges that may disrupt the normal electromagnetic meridians seen in good health. Additionally abnormal unhealthy electrical waves may lead to interference with proper neurological function of distant structures (foot paralysis, etc.). Unusual pain problems need to raise the possibility that the electromagnetic meridians are being disturbed by a root canal abscess or cavitation.

Mercury poisoning can be avoided by limiting the number of amalgam extractions done or one root visit and having the patient, dentist and dental assistant breathing air from a remote site containing oxygen through a mask during the procedure. The room where amalgams are removed is the most dangerous room in a dentist office. Ironic that mercury is considered a hazardous waste anywhere in the open environment, but once it's in your mouth it's considered safe-go figure! Mercury using dentists and their assistants have a high rate of suicides, depression, impaired orientation, and infertility because of chronic exposure to this mercury vapor. Biologic dentistry is concerned with selecting the therapy that will cause the least disturbance to the immune system. To locate a biologic dentist go to a search site like Google and enter Biologic Dentistry and click on amalgam directory. This directory provides names, addresses and phone numbers of biologic dentists in the US, Canada, Europe, and other parts of the world.

The Invisible Toothbrush

Let's start with three inescapable facts:

1) The principal site for chronic disease is the mouth

2) Ninety-five percent of the "civilized" population suffers with tooth decay and/or periodontal disease.

3) Judged by our current successes and failures, the present explanations and solutions are filled with contradictions. For example, more brushing and flossing doesn't necessarily guarantee less disease.

Turn on the tell-lie-vision and within minutes, you are likely to hear about a new fangled vitamin-stuffed cereal. Tune in the radio and discover that we now have fiber in convenience foods. All of this stems from the well-established fact that vitamins and minerals influence every cell, tissue, organ and site in the human system. It figures, therefore, that the mouth should also be part of the story. What is the connection between nutrition and susceptibility to oral diseases?

The centerpiece for stomatology (the medical study of the physiology and pathology of the mouth) is cleanliness. This, we are told includes good cleansing habits which will result in good oral hygiene while poor cleansing habits will result in poor hygiene. Much less clearly understood is the importance of the inner world, namely gingival (gum) tissue metabolism, to foreign and external accumulations. In the past, plague has been regarded as inert matter. Now it is recognized that this so-called debris is a microcosm containing myriads of living neutrophils (white blood cells) and other formed elements. Its environment is remarkably similar to human blood and tissue fluid.

Viewed in this perspective, the role of the organism's metabolic status as a possible contributor to plague formation becomes more understandable. Plague is indeed related to the internal milieu as judged by vitamin C metabolism. In other words, this can be viewed as a demonstration of non-mechanical brushing-an invisible toothbrush. The importance of Vitamin C is also emphasized as one of a number of contributing factors to the genesis of periodontal pathosis. It has been established that 20% of gingival collagen is turned over daily. Fibroblasts require Vitamin C to produce collagen. Hence, the high turnover of gingival collagen probably renders gingival remodeling and repair particularly vulnerable to Vitamin C deficiency. Bottom line gum disease is a Vitamin C deficiency.

The following are excellent sources of Vitamin C: Acerola berries, Red Chile Peppers, Guavas, Kiwi, Camu-Camu, Rose Hips, Red & Green Bell Peppers, Leafy Green Vegetables, Parsley, Broccoli, Brussels Sprouts, Watercress, Cauliflower, Persimmons, Red Cabbage, Strawberries, Papayas, Tangerines, Oranges, Lemons, Limes, and Calf liver. Of course all items must be organic and non-genetic.

If you choose a Vitamin C supplement it MUST be from a whole food source which contains the whole Vitamin C Complex (ascorbic acid, tyrosinase, rutin, bioflavonoids, copper, manganese, and other enzymes & minerals not known by man). All commercial ascorbic acid of Vitamin C is made from corn. All commercial corn is genetic. Companies that make a whole food vitamin C supplement are New Chapter and Mega Foods.

Oral Hygiene Protocols:

Receding Gums: Co enzyme Q10: 60mg/day

Rebuild enamel of teeth: Black Walnut or Blessed Thistle Extract: 3 or 4 drops on toothbrush while brushing.

Natural Toothpastes:

Baking Soda
Jason's Naturals
Uncle Harry's Natural Toothpaste
Sea Salt

ALERT:

Researchers have discovered that Triclosan, a chemical in products of commercial toothpaste, anti-bacterial cleaning products, dishwashing liquid & hand wash react with water to produce

CHLOROFORM gas (same gas used in Gas Chambers). If inhaled in large enough quantities, chloroform will cause depression, liver disease, and lung cancer.

The following products contain Triclosan:

Dentyl Mouthwash
Colgate Total Fresh Stripe
Colgate Total
Sensodyne Total care
Tesco
Mentadent P
Aqua Fresh

16. RITALIN: THE DRUG THAT IS KILLING OUR CHILDREN

Several authorities have reported that the short-term effects from the administration of Ritalin include "Ritalin Rebound", loss of appetite and resulting weight loss, insomnia, headaches, stomachaches, drowsiness, potential liver damage, facial tics, some bad character and apathy. Parents need to become more logical and study the applications and the effects of drugs in addition to screening school systems, teachers and pediatricians before they release their children under the care of these people. Why? Because in addition to the most commonly prescribed drug, Ritalin, other drugs are now permitted for so called ADHD symptoms which are, Adderall, Dexedrine and Metadate (long acting Ritalin), which all are forms of amphetamines or "speed".

Here are some compelling facts on ADHD:

- ADHD is a psychiatric diagnosis with no valid test to prove such a condition.
- ADHD was voted into existence by a show of evil hands
- Side effects of the drugs used for ADHD include psychosis, paranoia, aggression, heart attack, cardiac arrhythmias and high blood pressure.
- Ritalin has the same addictive nature as cocaine.
- Ritalin treatment predisposes takers to cocaine's reinforcing effects.
- America uses 90 percent of the worlds Ritalin supply.

The end result of this chemical administration is addicts and lunatics. Their brains are being fried and their body functions are malfunctioning. This is what Ritalin and a dozen other psychiatric drugs create in the human body. Attention Deficit Hyperactivity Disorder is a fraud being perpetrated on the parent, teacher, nurse and the child by the psychiatric industry that is in constant need of billions of dollars being projected yearly. Truthfully, there is no adverse distinction between the effects of Ritalin, amphetamines and cocaine in case you didn't know.

According to the DEA (Drug Encouraging Agency) statistics, emergency room admissions due to Ritalin abuse numbered 1,171 in 1994. The side effects of Ritalin addiction include strokes, hypothermia, hypertension, and seizure. Several deaths have been attributed to Ritalin abuse, including that of a high school senior in Roanoke, Virginia, who died from snorting Ritalin after drinking beer.

Ritalin affects the same receptor sites in the brain as cocaine, which triggers the same effect on the body when taken in the same manner. According to medical research, Ritalin and cocaine are used interchangeably. It is a known fact that Ritalin is currently used and sold by teenagers and college students as a street drug. The MediSin's Adderall and Dexedrine are straight amphetamines. The innocent children are also prescribed another MediSin called Clonidine or Catapres, which is an adult high blood pressure medication. Clonidine sounds like a clone on cloud nine. The medical sin about this is that these drugs have never been tested on humans under the age of 18.

Every child deserves the natural right to be free of pharmaceutical influence. There are many side effects to drugs prescribed for ADHD symptoms. One of the major problems with attention and behavioral disorders is the diet. If your pediatrician does not understand that allergies from wheat, corn, soy or dairy are rampant in the diet, then find another one. For years doctors and scientists have known that the human body requires minerals, trace elements, vitamins, enzymes, etc. in order to have optimum health. If the body lacks any of these sources the child will experience an imbalance. For example, if the brain does not get quality fats (yes, fats - the brain is 60% fat) test performance in school is below average.

There are many horror stories about the MediSin Ritalin, but one the most horrifying results from the use of psychiatric drugs occurred among high school students from different parts of the country. It is well known that most of the students who participated in the high school shootings were on mind-altering MediSin's or psychiatric drugs. T. J. Solomon, the 15 year-old from Conyers, GA, who shot six classmates in May 1999, was on Ritalin; 18 year-old Columbine killer of Colorado, Eric Harris was taking the antidepressant Luvox; and Kip Kinkel, the 15 year-old from Springfield, Oregon who killed both parents, two schoolmates, and wounded 20 other students on May 21, 1988, was being prescribed Prozac, one of the most widely prescribed among the anti-depressants.

These are not isolated cases. Of the estimated two million kids under 18 years of age in America who have been prescribe Ritalin, Luvox, Prozac, Paxil, and other antidepressants and psychiatric drugs, many have committed violent acts, killings or suicides. Many others are walking time bombs. In California (1995), a 16-year-old Jarred Viktor was convicted of first-degree murder for stabbing his grandmother 61 times. Ten days earlier, Jarred had been prescribed the anti-depressant Paxil for pre-existing problems—drinking, drug abuse, and suicide contemplation. A 13-year-old, Matt Miller committed suicide in Kansas by hanging himself after taking the antidepressant Zoloft for a week. Wake up People!

Articles in the U.S. magazine Health and Healing and in the British daily, the Observer, charge that Prozac, produced by the Eli Lilly Company, has the effect of producing akathisia, a condition of severe agitation and disorientation, which they describe as a fuse for a violent outburst. A Study conducted by Dr. David Healy, director of the North Wales Department of Psychological Medicine at the University of Wales, found that Prozac produced violent behavior in mentally healthy volunteers, and claims the drug may have been the trigger for many violent acts, including murders for which people are in prison.

In the last 20 years, the term depression has been promoted like a hit record. How can a normal child be depressed? Children are children, they go through growing pains, they get spankings, they get disappointed during the holiday season when they don't get their favorite gift. So why is the depression label being pushed upon the children and adults of American? You guessed it economics!

17. PROZAC: THE CRAZY THING ABOUT IT

Over 38 million people have been prescribed the MediSin Prozac. Unlike old prescription tranquilizers like Valium and Librium, Prozac was promoted as safe. With believable advertisement, the public began to accept Prozac as a safe drug. Now Prozac has become the General Practitioner's pacifier to teenagers and children. Eli Lilly's Prozac, the worlds most recognized MediSin, was supposed to be 20th century's answer to life complexities for those of the blue pill lifestyle. Prozac even made its debut in the original movie the "Exorcist." Maybe Reagan who was played by Linda Blair was on Prozac and not possessed by some old devil!

Eli Lilly's Prozac has become the world's most successful commercial drug. However, in spite of Prozac's global success, over 200 cases have brought Eli Lilly to the U.S. court since 1988 for the horrific side effects of suicide or violence. One of the first Prozac cases was Joseph Wesbecker, a Louisville printer, who took several automatic weapons to work one day, and killed eight and injured 16 of his colleagues before turning the gun on himself. Regardless of the courts outcome, Eli Lilly and the "big wig" attorney firms were able to either have the case dropped or they were allowed to silently settle out of court for a few million dollars. This type of penalty is only a pubic hair for a corporation like Ely Lilly. In most cases involving large corporations like Pfizer, GlaxoSmithKline and Monsanto, the corporations have utilized their power and revenue to brush off any case, by a mere fine that doesn't even touch their pocket books and is considered minuscule, at best.

As early as 1978, Eli Lilly's very own internal documents revealed a large number of adverse affects from Fluoxetine (Prozac) that included psychosis, restlessness, and akathisia in clinical trail patients. Akathisia is a very dangerous mind state triggered by anti psychotic drugs which is the primary cause of both suicide and homicidal-suicidal feelings. Also, anti-psychotics such as chlorpromazine while sometimes increasing the feeling of suicide also take away the will to fight. Lily was well aware of this effect and they issued no warnings about the possibility, even though the condition had been cited in some patients during the clinical trials before Prozac was even given a license.

The use of benzoiazepines was permitted, to cover up adverse effects of akathasia. From that point on, Lilly's trial subjects were placed on tranquilizers to get them over the akathasia. The human subjects that continued to develop akathisia or who had already developed suicidal potential were excluded from the trials; obviously because it would interfere with the future success of this particular MediSin. Yet once Prozac hit the market there was no warning label with it, so the General Practitioners prescribed it without any second thought.

On May 25, 1984, according to Lilly's internal documents, a letter from the Behavior Genetics Association (BGA) stated: "During the treatment with the preparation [Prozac], 16 suicide attempts were made, two of these with success. The patients with a risk of suicide were excluded from the study; it is probable that this high proportion can be attributed to an action of the preparation [Prozac]."

In 1985, Germany refused to license Eli Lilly's MediSin Prozac. Though most of Lilly's promoting was conducted in the U.S., they still persisted in Germany. By 1989 Lilly had complied to the BGA's strict policy of warning labels to GP's that there was a risk for suicide unless they are provided a supportive drug that would sedate the patient in case of a reaction from Prozac. In 1992, this warning was finally included on the German package insert. It states "For his/her own safety, the patient must be sufficiently observed until the anti-depressive effect of Fluctin [Prozac] sets in. Taking an additional sedative may be necessary."

What is amazing and worth considering is that for a MediSin like Prozac to cause dismay for so many families and individuals, it has been afforded strong protection. Maybe it's the 11.54 billion worldwide Pharma sales, which are too important to openly reveal to the general public. Eli Lilly and Company now issues a full list of side effects, which they must do under the law. There is, unfortunately, no law that mandates or enforces a list that is completely comprehensible by a layman (common person). We would extend ourselves by saying that there are many doctors, practitioners or nurses that are unable to complete the list of adversities with full comprehension. We could question that the list of side effects was deliberately written so that the average person would not comprehend the side effects. Nevertheless, you can be assured that the potential adverse effects are severe, including side effects like psychosis, breakdown of muscle control, heart attack, stroke, compromised immune system and even cancer. It is obvious that the manufacturer didn't want you to understand because you are just a "casualty of revenue."

18. THE WAR ON CANCER: NIXON'S BIGGEST LIE!

If you could complete your life span without developing cancer, you should consider yourself fortunate. Cancer is a disease that certainly has no bias, it attacks all people of all classes, and transcends all races and cultures. Cancer will strike you whether you are a Democrat or Republican, capitalist or communist, believer or disbeliever, saint or sinner, prince or pothead. There is hardly a family today that has not been infiltrated by cancer. When this disease makes its debut, whether it be melanoma, leukemia, colon, brain, lung or liver, there is almost never a happy ending regardless of how much money you possess.

Many of your prominent entertainers & sport jocks over the years have crawled into the ring with the cell from hell and lost! People like John Wayne, Walter Payton, Jackie Wilson, Michael Landon, Telly Syvlalas (Kojak), Gregory Hines, Jackie Kennedy, and Mickey Mantle. Yes, even names of the rich and the famous are among the over 600,000 cancer deaths annually in America. Not to mention the 1.2 million new cancer cases that will surface this year. In the 21st Century, 50 percent of the American population will develop some form of cancer in their lifetime. Thirty to forty years from now virtually everyone that indulges in the standard commercial dietary lifestyle will experience an episode of cancer sometime within his or her life.

Cancer is not the culprit behind the death that it causes. It is a self-infliction of dietary neglect, environmental toxins, and emotional baggage. The repeated consumption of MediSins like, white sugar, white flour, benzenes, sulfur dioxide, irradiation and industrial pollutants create enough toxicity and poisons in our blood stream to cause metabolic failure within the body. Eventually, the body produces a more acidic state, abnormal multiplication of cells, a clogged lymphatic system and pancreatic breakdown. The end result, cancer! It is important to understand that while cancer, like other forms of ill health is a condition of modern civilization as a whole, remember the individual is largely responsible for the development of the disease.

The Standard American Diet that is consumed is the underlying culprit of cancer. In fact, just about every so-called food item in the grocery chain has been produced with some form of MediSin. Most of the food items in your grocery cart are either dead, acidic or toxic. The by-products that you call food are also preserved, irradiated, synthetically enriched and sodium bombarded. Though these so-called food items may smell good, and look appealing, "don't judge your meal by its cover". Believe it or not, you might be better off buying Science Diet or some other mineral enriched pet food.

In America most people have no dietary principles. We allow ourselves and our children to indulge in cancer causing meals, like nitrate preserved hotdogs, and luncheon meats served with constipating white bread. One meal after another increases the risk of cancer; while, the other clogs your colon. Even though the human body has the capability to naturally keep cancer in check, it can become a "feeding cell from Hell" when one continuously indulges in a toxic dietary and stressful lifestyle. Some cancers are also generated by excessive radiation, pollution, biological and chemical weapons. No matter how sophisticated and intelligent the medical profession may appear, if they have not come to the realization that dietary neglect is the underlying cause of cancer then they need to choose another profession, period!

There are many theories about cancer and many excuses as to why they are still racing for a cure. It is time to replace the theories with the facts. First of all, in order to understand cancer we have to understand its genesis or what causes it. Though there are many types of cancer, they all have one thing in common and that is physiological imbalance from a toxic body. It is unfortunate that mankind developed this anti-life state of mind where he has produced foods of commerce like condensed milk, canned meats, white bread, white sugar and refined table salt (sodium chloride), and delivered this life taxing resource to the world. For example, in a 1968, there was an epidemiological study indicating that dietary habits of refined food consumption and environmental chemical agents became the underlying cause of the worlds increase in cancer, not genetic factors as western institutions have you believe. The data from the study showed over a course of three generations, Japanese migrants in the U.S. contracted colon cancer at the same rates as the average American because they incorporated the Standard American Diet (SAD).

Cancer is an indication that the lifestyle we practice is not in harmony with the "laws of creation." The combination of emotional imbalance, spiritual death, and tangible poisons create havoc in our immune system. Cancer, a disease characterized by the abnormal multiplication of cells, is largely the result of long-term physical, mental and emotional toxicity. Modern medical professionals cannot relate to this fact because their education is based upon theory rather than universal and divine law.

Over the last 45 years, modern medical science has mounted a tenacious campaign to solve the crisis of cancer, but they are still running. After you read this segment, it would appear as if they are running from the cure rather than for the cure. Modern medicine has pioneered advance techniques such as surgery, radiation therapy, chemotherapy, laser therapy, and hormone therapy. Maybe it's the professionals of this industry that need the therapy!

Dr. Albert Schweitzer, one of the world's most renowned medical researchers, who built a hospital in Lambarene, Central Africa, reported in his letter of October 1954, the following:

"Many natives, especially those who are living in larger communities, do not live now in the same way as formerly - they used to live almost exclusively on fruits and vegetables, bananas, cassava, ignam, taro, sweet potatoes and other fruits. They now live on condensed milk, canned butter, meat and `preserves and white bread." Within several years of replacing their traditional whole food diet the presence of cancer appeared among the natives. Cancer was non-existent prior to this lifestyle change. Research at that time showed that 20% of the Bantu population of South Africa experienced liver cancer, because of the consumption of dead, cheap carbohydrates, maize and commercial meals."

WHAT IS CANCER (IN LAYMAN) TERMS

Cancer is a mutated stage that is an absolute repercussion from the human body's unnatural chemical intake (radiation, environmental pollutants, nitrate, etc.), dietary neglect and emotional baggage. Cancer is not some foreign cell that falls out of the sky and enters the body. They are normal cells that eventually mutate out of control challenging and compromising the body's immune system. The human body can endure enormous dietary neglect and chemical abuse like smoking for years before it begins to succumb to cellular destruction or cancer mutation. Cancer can conquer the body in two ways (1) through tumor formation where the body's immune system is only strong enough to capture the cells and encase them which can remain for several years before it begins to spread, (2) The human body becomes so weak that it cannot inhibit the rapid spread of cancer cells due to organ damage, so cancer cells continue to metastasize from one area to another until there is nothing left. The immune system is the only internal force that can defeat cancer by challenging it with Natural Killers cells, T-cells and other immune system activity.

In 1996, more Americans died of cancer than in World War II, the Korean War and Vietnam combined, with 550,000 Americans dying of cancer. In 2005, it is predicted that 1,372,910 new cases of cancer in the United States will develop this year, and 570,280 deaths will occur. Will you, your spouse, friend or someone you know be among the number of new cases or deaths? It will be up to you to change that status. All these people will acquire cancer because of the over consumption of MediSins. Soon, over fifty percent of the population will be at risk for cancer.

TYPES OF TUMORS

Malignant tumors are cancer. Cancer cells can invade and damage nearby tissues and organs. Also, cancer cells can break away from a malignant tumor and enter the bloodstream or the lymphatic system. This is how cancer spreads from the original (primary) tumor to form new tumors in other parts of the body. The spread of cancer is called metastasis. Most cancers are named for the type of cell or organ in which they begin. When cancer spreads, the new tumor has the same kind of abnormal cells and the same name as the primary tumor. For example if lung cancer spreads to the brain, the cancer cells in the brain are lung cancer cells. The disease is called metastasis lung cancer (not brain cancer).

Benign tumors are not cancer. They can usually be removed, and if what caused the benign tumor is corrected, it will not return. Benign tumors do not spread to other parts of the body.

Conventional or Classical Understanding of Cancer

Classic medicine defines cancer as a colony of malignant cells (malignant tumor). Cancer is a popular generic term for malignant neoplasm, a group of diseases of unknown cause, occurring in all human and many animal populations and arising in all tissues composed of potentially dividing cells. The basic characteristic of cancer is the transmissible abnormality of cells that are manifested by a reduced control over growth and function, leading to serious adverse effects on the host through invasive growth and metastases.

Some feel that this theory is why classical medicine is losing the war on cancer, because it uses the wrong strategies. For example; focusing only on the tumor, and neglecting the rest of the body and its functions. The malignant tumor is really the best your body can do, given the circumstances. According to researchers, the tumor is a natural defense of our body developed through evolution. Unless you respond with something that will help redevelop the balance of the body, mind and spirit, you are going to die.

WHAT CAUSES CANCER

One of the specific causes of cancer development is the over acidic environment your body maintains from the over consumption of acidic foods, drug usage, environmental toxins, and emotional instability. The term acid and alkaline is when water (H2O) ionizes into hydrogen (H+) and hydroxyl (OH-) ions. When these ions are in equal amounts, the pH is a neutral 7. When there are more H+ ions than OH-ions, then the water is said to be "acid". If OH-ions outnumber the H+ ions, then the water is said to be "alkaline". The pH scale ranges from 0 to 14 and is logarithmic, which means that each step is ten times the previous. In other words a pH of 4.5 is 10 times more acid than 5.5, 100 times more acid than 6.5 and 1,000 times more acid.

When healthy, the pH of blood is 7.4. Thus, the pH of saliva parallels the extra cellular fluid .... The pH test of saliva represents the most consistent and most definitive physical sign of the ionic calcium deficiency syndrome. The pH of the healthy body is in the range of 7.1 to 7.5. If the range is from 6.5 to 4.5 the body is acidic. This represents the calcium deficiency of aging and lifestyle defects. Cancer patients are around a pH of 4.5, especially when terminal. Virtually all degenerative diseases, including tooth decay and gall stones are associated with excess acidity in the body. Though, the body has a homeostatic mechanism which maintains a constant pH of 7.4 in the blood, this mechanism works by depositing and withdrawing acid and alkaline minerals from other locations including the body tissues, bones, body fluids and saliva. Therefore the body can maintain a quality pH balance when properly nourished.

The Pancreas: the most over looked defense against cancer

Before the body can deteriorate into cancer, all the body's defense systems have to depress and shut down. If your pancreas is working properly along with the intake of enzyme loaded food, you will have a good chance of not developing cancer. Pancreatic enzymes, trypsin in particular, dissolve the protective protein coating which covers malignant tissues and makes it possible for the body's natural immune defenses to recognize the cancer cell as foreign and destroy it. Therefore, we suggest the consumption of pancreatic enzymes and foods live with enzymatic activity.

Beware of the commercial drugs and acidic foods

Constant consumption of dead acidic foods can make you a victim of MediSin. For example, American's have consumed more soft drinks than ever before with more than 15 billion gallons of soda pop consumed in 2000. This equates to one 12 oz bottle per day for every man, woman and child. According to the U.S. Department of Agriculture, children are heavy consumers of acidic soft drinks at unprecedented rates. This is probably why juvenile diabetes and obesity is becoming a major epidemic in America today. The active ingredient in most soda pop is phosphoric acid. The pH of most soft drinks is 2.8, which is very acidic. Many animal studies show that phosphoric acid, a common ingredient in soda pop, can deplete bone calcium. Studies also show that the over consumption of phosphoric acid can cause severe kidney and bladder damage. Most packaged goods in the grocery chain have very little nutritional value. They are mostly sodium bombarded and acidic pseudo-foods. So what happens if you continue to consume commercial soft drinks and commercial refined food products? You get a compromised immune system.

Adulterated foods are dead and have no activity that brings life to the cells of the body. Mucus forming foods (white rice and flour), nitrites (luncheon meats), sugars, all eventually cause decay within the body, ruining vital organs such as the stomach, spleen, kidney, liver and pancreas. By abusing these vital organs of the body, you will develop some form of cancer or degenerative disease. There should be a balance of alkaline and acid foods in the diet but eat mostly alkaline foods. Here is an example of alkaline and acid foods:

EXTREME AKALINE FOODS
Lemons and watermelons.

AKALINE FOODS
Cantaloupe, cayenne, celery, figs, limes, melons, papayas, grapes, pineapples, lettuce, asparagus, greens.

MODERATELY ALKALINE FOODS
Apples, avocados, grapefruit, peaches, peas, olives, okra.

NEUTRAL FOODS
Brown rice, barley, bananas, bran, maple syrup, beans.

ACIDIC FOODS
Corn, canned fruit, lentils, rye, noodles, oats, meats, dairy.

EXTREME ACIDIC FOODS
Coffee, prescription drugs, white sugar, white flour, dyes.

Note: There are some whole foods and grains that are considered neutral like whole brown rice, which should be eaten often.

THE TYPES OF CANCER

In modern medicine, cancer is classified into five major groups:

I. **Carcinoma**-a cancerous tumor or lump manifesting in the surface tissue of the body organs. It is the most common form of cancer, responsible for over 80% of the cases.
II. **Sarcoma**-a cancerous tumor originating in the bone, cartilage, muscle, fibrous, connective or fatty tissue.
III. **Myeloma**-a cancerous tumor originating in the plasma cells of the bone marrow.
IV. **Lymphoma**-a cancerous tumor originating in the lymph system.
V. **Leukemia**-cancer originating in the tissue of the bone.

MICROWAVES AND ELECTROMAGNETIC EXPOSURE

Another MediSin that has placed even more danger upon the human family is microwave ovens. It seems most households have microwaves, which competes with the idiot box (television) for operational use. Many people use microwaves not because it makes food taste better, but due to quickness in cooking. Russians knew something was wrong with microwaves, because in 1976 they were banned for use due to the fact that they caused cancer. However, your FDA assures you microwaves are safe, but the Russians found out that microwave food has these negative health consequences:

1) Microwave foods lose 60~90% of the food value
2) Micro waving alters elemental food substances causing digestive disorders
3) Micro waving alters food chemistry which can lead to malfunctions in the lymphatic system and degeneration of the body's ability to protect itself against cancerous growths.
4) Microwave food leads to a higher percentage of cancerous cells in the blood stream.

With just a few of these known consequences, why would you cook your food in a microwave or even have one in your home? Your best choice is to find a trash can and then go purchase a juicer.

Television, though it is a luxury of modern day society and our eyes to the world, also has potentially adverse effects, especially color television. Televisions contain a CRT (Cathode Ray Tube) that zigzags 15,000 times a second down the screen, projecting a large electromagnetic field. Several decades ago a British epidemiologist claimed in a medical journal that constant exposure to television contributed to cardiovascular and various forms of illnesses including cancer. So, if you have cancer, it is recommended that television should be avoided or at least limited to a half hour a day, seated at least 10 feet away from the screen. Then again, there are some television programs that are pleasant like Oprah, Montel, Tony Brown's Journal, Larry King, the Tonight Show, PBS, Discovery or A&E which may help stimulate some endorphins (healing chemicals in the body).

CLOTHING AND PERSONAL ACCESSORIES

Be mindful of synthetic clothing, such as nylon, polyester, acrylic, chemically treated cotton or genetically engineered fabrics. They impede and interrupt the chi (life force) or energy that flows throughout the body. This includes synthetic sheets, blankets and underwear. All natural or organic clothing is becoming more accessible, even hemp clothing is now available.

BODY CARE

Commercial soaps, deodorants, shampoos and other body care products may be harmful and slow the progress of cancer recovery or increase the spread of cancer. Some of the most harmful body care ingredients are sodium laurel sulfate, cocomide DEA and propylene glycol. These chemicals accumulate in the brain, heart, liver, kidneys, and eyes causing long-term damage. Choose more natural plant base products. Your local health food store carries a wide variety of wholesome body care products.

Way of Life	Healthy	Degenerative
Daily food	Whole	Processed
(Primary factors)	Natural	Artificial
	Organic	Chemical
	Unrefined	Refined
	Balanced	Extreme
	Seasonal	Un-seasonal
	Local grown	Transcontinental
	Home	Precooked
Environment & Lifestyle	Clean	Polluted
(Contributing factors)	Orderly	Disorderly
	Active	Sedentary
	Real	Synthetic
Outlook		
(Contributing factors)	Peaceful	Complaining
	Grateful	Arrogant
	Flexible	Rigid
	Cooperative	Competitive

AIR CIRCULATION

Free circulation of air and adequate sunshine is very important. People that tend to stay in the house most of the time will develop a compromised immune system, because of the household chemicals, dust, and human carbon dioxide. Legitimate scientific studies have shown that 19 common household plants like Chrysanthemum, Bamboo Palm, Moss Cane, English Ivy and Gerbera Daisy increase oxygen and help eliminate chemicals from the household air that may contribute to cancer. These chemicals include formaldehyde (carpets) and benzene (cooking oils) that activates the sheep liver fluke, a parasite that produces cancerous conditions. Purchase an Air Purifier from Alpine Air to eliminate mold, dust mites and pollution from the home.

DOCTORS WHO HAD THE ANSWER, but WERE ATTACKED

One of the most eminent geniuses of the 20th century was Dr. Max Gerson. In 1946, Dr. Gerson demonstrated medical proof of complete remission of cancer in over one-third of his patients before the Pepper-Neely Congressional Sub-committee for Hearings (S. 1875). Dr. Gerson entered the U.S. in 1933 from Germany and introduced one of the most astounding applications known in medical history today. He developed a clinical dietary approach to the treatment of a number of chronic diseases such as tuberculosis, asthma, arthritis, diabetes, heart disease, MS and even many types of cancer.

Dr. Gerson implemented a dietary protocol that consisted of detoxification with raw vegetable and fruit juices, raw calf liver juice (now discontinued because of the toxic chemical residue now found in calves), a vegetarian diet and caffeine implants in the form of coffee enemas to purge the liver of toxins and open the bile ducts. This holistic application was proven to expel toxins accumulated from the manifestations of illness as well as "dissolve tumor masses," which, once caught in the liver, would be released in the bile and exit through the kidneys. After the initial stage of organic juice fasting and enemas, patients would follow a long-term dietary regiment; involving low-sodium/ high potassium foods to maintain cellular balance.

Dr. Gerson demonstrated that cancer patients who had been given up for dead by hospitals could recover by his natural protocols. In spite of the anticipated reception of a Nobel Prize for his medical research, lobbying forces for surgery, radiation, and chemotherapy defeated his natural dietary protocol through intensive lobbying efforts. A Senate Bill that could have instituted research on dietary protocols that not only would prevent cancer but actually reverse it failed by only four votes. Through medical arrogance and political greed, Dr. Gerson's program was destroyed in 1946.

According to Dr. Spain-Ward's research; which, revealed systematic harassment and political suppression towards Dr. Gerson by the New York State Medical Society and the NY State Licensing Board, Dr. Gerson's publications were suppressed and reputable journals would not accept his articles. Soon thereafter, his hospital privileges at Gotham Hospital in New York were revoked. Dr. Gerson's license was completely denied and was forever banned from practicing medicine in the state of New York. So, thanks to the provocateurs of the AMA, the suppression of

Max Gerson became a tragedy in medical history. Emotionally crushed and concerned for his patients, he published "A Cancer Therapy - Results of Fifty Cases" in 1959 before his death.

The AMA, the same agency that was run by a circus clown on the pretext of protecting the FDA, and in violation of their legislation, mandated/eradicated what might have been the turning point in cancer research. The industry succeeded in not only destroying the professional career of this prominent clinical researcher, but turned away perhaps one of the only hopes for Americans and the world to win the "War on Cancer." Today, the idiots of western medicine, along with their brainwashed students proudly exercise their arrogant ignorance of the role of nutrition and diet in the eradication of cancer.

HOXSEY HERBS : ANOTHER SUPPRESSED DISCOVERY

Another battle between the Knights of Med Table and natural medicine was the dramatic episode between Dr. Fishbein *(the former circus clown)* of the AMA and Dr. Hoxsey.

Dr. John Hoxsey, a veterinarian, who had no intention on claiming that he was a medical physician, developed herbal formulas that turned out to be so effective that it reversed certain forms of officially diagnosed cancers. He discovered these herbal formulas through his expertise of veterinary medicine. His discovery occurred when his horse developed a cancerous lesion on the foreleg. He turned the horse out to pasture and within several weeks, the horse was fully recovered. Dr. Hoxsey credited the horse's recovery to certain herbs and grassy plants found in the unused pasture. He decided to investigate the science between the plants and the horse's cancer.

Dr. Hoxsey used his observation to develop two tonics, one taken by mouth and the other topically applied to skin malignancies. After durations of effective results, he began administering a series of applications to local people with medically diagnosed cases of cancer. After several applications, the malignancies decreased in size and some even disappeared.

Dr. Hoxsey organized a licensed medical staff and opened several clinics, the most famous in Dallas, Texas. He ran an advertising campaign on radio. Soon people traveled to Dallas from all over America and other western countries. Numerous patients that received the "Hoxsey application" attained long-term remission, and even cancer eradication. Dr. Hoxsey eventually wrote a book, aptly entitled "You don't have to die!"

If the medical community was fair and receptive to change, they would have observed that the mixtures of Hoxsey's formulas had anti-tumor and anti-cancer activity. They would have welcomed the fact that these natural formulas contained ingredients that stimulate the human body's natural immune defenses. Many of the specific plants were a part of the medical system that was indigenous to the American Natives (whom the westerners call Indians). These herbal remedies were researched and confirmed by the National Cancer Institute.

Needless to say it was Morris Fishbein who exercised medical arrogance, ignorance and stupidity to launch an anti-Hoxsey campaign. According to research it turned out to be a personal/business vendetta. Harry Hoxsey had allegedly rejected a financial and business offer from Fishbein and the drug industry to monopolize and commercialize Hoxsey remedies on a national scale. The AMA attempted to negotiate a proposal to get Hoxsey also to turn over the rights of the formula to an unnamed pharmaceutical company excluding Hoxsey from any decision making role. Plus, Hoxsey would not receive any royalties for the next ten years. Guess they thought Hoxsey was born the day before they made that proposal. Anyone with common logic could see right through the trickery and deception, so he refused. The next campaign was obvious, if they couldn't have the formulas then no one would! Fishbein along with the FDA waged a propaganda war against Hoxsey, his clinics and his licensed health staff. The FDA forced the clinic to close and they took refuge in Tijuana, Mexico where it still operates to this day.

ANOTHER GIFTED MAN IS ATTACKED

Royal Raymond Rife should be considered the master of microtechnology. He is responsible for today's electronic radiochemistry, biochemistry, microbiology, even ballistics and aviation.

Some of his inventions included the heterodyning ultraviolet microscope, a micro dissector, and a micro manipulator. Royal Raymond Rife was a student at John Hopkins; he received 14 major awards, and was honored with an honorary doctorate from the University of Heidelberg. He was most notable for manufacturing roller bearings, but what he was really famous for was the Rife scope.

Rife's microscope contained approximately 5,682 pieces and could magnify microscopic objects 61,000 times their normal size, making it easy to examine living blood tissue and identify cellular diseases. It was a two-foot tall microscope and weighed approximately 200 pounds. He became the first in modern science to actually see a live virus and until recently the Rife scope was the only microscope that could do this. So why hasn't any medical student or physician heard of Dr. Royal Raymond Rife? The same reason they have never heard of Antoine Be'champ, Harry Hoxsey, or Max Gerson, it's about control & and profits! In order for unnatural expensive medicine to succeed, natural economical medicine has to fail.

Rife could actually see various microorganisms or particles in blood, which are able to change form or shape and are therefore pleomorphic. Rife was also able to use ultra violet light to illuminate these forms or changes in cell formation. He was also able to produce frequency waves to match the frequency at which a microorganism vibrates. This science by Rife induced resonance and subsequently eradicated the targeted organism by frequency in the same way that a sound vibration can shatter a crystal glass. The famous Royal Rife used these innovative scholarly techniques to treat degenerative disease ranging from pneumonia to cancer.

Rife's expertise and scientific breakthrough was first introduced to the public in 1929 by the San Diego Union Newspaper. As early as 1920, Rife had identified a virus that he believed caused cancer. It was named the "BX virus." After 20,000 unsuccessful attempts to transform normal cells into tumor cells, Rife decided to irradiate viruses, catch them in a porcelain filter, and inject them into lab animals. Four hundred consecutive tumors were created from this procedure. He began subjecting the viruses to different radio frequencies to see if it was affected by them. It was found that all viruses had responded to the frequencies.

Rife discovered a frequency he called "Mortal Oscillatory Rate" (MOR) that could destroy targeted viruses by the wavelength of the frequency (770 Hz, 880 Hz, etc.). This frequency could destroy targeted viruses without harming the surrounding normal tissue. It was discovered that everything has its own frequency. In fact, there are literally hundreds of trillions of different resonant frequencies. From this scientific discovery, Dr. Rife successfully eradicated cancer in 400 animal experiments prior to experimentation on human subjects. Rife discovered frequencies, which specifically destroyed herpes, polio, spinal meningitis, tetanus, influenza, and an immense number of other degenerative disease organisms.

On November 20, 1931, Dr. Royal Rife was honored by forty-four of the Nation's most respected medical authorities with a banquet billed as "The End to All Disease" at the Pasadena estate of Milbank Johnson *(see above picture)*.

In 1934, the University of Southern California appointed a Medical Research Committee to transfer from Pasadena Hospital to Rife's San Diego Laboratory and Clinic for treatment. Within 90 days of treatment, if the terminally ill patients were still alive, then the doctors and pathologist would examine the patients. Amazingly, after the 90 days of the Rife treatment, the Committee concluded that 86.5% of the patients had been completely cured! The treatment was then modified and the remaining 13.5% of the terminally ill patients also responded within the next four weeks. The Rife technology recovery rate turned out to be 100%! In 1937, The Beam Ray Corporation manufactured fourteen of the Rife's Frequency instruments.

Now, the real drama. You've guessed it, Morris Fishbein, the former circus clown (with no formal medical education or compassion for preserving human life) got wind of Rife's invention and sent a "bootlicking" attorney to strike a buyout deal with Rife. Again, like any other pioneers with integrity, Rife could sense the trickery of Fishbein, and he refused. After Rife spent decades of accumulating meticulous evidence of his discoveries, including film and stop motion photographs, an arson fire destroyed the multi-million dollar Burnett Lab in New Jersey, the lab that validated Rife's work. Soon after, someone poisoned Southern California's AMA President, Dr. Millbank Johnson just before he was going to prepare a statement announcing to the world that Dr. Rife's electronic therapy had a 100% accuracy rate by curing 16 of 16 patients. The most dramatic episode occurred when police were ordered to illegally confiscate the remainder of Rife's 50 years of research. Fishbein's political pull continued to create court battles that generated enough legal bills to bankrupt Beam Ray forcing it to close. After that, Fishbein used his power within the AMA to stop further research of Rife's work.

By 1950, Dr. Rife partnered up with John Crane, an electrical engineer and for ten years they worked together to build more advanced frequency machines. However in 1960, the AMA shut them down. The agents even went to the extreme and destroyed all of Dr. Rife's machines and notes; most were never recovered. John Crane was sent to prison for a little over three years in spite of the favorable testimonials of fourteen patients. Discouraged and emotionally crushed, Rife became an alcoholic in the latter days of his life. Rife finally died from a combination of Valium and alcohol.

So what happened to the physicians that honored the discovery? Well, the AMA sent a letter to all the physicians that attended the banquet forcing him or her to deny that they ever knew of Rife or his work.

SURGERY: RADIATION AND CHEMOTHERAPY: YOUR ONLY CHOICES IN AMERICA

We are approaching the 4th decade of former President Nixon's "war on cancer." We can't say exactly how many billions of dollars have been wasted on cancer research, education, and treatment. However, we can say it doesn't look like they are any more interested in natural or alternative treatments than 38 years ago. The medical institutions claim that they want to protect us from quackery, but who's fooling whom? How many years are Americans going to endure MediSins of poisonous and butchering therapy? The industry has our women in fear of losing their self-esteem, sexuality, their breast and their womb, while the men fear physical and chemical castration. Despite the institutional cheers and hospice support, potential victims are rarely free of the fear that someday the cancer will return. This is because there is no true story being told about real cancer survival. "Five year survival" is a conventional milestone for cancer patients and a realistic achievement for allopathic doctors.

The cancer industry is practically a goldmine for the pharmaceutical and medical industry. The National Center for Health Statistics figured the total costs of cancer at $71.5 billion in 1987. At that time, the direct cost of all illnesses in the U.S. was $371.4 billion (ibid). Direct costs are well over $500 billion and will continue to increase. Indirect costs are expected to reach $200 billion, if it has not already.

SURGERY

The most common method of treating cancer conventionally is with the surgical blade. Surgery has been practiced since the dawn of medical history to remove malignant tumors. Hippocrates (460 B.C.- 370 B.C.), who according to ancient text understood well and even coined the term carcinoma, urged physicians "Above all, does no harm." But treatment for certain types of cancers would do just the opposite.

The so called "ingenious surgeons" devised an operation for the head and neck called the Commando. This involved the removal of the patents mandible, or jaw. For pancreatic cancer it involved the removal of many organs adjacent to the affected gland on the theory that they might be harboring a nest of cancer cells. However, despite this radical application, the survival rate for pancreatic cancer remained persistently at a low 5% five-year survival for localized pancreatic cancer and 0-3% if the cancer had already metastasized.

Another operation called total exoneration designed by Dr. Alexander Brunschwig involved the removal of the rectum, the stomach, the urinary bladder, and part of the liver, the spleen, colon, pelvic floor wall, and all the internal reproductive organs.

Patients were unfortunately being gutted out like a rehabbed house with the hope that the cancer would be eliminated. Brunschwig himself admitted that the operation was "a brutal and cruel procedure" (New York Times, April 8, 1969).

The ultimate butcher operation was the hemicorporectomy-literally, the removal of half the body. This amazing circus surgery was originated by Theodore Miller, a memorial surgeon involved in the amputation of everything below the pelvis in the treatment of advanced bladder or pelvic region malignancy. Not surprisingly, many patients preferred to let cancer take its toll rather than be butchered like that (New York Times, November 30, 1969). Needless to say, that surgery had gone as far as it could go, unless they could dissect the entire body and put it back together. Don't be surprised if something like this has been attempted; if they thought about it, they probably tried it!

RADIATION THERAPY

The second so-called effective method of treating cancer is radiation therapy or the "beam." Radiation therapy is a branch of radiology that involves the use of radioactivity (ionizing radiation such as Gamma Rays or X-ray as therapy). The American Cancer Society claims that out of seventy-five years, radiation therapy is more sophisticated, accurate and effective with fewer side effects. Radiation therapy has become the standard application, especially with cancers of the neck, the uterine cervix, and the beginning stages of bladder, prostrate, skin, bone, and certain types of brain cancers.

According to Jane Brody of the NY Times who co-authored with the America Cancer Society VP, Art Holleb, Senator Hubert Humphrey, was a "famous beneficiary of modern radiation therapy who died of bladder cancer despite his extensive surgery, chemo and radiation therapy. Radiation therapy was the initial application used in the defense of his bladder cancer, but failed to intercept the massive growth of the bladder tumor." According to Brody and her co-author, Senator Humphrey was considered a beneficiary because he remained well for three years until he developed new and more advance cancers.

Though radiation is claimed to be a very effective application, only a few cancers have successfully responded to the radiation procedures. For example, radiation therapy to lung cancer may cause extensive inflammation followed by scarring of nearby normal lung tissue, thus causing damage to the treated lung even though the tumor is completely eradicated. According to Prof. John Cairn's, "cancer cannot be cured by radiation because the dose of X-ray required to kill all the cancer cells would also kill the patient" (Cairns, 1985).

According to studies of patients treated with radiation therapy, they have a 76% recurrence rate of bladder cancer following the treatment. Radiation therapy is comprised of electromagnetic radiation and radioactive isotopes. Electromagnetic radiation utilizes gamma rays and x-rays during the therapy while radioisotopes Cobalt-60 and Iodine-131 is often employed as the modus operandi for delivering radiation therapy.

Many doctors are so protective over radiation therapy that they overlook the side effects. Radiation can damage the cardiovascular system causing internal bleeding and destruction of the villa (the minute projections from the intestinal wall that is the primary site for nutrient absorption). Radiation therapy also greatly compromises the immune system by damaging the bone marrow, causing lipid per oxidation. Other serious toxic effects from radiation include shrinkage of the spleen (the master of digestion and blood reservoir), and the shrinkage of the thymus gland (the gland responsible for protection of bacterial and viral invasion, production of T-lymphocytes and it also is responsible for receiving stem cells from the bone marrow). Radiation therapy also causes cachexia (muscle wasting), loss of Vitamin C and corrupts the balance of sodium and potassium.

If these adverse effects are known, then why is radiation used so extensively? There are several factors as to why this therapy has not been reviewed or analyzed with integrity. One reason is that doctors are in serious denial, maybe due to a brainwashing technique in medical school, remember the "Manchurian Candidate"? Second, it is almost impossible to get a "peer review" that will accept a study of iatrogenic (doctor-caused) disease. You just can't walk up to a professional of the medical industry and convince them to accept the possibility of a doctor-caused cancer. "For nearly 40 years radiologist's have been engaged in massive malpractice-which is something that one doctor will not mention to another." (Bross, 1979)

In summary, radiation therapy appears to be of limited value in the treatment of cancer, although it may be preferred over other applications, depending on the cancer. One of the main problems with this application is that it compromises the immune system, period! Doctors need to become more educated in preventing the adverse affect of this therapy by using natural substances that may increase the effectiveness of radiation therapy by supporting the body's own immune system.

Substances like the amino acid glutamine, vitamin A, and the carbohydrate acemannan either increase the susceptibility of cancer cells or improve the effectiveness of radiotherapy. Other substances or supplements like beta 1, 3 glucans, hyaluronic acid, and selenium protects the body against the toxic effects of radiation therapy. This also includes papain, super oxide dismutase, essential lipids, and pancreatin. According to "alternative studies", codonopsis, ginseng and the world famous Reishi mushroom counteracts the suppression of the immune system caused by radiation therapy. Supplements like the world-renowned fermented yeast formula Bio-Strath or Haelen 951 has been shown to help prevent the cachexia and depletion of hemoglobin.

CHEMOTHERAPY

The third and most ludicrous application of all is the famous chemotherapy. This so-called proven cancer therapy is supposed to kill cancer cells without harming normal tissue. In reality, the orthodox chemotherapy has yet to be considered a safe application because it cannot just neutralize cancer cells. The activity of many chemotherapy agents blocks the essential metabolic step in the process of cellular division. Since cancer cells often divide more rapidly than normal cells, this lethal "anti-metabolite" action should specifically target the cancer cells, but most of the normal tissues have cell dividing activity, therefore chemotherapy destroys all healthy tissues along with the cancer cells. As a result, loss of hair, bone marrow and intestinal tissues are common.

Chemotherapy often brings a series of blood diseases (such as leucopenia, thrombocytopenia and plastic anemia). Chemotherapy on the gut can also be disastrous. This is why cancer patients have difficulty eating or absorbing their food as a result of nausea, bleeding sores around the mouth, soreness of the gums and throat and the destruction of the entire mucosa of the gut.

Although chemotherapy is used for the treatment of cancers like breast, colon and lung malignancies, these cancers generally do not respond to this form of treatment. According to researchers Maugh and Marx, chemotherapy is not effective against tumors that have metastasized, because the immune system is already compromised. If chemotherapy has any effectiveness it would be against small tumors that have only recently developed. Just recently (January, 2005) former McDonalds CEO, Charlie Bell died of colon cancer. Chemotherapy was his choice of treatment (or maybe his doctor's), but to no avail, he did not make it past six months since his diagnosis, trading in his Big Mac for a six-foot hole in the ground at the age of 44.

In the 1950's, the introduction of Interferon appeared to be a "genie in a bottle", even the financial runners at Wall Street were placing bets that this was the one: a real winner. However in 1982, it was discovered that this too had toxic side effects. In that same year four patients that were treated with Interferon died, as one reporter put "From wonder drug to wallflower," (ibid). Currently, Interferon is approved to be used in the treatment of hairy-cell leukemia and juvenile laryngeal papillomatosis and now Hepatitis C, but Interferon has failed to live up to its promises.

Many more drugs were thrown into the cancer arena. Back in 1955, the center of drug testing shifted from the Sloan-Kettering Institute to the National Cancer Institute's (NCI) Cancer Chemotherapy National Service Center in Bethesda, Maryland. Our Congress allocated $25 million to test 20,000 chemicals a year at "The Wall Street of Cancer Research," in the words of the center's director Dr. Kenneth M. Endicott (Newsweek, January

20, 1958). Companies began manufacturing chemotherapy drugs as if it were candy. In 1984, Bristol-Myers alone sold $153 million in chemotherapeutic drugs, Krestin one of the best selling cancer drugs out of Japan had $359.1 million in sales. According to U.S. government figures, the market went from $270 million in 1983 to over $564 million in 1987 (U.S. Department of Commerce, 1983-1987).

The money that is being spent and the treatments that are being used on patients are appalling. The health of the American people is being destroyed by the millions on expensive life threatening MediSins like, chemo, radiation and surgery. They are being destroyed by the clique that calls him or herself an "oncologist." An oncologist is the only medical politician-profession who has a vested interest in preserving the toxic applications with no change other than making more money. They maintain a multi-billion dollar confidence game. They pretend that the treatment is working, and then they have a very persuasive way to convince the masses that it is working.

We have allowed the provocateurs of medicine to dictate the applications of cancer. Anyone who even conceives the notion of opposing the status quo and advocating something efficacious, non-toxic and divine is prosecuted. So ask yourself, why are you allowing the agents of devilment to destroy you, your family and your future? Remember what Thomas Jefferson said, "When the government fears its people you have liberty, when the people fear the government you have tyranny." You have a choice, either to die in vain from medical trickery or to live in optimum body and spirit.

The Cancer Battle Plan

With all the chaos, persecution and mis-education about cancer, the best thing to do is to start taking your health into your own hands and prevent it. These are the following steps to take in order to prevent cancer:

- The first thing to address as with any other disease is the diet. It is imperative to consume whole grains such a brown rice, millet, oats and other forms of grains from an "organic source".
- Organic fruits and vegetables should be the first choice of produce. If you cannot afford all organic produce purchase a good produce wash that you will find in either the grocery or health food store.
- Purchase reverse osmosis or distilled water only, but be mindful of the brands that you select. There are still some con artists in the water industry.
- Eat salads (not head lettuce) on a daily basis especially if your body is retaining toxins. Avoid salad dressings that contain canola oils or any refined oil.
- Conduct a periodic colon cleanse and a blood detoxification.
- Exercise of course is very important to help cleanse the lymphatic system.
- Mental outlook positive
- Emotionally stability
- High spiritual connection to the Creator

These are just some of the basic fundamentals to follow that will keep your body in an optimal state. Please read in Chapter 36 "Solutions to MediSin" for more information.

Great Immune System Builders

Since there are so many products, claims and hype in the alternative medicine and health food industry, we will give you a list of a few applications with proven efficacy based on primary research, not borrowed science:

Astragalus: a root that contains polysaccharide (essential complex sugars) and can be taken in extract, tea, or capsule form has been proven to build immune system immensely, by stimulating the production of T-cell lymphocytes, also has been shown to protect the liver. Astragalus can be taken safely by adults and children without adverse effects on the immune system.

Bovine Cartilage: Dr. John F. Prudden is the foundation for the research and application for all cartilage products including shark cartilage. Bovine cartilage was scientifically and clinically studied by Judah Folkman, M.D., while working at a Children's Hospital and Harvard medical school. A study was also conducted by Brain G.M. Durie, M.D. with the Department of Medicine at the University of Arizona. It was found that the bovine cartilage had a direct anti-mitotic effect of human ovarian, pancreatic and colon mutations. Apparently, the bovine cartilage proved to have the ability to inhibit cell division in several kinds of cell mutations. It was demonstrated to be more effective than the popular shark cartilage.

Essiac Tea: This Native American formula is a special blend of sheep sorrel, red clover, Indian rhubarb, and burdock root. Though there are many copycats and counterfeits, the original Essiac formula adopted by Registered Nurse Rene Cassie has been reputedly demonstrated to not only completely detoxify the entire body, but stimulate the immune system as well.

Ellagic Acid: a type of phenolic acid that helps prevent various forms of cancer by counteracting many synthetic, naturally occurring carcinogens preventing them from converting normal, healthy cell into cells of mutation.

Systemic Enzymes: this proprietary blend of powerful enzymes has been clinically shown to attack the outer coating of cancer cells. This coating disguises and protects the mutated cells from being recognized by the Natural Killer (NK) cells of the immune system. According to clinical research, systemic enzymes also help the body to stimulate T-cells and NK lymphocytes.

Inositol Hex phosphate(IP6) (phytic acid): Has been clinically proven to be very supportive for the immune system. Inositol Hexaphosphate (phytic acid) has been shown to reduce tissue damage during inflammation. Not only does the naturally derived substance made from brown rice neutralize inflammation but increases the production of T and NK cell by several hundred percent. These immune system cells are responsible for protecting the body from cancer mutation.

Mushrooms: There are many medicinal mushrooms like Shitake, Maitake, and Reishi that help build a very strong immune system by building helper T cells, memory T cells, and NK-lymphocytes. Some mushrooms stimulate the production of interlukins 1-2 and 3. It also activates macrophages and prevents foreign cell mutation.

Ginseng: One of the most powerful adaptogens and anti-stress agents. Ginseng has been clinically proven to help regulate many functions of the body. There are a wide variety of ginseng such as American, Korean, wild mountain and pseudo ginseng like Siberian, Ashawaganda and Rhodiola. Studies have also shown that ginseng suppresses mutated cell growth by activating NK cell lymphocytes. The quality of ginseng may vary from brand to brand. But if using a good quality ginseng, the health benefits can be promising. Ginseng should be taken for 45-60 days consecutively for optimum results.

Coenzyme Q10: Considered as one of the most powerful antioxidants and essential nutrients of life. Scientists believe that low levels of coenzyme Q10 is directly linked to congestive heart failure and cellular damage. In a study published in Clinical Investigator, Dr. K. Folkers found that the immune function was dramatically increased with a daily dose of 60 mg of CoQ10. So dramatic was the increase, Folkers felt that age-associated decline in immune function could be reversed with CoQ10.

Parasite cleanse: a parasite cleanse is necessary to eliminate the various forms of protozoa, worms and flukes that invade and interrupt the healing processes in the body. Naturopathic physician Hulda Clark, N.D., Ph.D., author of the book " A Cure for All Diseases", recommends using a blend of three herbs to flush the parasites out of your body: Primary research has shown that black walnut, wormwood and ground cloves eliminate parasites and their eggs. This will reduce cellular mutation.

Whole foods and Spiritual Balance: Chemical free food is essential for optimum health. Make sure that you are buying and consuming foods that are in their natural state, meaning "organic" according to the health food industry standards. The less chemicals the body has to neutralize the greater the chance that you become disease free. Read more on the varieties of fruits, vegetables, nuts, seeds and grains and how to properly combine and prepare them. Most natural and organic items can be found at your local health food stores which includes Wild Oats Markets.

Stay as spiritual as possible, greatly reducing the amount of television, negative people and stress. Make every attempt to meditate and pray whatever your spiritual faith may be. Remember to love yourself, your family, friends and the environment that you live in.

These are just a few ways to build your immune system and protect your body from cellular mutation. Once you eliminate all the MediSins from your diet, and reconnect yourself with the universal laws of divine life then you will begin to reach a healing plateau that will award you with a disease free life.

10 questions you absolutely must ask your Cancer Specialist (specialist in killing) before undergoing treatment:

1) Doctor-after you remove my tumor with chemotherapy, radiation or surgical procedures, what are you going to do to address my cancer?

Comment: Being that cancer is a whole body metabolic disease from head to toe due to a weakened immune system, weakened organs, tissues and cells, low cellular energy, acidic pH, low oxygen tissue environment, toxic emotions, nutritional deficiencies, etc., the only treatment protocol to reverse cancer permanently and to prevent secondary tumors from manifesting is to address the primary causes of cancer.

There is not one cancer treatment in mainstream medisin that administers non-toxic treatments to boost and modulate the immune system, correct nutritional deficiencies, strengthen organs, cells and tissues, remove cancer causing toxins from the body, alkalize the pH, increase metabolic energy or strengthen the emotional and spiritual state of the patient, which are all necessary for ridding cancer. Oncologists are brainwashed into believing that the tumor is the cancer while the tumor is just the side effect of cancer, which is a whole body metabolic disease. Their whole medical education is based on a false premise of tumor removal not cancer removal. If the cure for cancer were in the tumor removal, they would have cured cancer 60 years ago.

2) What non-toxic treatments do you have in your medical toolbox that can repair the cellular DNA damage done by chemotherapy and radiation to prevent leukemia, secondary tumors and future tumor sites from occurring?

Comment: Unfortunately there is no drug, chemo agent, radiation or surgical procedure to date that will repair cellular DNA damage done by their treatments. All mainstream cancer treatments damage, not repair, cellular DNA. All non-toxic treatments that repair cellular DNA damage are found in alternative medicine outside of mainstream medicine.

3) The reason I have cancer is that my organs, cells and systems, especially my immune system, are in a severely weakened state due to an overexposure of accumulated toxins throughout the years. What can you do to remove the cancer causing chemicals and toxins that are imbedded in my organs, tissues, bloodstream and cells?

Comment: Mainstream medicine has no detoxification procedures to cleanse the liver, kidneys, blood, and colon, lymph, which limits their long-term success and allows the cancer to return because they leave the growth medium for cancerintact. You have to go outside of mainstream medicine for detoxification methods using herbs, homeopathic remedies, colon irrigation, coffee enemas, botanicals, etc. to remove cancer causing toxic residues.

4) Since nutritional deficiencies are a major factor in contributing to my cancer, what nutritional assessments do you use for diagnosing nutritional deficiencies and imbalances?

Comment: Because of their limited knowledge of nutrition in medical school training (less than two hours in most medical universities), nutrition, diet, or even nutrient assessment testing procedures are obsolete in allopathic medicine. Due to their ignorance in the direct correlation of diet to cancer origin, you will not even see it addressed in mainstream medicine. However, nutrition is absolutely necessary to reverse and prevent not only cancer, but all disease. The building blocks of every organ, cell, tissue and even your immune system come from nutrition, not toxic pharmaceuticals, chemo or radiation. The only way to address deficiencies is outside of mainstream medisin.

5) With sugar being the main fuel source for tumor growth, called sugar fermentation or sugar glycolysis, what dietary regimen will you give me that address the foods and beverages that I should avoid so as not to feed my tumors?

Comment: Mainstream doctors are totally oblivious to the sugar/cancer connection. Therefore, the best advice you will receive is to eat anything to prevent yourself from losing weight. In their ignorance, doctors are actually feeding the tumors with sugar, cancer-causing chemicals, preservatives and additives found in the Standard American Diet (SAD). Just take a look at the menu in all the top cancer institutes such as M.D. Anderson. You will find cheesecake, sodas, margarine, and sugar laden beverages on their menu. THIS IS A DISGRACE TO MODERN MEDICINE WHO IN THEIR PRIDE THINK THEY HAVE ALL THE ANSWERS.

6) Do you have any treatment methods that are non-destructive and beyond the strategies of tumor removal or containment?

Comment: The answer is no. While mainstream medicine seeks a quick fix, magic bullet, linear approach, to cancer treatment, there is no single treatment, linear approach for cancer treatment and there never will be. All mainstream cancer treatment protocols are focused on tumor removal or tumor containment, not your cancer. They are limited to four destructive tools: cancer drugs (pharmaceuticals), cut (surgery), burn (cobalt radiation), or poison (chemotherapy). Take your pick. You will receive one or more of these primitive, destructive treatments. These treatments are analogous to giving a gorilla a hammer to fix a computer; chances are he'll do more harm than good.

Because cancer is a multi-faceted disease, it demands multi-faceted treatment protocols that can only be addressed outside of mainstream medicine. There is no non-toxic treatment to date in mainstream medicine that can reverse the cancer process.

7) Because there is an emotional and spiritual component to cancer, what will you do to release the emotional toxins such as anger, stress, unforgiveness, anxiety, etc? I've harbored subconsciously that have influenced my cancer growth?

Comment: Because physicians are taught in med school that if you can't see it in pathology or lab assays, if you cannot hear it in a stethoscope or feel it in a palpitation, it's not reality or an integral part of the disease process. Because of the atheistic mind-set drummed into them from university indoctrination, the unseen plains of the spirit and soul (emotions) are totally regulated as an intricate part of cancer treatment and yet emotion is a main component in all cancer patients. At best, you will get a referral to see a psychiatrist or a psychologist.

8) Since all organs and tissues are necessary for establishing and maintaining health from cancer, how can cutting out lymph nodes and body parts reverse my cancer?

Comment: It can't. The removal of cancerous organs and tissues will only cause a weakened state to the body and immune system. Every organ and tissue is accounted for-even your lymph tissues, appendix, tonsils and adenoids. By removing organs and tissues, other organs have to work double overtime to compensate for the missing organs, which throws off homeostasis (balance) and allows secondary tumors to manifest. God did not create us with excess body parts.

9) What is the long-term success rate of defeating cancer with chemotherapy, radiation, surgery or pharmaceuticals?

Comment: They tout a 42% success rate, which is based on a five-year yardstick or five year survival rate. However, they do not take into account the people dying from secondary tumors. The statistics are deliberately manipulated to mask the real holocaust that is taking place within mainstream cancer treatments. The true statistic is less than 10% when all factors are taken into consideration. Let me just give you an example of how these numbers are manipulated. Suppose someone is diagnosed with colon cancer and decides to go through with all of the treatments offered by mainstream medicine. After eight months, their doctor determines through cancer markers, CAT scanning, MRI scanning, etc. that the cancer has gone into remission. That patient is considered a statistical cure. However, if a secondary tumor pops up in a distant organ or another region of the body in two years due to their previous treatments, the secondary tumor is considered a new cancer statistic. If this patient survives for five more years he/she is again listed as a statistical cure. However, if he/she dies in the first day after the fifth year, there is no record of this being a cancer failure. Mainstream cancer statistics are a sham.

10) One final question for your doctor-if you were in my shoes (having aggressive malignant cancer) after what you have witnessed for years in your practice (think of that word "practice"), would you choose to treat yourself with chemotherapy or radiation?

Comment: If your doctor were truthful with himself and you, he or she wouldn't even hesitate to say "absolutely not." Could you imagine seeing cancer victims day after day? Most if their patients look like death warmed over. They are emaciated, their skin is pale, many suffer from severe vomiting, their hair has usually fallen out, and they live with excruciating pain and are dying slowly, all because of the treatments, not the cancer.

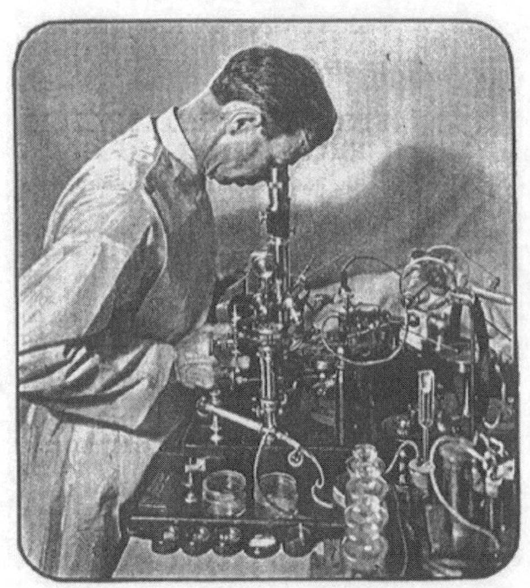

MOST POWERFUL MICROSCOPE

Most powerful in the world is a microscope designed and built by a San Diego, Calif., chauffeur. Its magnification of 17,000 diameters would be sufficient to make the head of a pin appear more than five feet wide. With its aid Dr. Arthur I. Kendall, noted Northwestern University bacteriologist, has observed forms of typhoid germs hitherto invisible. The microscope has six quartz lenses packed in glycerin, uses polarized light, and dispenses with the usual need of staining specimens for observation. R. R. Rife, the inventor, has for years indulged his hobby of microscope-building and germraising (P.S.M., June '31, p. 27).

19. THE MEDISINS BEHIND HORMONE REPLACEMENT, HYSTERECTOMIES, MAMMOGRAMS, and PSA

Since the 1930s, American women have been trained and bullied into thinking that a natural normal event in their life-menopause-is a diseased condition requiring treatment. Strange, how did all the millions of women throughout history up to the present time muddle through it? How do less fortunate nations or non-HMO lifestyles survive the ordeal? Always keep those two questions in mind when you read anything mainstream: whether it is advertising or articles regarding women issues. The "new" "medical condition" requires drug therapy, which coincidentally has just recently been "discovered": synthetic estrogen-hormone replacement therapy.

The story really begins in 1938 with the discovery of Diethylstilbestrol (DES) by Charles Dobbs. DES was supposed to be the first "synthetic estrogen." Dobbs first thought DES would solve the problems of menopause, but the AMA immediately began to make extravagant predictions for "preventing miscarriages" and solving all problems of pregnancy as well. After many years, DES was being prescribed for a "safe pregnancy" and to "prevent miscarriages." By 1960, it was found that between 60 and 90% of DES daughters had abnormal sex organs, leading to high rates of infertility, miscarriages, and cervical cancer. (Sellman, P.28) DES sons commonly had testicular dysfunctional and were often sterile. The drug was not taken off the market until 1971! (Kamen, p.99) By that time the industry didn't need DES any more for its bottom line, because estrogen replacement therapy (ERT) was around the corner.

Public attention was then diverted away from the disasters of DES by a 1966 best seller called "Feminine Forever," by Robert Wilson, a New York gynecologist. Wilson's thesis was that menopause is an estrogen-deficiency disease. Not missing a beat, the drug industry immediately donated $1.3 million to set up the Wilson Foundation for the sole purpose of developing and promoting estrogen drugs. Within a few years, with no real proof that Wilson was right and with superficial clinical trials, synthetic estrogen was being popularly prescribed and a new industry was off and running.

A little problem developed in 1975, and sales plummeted. The New England Journal of Medicine (Dec. 1975 p. 1199) published its findings after studying the causes of endometrial cancer. They showed that women who took the new estrogen drugs had just increased their risk of endometrial cancer by a rate of five times If they used the drugs longer than seven years it jumped to 14 times the normal incidence. Since the manufacturers of these synthetic hormones think nothing about your health but only of profits: it was found, though not conclusively, that rates of endometrial cancer could be reduced if synthetic progesterone were added to the synthetic estrogen. Synthetic progesterones are called progestins. So they changed the name from Estrogen Replacement therapy to Hormone Replacement Therapy (HRT), and the show went on. Sales climbed back up and then continued to grow.

As the HRT industry gained strength, the manufacturers began to make additional claims about the benefits of HRT, claims that were again unsupported by solid research:

-HRT could prevent osteoporosis
-HRT could prevent heart disease

As a matter of fact the American Cancer Society conducted a huge 13-year study of some 240,000 postmenopausal women to determine the relation between HRT and cancer. Their finding showed a 40% higher incidence of ovarian cancer. After 11 years of HRT, the figure jumped 70%!

Side Effects of HRT:
-increased risk of breast cancer
-increased risk of endometrial cancer
-osteoporosis
-blood clots
-high blood pressure
-vastly increased rate of heart attack
-skin reactions
-hair loss
-fluid retention, bloating
-vaginal bleeding
-rash, acne
-weight loss or gain
-breast tenderness
-depression
-stroke
-lupus

It should be obvious that effects like these are systemic (everywhere the blood goes) and as such can affect practically any weakened tissue in the body. To say that drugs and chemicals cause a downward spiral of health is not just a metaphor. A growing number of medical researchers who do not represent the interests of the drug cartels are stepping forward to show that the symptoms of menopause are not caused by too little estrogen, but by too much. We are looking at mastery in control of information. The motivation is simple: $1 billion per year.

John Lee, MD, an ethical endocrine researcher, explains why HRT does not work. Simple: HRT's synthetic progesterone is completely altered after going through the digestive system, when its gets to the liver. The liver changes in into three metabolites. Any benefits are thus cancelled. Dr. Lee's view and that of other proponents of natural progesterone products is that the problems experienced during menopause are not caused by a lack of estrogen, but a lack of progesterone.

REMOVING YOUR PRIZE POSSESSION

At the rate hysterectomies are performed in America it would seem to an OB-GYN that this type of procedure is a cash cow. Over 600,000 hysterectomies are performed each year on gullible women who are brainwashed into believing that their womanhood is no longer needed. To this day, about 20 million women have met the knife, and 1 out of three women have had surgical menopause before the age of 49. More than 40% of the time, the ovaries, fallopian tubes, and cervix are removed during the course of this surgery. There are three surgical approaches to a hysterectomy. The most common method is abdominal hysterectomy, which involves an eight-inch incision across the lower abdomen, just above the hairline, to remove the womb through the abdominal wall. About 20% of hysterectomies are vaginal procedures.

So what is the benefit of this butchering surgery or is it the medical industry that's actually benefiting? It is a known fact that hysterectomies will lead to postoperative physical and psychological problems described as "post-hysterectomy syndrome". This syndrome includes low libido, depression, hot flashes, urinary problems, fatigue and joint problems. It was found that at least 70% of women that went under the knife experienced these episodes. Women also experience hormonal disruptions which affect chemical reactions called beta-endorphins that encourage a sense of well-being.

These are several of the complications that would pose a problem in a woman's future after the surgery:

1. **Bowel injury:** If the bowel is accidentally cut, clamped or severed, the contents of the intestine can spill into the abdominal cavity causing infection of the peritoneum, a transparent cellophane-like sac that surrounds the abdominal organs. If infection occurs and is not properly addressed, it could be fatal.

2. **Bladder injury:** Though there is a possibility that this could happen, the injury can be corrected. If the injury is not corrected, there is a risk of peritonitis as with the bowel injury.

3. **Injury to the urethra:** The urethra is a tube connecting the kidney to the bladder. It is next to the cervix and can be easily damaged. If this happens, an outflow of urine from the kidney to bladder will be blocked leading to kidney damage.

4. **Postoperative bleeding:** This occurs when the surgeon fails to secure the major artery, which can lead to hemorrhaging and death. The draining of the blood will lead to the formation of adhesions.

AT WHAT POINT IS A HYSTERECTOMY RATIONAL?

The hysterectomy is offered as a treatment for several female complications. In America, surgery is the primary application for uterine fibroids, and benign tumor growth even though these complications are not life threatening. Fibroids account for at least 40% of all hysterectomies. Endometriosis contributes to about 34% of all hysterectomies, and a prolapsed uterus takes the remaining 26% of the surgeries.

The crazy thing about the medical profession is that it continues to reassure and convince women that it's ok to live the rest of their life without a womb or uterus. However, what they fail to mention is that uterine fibroids, cysts, and endometriosis can be reversed or all together avoided. Estrogen dominance is one of the primary causes of these complications. The bottom line is that a hysterectomy is never rational.

UNDERSTANDING ESTROGEN AND PROGESTERONE

Estrogen isn't really a single hormone. Estrogen is a spectrum of a class of hormones with estrus activity, which includes Estuarial and Estrone, both of which are implicated in activating abnormal cell growth when abnormally produced in the body. The other hormone component is Estriol which is known to be cancer inhibiting. All three of these hormones, Estradiol, Estrone and Estriol perform different activities. They are primarily produced in the ovaries though small amounts are secreted from the adrenal glands during pregnancy. Even though the estrogen components have several biological benefits within the human body their overproduction will create very adverse effects. Even in males excessive estradiol will produce an enlarged prostate and increase the risk of a heart attack. In women, excess estrogen will increase the risk of breast, endometrial, and ovarian and uterine cancer.

Progesterone is produced in the ovaries. It is the precursor for estrogen and testosterone, as well as all other natural steroid hormones. Progesterone is directly involved in burning fat energy, protecting against fibrocystic breast disease, normalizing blood clotting, restoring sex drive, normalizing blood sugar, fat conversion, regulates estrogen production, and new bone formation.

If you can recall your health science class in high school, an egg is presented once a month from the ovaries, wrapped in an envelope called a follicle. After the follicle lets go of the egg, the egg journeys down the fallopian tubes on its way to the uterus where it awaits possible fertilization. The burst follicle still has an important job to do: it begins to produce progesterone, for the next two weeks. Progesterone's job is to maintain the uterine lining until one or two things happens:

-Pregnancy
-No pregnancy

If pregnancy occurs, progesterone production is taken over by the developing lining itself-the placenta. The burst follicle simply can't make enough progesterone for the demand, since the uterus will expand from the size of a lemon to the size of a basketball during the next nine months. If no pregnancy occurs, the follicle stops producing progesterone, which triggers the collapse of the blood-rich lining, which is then expelled as the woman's monthly flow. So the interplay between these two hormones estrogen and progesterone controls the entire infrastructure of reproduction, on a daily basis, after the onset of menarche (first flow) in adolescence. Estrogen creates the lining each month; progesterone maintains it.

American scientists started studying hormones in the 1930's. One of the first foods studied was the wild Mexican yam for birth control and the development of synthetic hormones. By the

1940's, western scientists had finally figured out the importance of hormones in the female reproductive system. **Note that this is western science.** The science of hormone balance was intuitively divine in the days of ancient Africa, India and China. Once western science isolated progesterone and figured out its chemical structure, the move was on to explore the possible therapeutic treatments using the hormone. Researchers had aspirations in using progesterone for women suffering from gynecological disorders, especially from the chemically and commercially induced PMS.

There were obstacles to overcome in manufacturing a drug suitable for the general public. Natural progesterone was rarely accessible. Extracting it from animal sources was difficult, time consuming and prohibitively expensive. For example, Primarin is urine extracted from pregnant horses, yes ladies next time you are at the races just stop by and shake a horse's hoof! Natural progesterone therapy would require large doses to be effective, at a cost of anywhere from $80 to $1,000 per gram; an amount that only the wealthy could afford. Aside from the expensive cost, the drug had to be administered by needle, and the shots were painful and not easily metabolized. Until a researcher could find a better application, the treatment would remain impractical.

Estrogen Dominance was first coined by Dr. John Lee. For two decades, Dr. Lee had been exploring the basis for the proliferation of PMS, endometriosis, ovarian cysts, fibroids, breast cancer, infertility, osteoporosis and menopausal symptoms. Based on thorough research, some professionals find that various stress factors, malnutrition, and xenoestrogens (foreign estrogens) are the contributing factors to estrogen dominance.

ESTROGEN DOMINANCE

Estrogen Dominance not only causes menopausal symptoms or PMS, but here is a list of other complications:

Allergies	**Endometriosis**	**Brain fog**
Depression	**Excess blood clotting**	**Uterine fibroids**
Dry skin	**Fatigue**	**Uterine cramping**
Cancer	**Mineral depletion**	**Memory loss**
Gallstones	**Miscarriage**	**Vaginal dryness**

Fluid retention **Bone loss** **Femininity in Men**

Environmental (xenoestrogens) estrogens are beginning to take its toll on many young women. Due to industrial, environmental and household chemical exposure along with synthetic and refined foods, women unconsciously create these xenoestrogens. Thirty or more years ago young women getting partial hysterectomies due to ovarian cysts or uterine fibroids was practically unheard of. So what is going on? The violations of natural health are being abused and taken for granted.

No matter how much science goes into the technology of OB-GYN, if the foundation of biological law is broken, then technology and advanced medicine will only serve as a band-aid. The body cannot metabolize synthetic hormone replacement because it was never programmed in your "biological hard-drive" during creation. "Man-made anything" can never provide the essence of the natural, pure and the divine.

African-American women are experiencing the full spectrum of hormone hell! One of the problems is dietary neglect and chemical dominance within the body. The large consumption of commercial meats, caffeinated beverages, white sugar, white flour, hydrogenated oils, fast food and high sodium foods, just to name a few are creating very acidic and inflamed conditions within the body. In addition to the wrecking crew of the food chain, commercial and synthetic hair care products, cosmetics, shampoos and even tampons will eventually create a "hormone frenzy" or "hormone hell" within the body.

As with any health issue, there are laws that need to be obeyed in order to have equilibrium and hormonal balance. Endometriosis, uterine fibroids, ovarian cysts and PMS are practically absent in women from countries like Asia, Africa and India. Most women from these countries eat to live and follow their own ancestral diet, which corresponds with their physical constitution, blood type, and biological makeup. Whole foods, like brown rice, millet, barley, vegetables, fruits, properly raised and slaughtered meats play a key role in hormonal balance. Foods like hormone treated meats, preservatives, canned goods, frozen foods and greasy potato chips break the laws of equilibrium.

MAMMOGRAMS

Since 1928, physicians have been warned to handle "cancerous breasts with care for fear of accidentally disseminating cells" and spreading the cancer. Nevertheless, mammography entails tight and often painful breast compression, particularly in pre-menopausal women, which could lead to distant and lethal spread of malignant cells by rupturing small blood vessels in or around small undetected breast cancers.

Recent confirmation by Danish researchers of long-standing evidence on the ineffectiveness of screening mammography has been greeted by extensive nationwide headlines. Entirely missing from this coverage, however, has been any reference to the well-documented dangers of mammography:

1) Screening mammography poses significant and cumulative risks of breast cancer for pre-menopausal women. The routine practice of taking four films of each breast annually results in approximately 1 rad (radiation absorbed dose) exposure, about 1,000 times greater than that from a chest x-ray.

2) Radiation risks are some four-fold greater for the 1 to 2 percent of women who are silent carriers of the A-t (ataxia-telangiectasia) gene; by some estimates, this accounts for up to 20 percent of all breast cancers diagnosed annually.

3) The widespread acceptance of screening has lead to over diagnosis of pre-invasive cancer (ductal carcinoma in situ), sometimes treated radically by mastectomy and radiation, and even chemotherapy.

4) The dangers and unreliability of screening are compounded by its growing and inflationary costs. Screening all pre-menopausal women would cost $2.5 billion annually, about 14 percent of estimated Medicare spending on prescription drugs.

The ineffectiveness and dangers of mammography pose an agonizing dilemma for the millions of women anxious for reassurances of early detection of breast cancer. However, the dilemma is more apparent than real. As proven by a September

2000 publication, based on a unique large-scale screening study by University of Toronto epidemiologists, monthly breast self-examination (BSE) following brief training, coupled with annual clinical breast examination (CBE) by a trained health care professional is at least as effective as mammography in detecting early tumors, and also safe. National networks of BSE and CBE clinics staffed by trained nurses should be established to replace screening mammography. Apart from their minimal costs, such clinics would empower women and free them from increasing dependence on industrialized MediSin and its complicit medical institutions.

Women who want a non-invasive and non-toxic approach to breast wellness can select the services of a trained MD in the field of Thermography. This system of screening is very effective in giving a 10 year projection on the health of your breasts and its non-toxic. To locate a certified Thermographic specialist in your area go online to: www. BreastThermography.com

The attack on women is a very complicated subject. It will continue to remain complicated unless both women and men reconnect themselves with the divine laws of living. Again there is nothing in scripture about the most important cradle of life, the woman's womb being surgically removed from her body or her breasts smashed like a pancake to determine the health of those glands. The women's reproductive system was created for a multitude of functions just like any other organ or gland is within your body. It is not a "disposable trash bag" to be used and thrown away. We have no respect for any doctor or OB-GYN that endorses or encourages hysterectomies.

Changing your lifestyle, diet and spirit along with incorporating more holistic applications; will bring your body back to a state of equilibrium, not a prescription medicine. In regards to natural progesterone use, the herb Chaste Berry (Vitex) or Maca.

<u>Other Protocols</u>

Fibroid Tumors/Cyst/Fibrosis of the Breasts: Myomin (4 caps/day) from Chi Enterprises (714) 777-1542, Lugols Solution of Iodine (2 drops/day) from www.jcrows.com

Hormonal Balance: Chi-F by Chi Enterprises (714) 777-1542
PSA: Friend or Foe?

In the early 1990s, panic over the spiraling growth of prostate cancer and the sudden availability of the new test caused doctors' offices to be flooded with calls from the middle-aged and elderly: a mature man might feel perfectly fine yet would now have yet a new number to worry about-an increase in the prostate specific antigen (PSA).

While the jury is still out on just how many lives will be saved by the mass terrorizing of men over 50 by PSA tests, what is clear is the national campaign for PSA tests had an interesting origin.

As the Wall Street Journal (WSJ) reported in 1993:

> Some troubling questions have emerged about the role the healthcare industry played in influencing the [American Cancer] society's recommendation [that men over 50 have PSA tests]....and about the reliability of the test itself, which costs from $30 to $70. Aside from the charge, possible related expenses include biopsies, ultrasound tests, repeat biopsies, treatment for complications from treatment. Thus, the total cost of mass screening has been estimated at $28 billion a year in the US alone.

The WSJ noted that "the crucial step" prior to the American Cancer Society recommendation had come in October 1991 at a urological conference held by the American cancer Society to discuss the experimental PSA test. Reported by the WSJ:

> The healthcare industry picked up the entire $86, 649 hotel tab for that four-day symposium at The Cloister, an elegant Sea Island GA resort. Among those paying for the hotel stay were the Hybritech inc. unit of Indianapolis's E-lie Lilly & Co. and TAP Pharmaceuticals, a joint venture of Japan's Takeda Pharmaceutical Co. and Abbott Laboratories. Hybritech and Abbott... are the only two companies with prostate blood tests approved by the US Fools and Demon Administration (author's emphasis). Others helping pay the bill were major players in the business of treating prostate disease: Bruel & Kjaer Instruments, which makes ultrasound equipment; and prostate drug sellers Merck & Co., the Kabi Pharmacia unit of Sweden's Procardia AB,

the Schering Laboratories unit of Schering-Plough Corp. and the ICI Pharmaceuticals unit of Imperial Chemical Industries PLC of Britain. FOLLOW THE MONEY (Author's Emphasis)!

Now, a study in the Oct. 6 issue of the Journal of the National Cancer Institute (JNCI) reports that the PSA may actually be one of the means; by which, the body fights cancer. The researchers, a group of scientists from Entremed, a Maryland biotech company, had noted previous studies that found elevated levels of PSA in the blood of women with breast cancer. Not only was it present, said Dr. John Holaday, one of the authors of the JNCI study, but the higher its concentration, the better the women did. The new study reveals that PSA acts as an "angiogenesis inhibitor," slowing or preventing the growth of blood-vessel cells in test-tube experiments using human cells.

"Rather than being a harbinger of bad news, as in prostate cancer, PSA represents the body's own attempt to fight cancer by producing PSA, and possibly other anti-angiogenic factors," Dr. Holaday continued. Angiogenesis is the process by which cancerous tissues cause the formation of blood vessels that bring nutrition to tumor cells. Anti-angiogenesis is one of the newer methods scientists are using to try to interfere with a tumor's blood supply, thereby killing it without damaging normal tissue. This technique is being actively investigated by researchers in many centers.

The PSA test alone is not an adequate basis for determining treatment. Sometimes the best treatment for Prostate cancer is no treatment at all. The reality is that a number of factors need to be considered before treatment options are selected, and treatment itself may cause complications, such as urinary incontinence or impotence.

An elevated PSA test does not automatically mean that cancer is present. Like the digital rectal exam, a PSA test can erroneously indicate prostate cancer and fail to detect it. So while the screening may lead to earlier diagnosis, it can also lead to treatment of cancers that don't need to be treated, because of very slow growth. In older men, prostate cancer often develops so slowly that they will die with it, not because of it. And despite more than 10 years' experience with PSA screening, there have been few controlled studies on whether PSA testing reduces the prostate cancer death rate.

The PSA detection business has thus added hundreds of thousands of prospective clients to the cancer-treatment pool. We are aware of numerous cases of elderly asymptomatic men who spent small fortunes on therapy whether it was necessary or not-lured into the medical loop by a "suspicious" PSA and delighted to see its numbers drop whether this had anything to do with cancer or not.

We also became aware of an iatrogenic problem involved with the PSA obsession-a "suspicious" PSA number is usually followed by a biopsy of the prostate, the only authentic confirmation of cancer. In some cases, the massive spread of prostate cancer occurred after the biopsy. This chain of events would almost certainly not have begun if there had been no PSA test in the first place.

In 1995, Washington University-St. Louis researchers told the American Urological Assn. that detection of a "free" PSA fragment could detect 90 percent of prostate cancers and thus greatly lower guesswork and reduce the number of unnecessary biopsies. The news was timely in that USA Today was reporting at about the same time that the standard PSA test was falsely diagnosing the disease in an amazing two out of three cases, which the UK confirmed later. Yielding to such data, the 100,000-member American College of Physicians (ACP) in 1997 broke with Cancer Inc. and recommended against routine cancer screening for all men. We feel that this recommendation still applies today.

Recommendations for prostate health:

Eat a handful of raw pumpkin seeds daily (Japanese men eat one handful everyday and prostate cancer in non-existent in Japan)

Eat foods high in Zinc & Selenium: all raw nuts, all whole grains, grass-fed organic meats, wild ocean fish, organic leafy vegetables, and sea vegetables.

Herbs: Eyebright, Echinacea, Bilberry, Ginger, Burdock, Sarsaparilla, and Cayenne.

Products: Zylamend by New Chapter: clinically tested to eliminate prostate problems.

Prosta-Chi & Myomin by Chi Enterprise: high PSA scores and cancer of the prostate.

Jim Hats: Uterine & Cervical Cancers

An article in the March 17, 1997 issue of U.S. News & World Report magazine begins its article called PROBLEM POWDER by warning that according to a study "A possible tie between talcum powder and ovarian/cervical cancer, long suspected because of talc's chemical similarity to asbestos.....exists".

The study which was published in the American Journal of Epidemiology found that "women who used talcum powder in the genital area had an increased ovarian/cervical cancer risk of 60%; women who used feminine deodorant sprays had a 90% increased risk. Although not addressed, there are many ways in which talcum powder is used. It is used in condoms, balloons, surgical gloves to keep the latex from sticking together. Many dentists are developing life threatening immune disorders due to poisoning from latex gloves. It is found on many panty liners and feminine napkins. It may even be found in your facial tissue.

The purpose of this section we will focus on latex condoms. People all over the world are using latex condoms. Their days are numbered if they do not use any (according to the media). Girls and boys double their condom usage because they have been taught to believe it is safe. Their parents and teachers ask each day if they remember to use latex condoms. What is really mind blowing is that at present there is no proof that latex condoms are even able to prevent sexually transmitted diseases!

Latex condoms contain denatured oils. Thus condoms containing oil have higher amounts of toxic particles than condoms containing water. Lubricated latex condoms are coated with silicon and talc. Talc is a chemical similar to asbestos and is a known cancer causing substance. Also, talc on condoms could result in fallopian tube fibrosis with resultant infertility. Silicon in the Benzene family produces a substance that suppresses the immune system in the body.

Benzene is used worldwide. Industries use and apply Benzene when they make synthetic fibers, nylon, plastics, rubbers, drugs, explosives, dyes, detergents, soaps, pesticides, lubricants, preservatives, photographic chemicals, and much more. When people are exposed to Benzene they get the following symptoms: Abdominal pains, abnormal bleeding, anemia, bone and joint pain, fatigue, infections, fever, lymphoma, damaged liver, and many more. Benzene kills by decimating the blood bone marrow in which it burns the endocrine system out causing hyperproduction of different hormones like cortisone and cortisol. In this process ones age is speeded up, the person looks older as the body is severely inflamed from Benzene intoxication.

Solution: If you're single, abstinence is always your best choice. It isn't always easy, but it always works. By abstaining from sex, you eliminate the possibility of pregnancy and sexually transmitted disease. If condoms are your method of 'protection' then seek out non-latex condoms.

20. CHOLESTEROL AND STATINS: WHICH ONE REALLY KILLS?

Due to medical and commercial propaganda you have been brainwashed into thinking that cholesterol is an evil substance that should be avoided at all cost. Cholesterol is a valuable biochemical, it forms, for instance, the basis of steroidal hormones and vitamin D and is highly concentrated in the brain as well as the liver, adrenal glands and nerves. It is also a necessary steroid that contributes to the manufacturing of key male and female sex hormones such as pregnenolone, testosterone, estrogen, progesterone, and cortisol. These components are critical for mineral-regulating functions of the kidneys, the immune system and every cell of the body particularly the brain and nerve cells. Cholesterol started to get its bad rap after WW II because the corporations that make refined vegetable oils needed a villain so they could promote their poisons to an unknowing and gullible American public. However, the rise in cardiovascular disease was next to non-existent prior to WWI, but after WWII it skyrocketed 400%.

Today, heart attacks and strokes are the two leading causes of death among people in the U.S. They accounted for 40% of all deaths in the 1990's, kill about 850,000 people in the U.S. each year, and cost about $70 billion in treatments and lost work time (U.S. Surgeon General's Report on Nutrition and Health 1988). The cholesterol theory of disease and the treatments based on it are failing too many of us. We need to take a closer look at this theory (UNPROVEN FACT).

For the last 60 years, elevated serum (or blood) cholesterol levels have been blamed for fatal diseases of our heart and arteries (Cardiovascular diseases or CVD), which include heart attack, pulmonary, peripheral arterial disease, stroke, high blood pressure, heart failure and kidney failure. According to the cholesterol theory, high total cholesterol and high low-density lipoprotein (LDL) levels predispose us to CVD. Many studies to support this theory have been carried out, and all are open to other interpretations.

The average total cholesterol level for Americans is 220mg/dl. At 240 mg/dl, the death rate from CVD is two times higher than the average; at 260 mg/dl, it is six times the average. People in less fortunate countries (Sudan, Nigeria, etc.) who eat a simple diet containing whole grains, vegetables and little food of animal origin, have cholesterol levels in the 120 to 160 mg/dl ranges, and CVD is rare. Vegetarians die from CVD only 25% as often as the average American. Furthermore, CVD was rare before 1900. During the first and second World Wars, when less commercial animal products and more fruit and vegetables were eaten, the CVD death rate fell dramatically. From the evidence, it looks like cholesterol levels predispose us to CVD, and low cholesterol protects us. Looks can be very deceiving! Foods containing cholesterol are blamed, along with the cholesterol they contain.

The cholesterol theory of CVD has many flaws. Medical doctors have little success in preventing and curing CVD with treatments based on this theory. They can neither predict accurately which individual will fall prey to this epidemic nor when, because risk factors are statistically, rather than individually defined. For example, the "French" paradox refutes the cholesterol myth. Even though the French have a high intake of fat, the French have a low incident of coronary heart disease. The Eskimos who consume large amounts of dietary cholesterol, have high blood cholesterol, yet experience very little coronary heart disease. Another group, the Asiatic Indians consumes a high percentage of dietary cholesterol, mostly from butter, yet has an exceptionally low incidence of heart disease.

Cholesterol consumption in North America has remained constant since 1900, when CVD increased greatly between then and now. As we look back in time, fat consumption was lower. Refined sugar consumption was lower. Intake of minerals and vitamins was higher in diets containing vegetables, fruit, whole grains and less commercial meat. During two World Wars, people ate more vegetables, less margarine and shortenings, and consumed the grains fed to grazing animals, before, between and after these wars. Although fat and cholesterol consumption was the same, the consumption of minerals, vitamins, essential fatty acids (EFA), and fiber was higher. Animal protein and refined sugar were also lower during these war times. All of these factors – not cholesterol alone – have to be considered when pointing the finger at cholesterol for the rise in cardiovascular disease and other degenerative conditions.

Stress was (presumably) higher during wartime as well, resulting in increased cholesterol production, which, if the cholesterol theory was correct, should have also increased the incidence of CVD.

William Lee Cowden, M.D., an internist and cardiologist based in Richardson, Texas, cites one of the many medical examples which refuted the notion that all cholesterol is bad and high levels will lead to heart disease. "I have a man in my practice that had a cholesterol count of 300 to 400 for many years," reports Dr. Cowden. "But because he's taking high levels of antioxidant nutrients and avoiding processed foods high in oxidized cholesterol, he's had no plaque formation and has even had plaque regression." Clearly, you would be well advised to consider these facts before turning to a cholesterol-lowering drug as the solution to your cardiovascular condition.

It has been shown that a high intake of polyunsaturated oils (corn, soy, and safflower, etc.) has led to an increased risk of cardiovascular disease. Refined sugar foods contribute to the development of cardiovascular diseases, because sugar ingestion raises insulin levels, which block a key enzyme, that synthesis cholesterol. As with diabetes, the higher sugar intake the higher the insulin level, which causes the cholesterol to synthesize in the liver, raising cholesterol levels in the blood. In animal experiments, it was found that high sugar diets were less damaging in the presence of saturated fats such as beef tallow or coconut oil. As a matter of fact beef from free-range grass feed cows provide CLA (conjugated linoleic acid), which not only stabilizes cholesterol, but also alleviates atherosclerosis, prevents diabetes mellitus type 2, and potentially inhibits some forms of cancer.

Despite the huge effort to bring valid research to the table, western medical research so far has not conclusively shown that a high cholesterol diet or high cholesterol levels actually contribute to heart disease. As you will see from the following published scientific facts, it is often the contrary:

- Medically supervised trials with low-cholesterol diets were unsuccessful in significantly lowering blood cholesterol levels or reducing the risk of heart disease.
- Low blood cholesterol does not mean freedom from heart disease. Some drug treatments to lower cholesterol have resulted in increased rates of heart disease.
- About 50% of men under the age of 55 who die of heart attacks do not have elevated cholesterol levels or any of the other risk factors such as hypertension, smoking, obesity or diabetes.
- Other cultural groups have a low risk of heart disease despite a high intake of cholesterol. This changes when they adopt processed commercial foods with compulsory pasteurization of milk products and chlorination of water supplies.

Recent discoveries show that oxidized cholesterol; as well as, oxidized fatty acids damages the arterial walls leading to CVD. If this is true, we must ask why cholesterol and fatty acids in the bloodstream become oxidized. A large part of the answer is that when antioxidants (AO), which prevent this oxidation from occurring, are lacking in foods due to poor choices or processing, then lipids and cholesterol are attacked by oxygen. The oxygen reacts to lipids/cholesterol causing them to turn rancid. For instance, when certain metals (iron or brass) have had long exposure to air they begin to rust or oxidize. This same process occurs in the body when no antioxidants are present. The deficiency of nutrients suggests that deficiencies of vitamins and minerals (including AO), fiber, and EFA are the key causes of degenerative diseases, including CVD. Refined sugars, refined oils, and refined starches are all absent of minerals, vitamins, EFA, fiber, enzymes and AO.

Famous Doctor of Dentistry Weston Price who traveled around the globe in the 1930's, examined many traditional diets, and discovered that all traditional diets maintained the health of the local people. However, within a single generation of introducing refined sugar and refined flour through trade with Europe and the Americans, incidences of the degeneration of teeth (decay), dental aches, and loss of bone structure was as high as industrialized countries. Dr. Price pointed to refined sugar and refined flour as the sources of their physical degeneration.

The research showed that the increased intake of vitamins, minerals, EFA, and fiber can lower cholesterol and triglyceride levels in our blood, and lends weight to the deficiency-of-nutrients application. Dr. Matthias Rath and Dr. Linus Pauling proposed a unified theory for the cause and cure of human cardiovascular disease. They suggested that its primary cause is a deficiency in Vitamin C, leading to the deposition of repair proteins in the arteries.

Vitamin C is necessary to form the protein bonds that keep arteries elastic and strong. Vitamin C is also the strongest AO normally present in our body, and recharges other AOs such as Vitamin E and carotene. When there is not enough Vitamin C in our diet, its level in our blood decreases, leading to a mild subclinical scurvy. Under this condition of Vitamin C deficiency, arteries that are weak bleed into tissue spaces and oxidation of fats and cholesterol increases.

To protect itself, our body increases its production of healing proteins. These thicken our arteries, thereby protecting us from bleeding into tissue spaces. However, thickened arteries also slow down blood flow. In short term, thickened arteries protect us from the lethal effects of Vitamin C deficiency. In the long term, thickened arteries may become blocked and kill us. A steady optimum intake of Vitamin C will reverse arteriosclerosis. Other nutrients that help prevent arterial damage and thickening include niacin and sulfur containing N-acetyl cytokine, carnitine, lysine, and praline which are all helpful in peripheral arterial disease, but Vitamin C holds the key.

The beauty of Vitamin C research is that it explains all of the observations in cardiovascular disease research. The cholesterol theory does not do this. The vitamin C suggestion is also consistent with the observations that led to the other suggestions about the cause of cardiovascular disease. Refined sugar interferes with Vitamin C activity. Interference with Vitamin C actually increases oxidation of both cholesterol and triglycerides. Lack of Vitamin C fits the deficiency of nutrients main point.

THREAT OF STATINS

Like all pharmaceutical drugs, statins entered the medical market with great promise. There are least 12 million Americans taking cholesterol-lowering MediSins, mainly statins. Statins were first given pre-market approval in 1987. A statin called Crestor (generic name rosuvastatin) though less expensive than Pfizer's Lipitor brought in about $8 billion of the $13 billion for total sales in 2002. This is quite expensive for a drug that contributes to adverse effects such as heart and kidney damage. Like all other drugs that have a man-made chemical structure, statins pose other very dangerous risks such as an increase in liver enzymes, the suppression of the immune system, and increasing the risk of some forms of cancer. One of the major problems with statins is that it contributes to congestive heart failure due to its interference with Coenzyme-Q10 (Co-Q10). The heart as a muscle cannot maintain optimum activity if there is a depletion of Co-Q10.

A cardiologist named Peter Langsjoen studied 20 patients with a completely normal heart function. After six months on a low dose of 20 mg of lipitor a day, two-thirds of the patients developed abnormalities in the heart's filling phase (when the muscle fills with blood). According to Lansjoen, this malfunction is due to a Co-Q10 deficiency. With the absence of this co-enzyme, the cell mitochondrial fails to produce energy, leading to muscle pain and weakness. The heart is especially susceptible because it uses a great deal of energy. Still, virtually all patients with congestive heart failure are put on statin drugs, even if their cholesterol is already low. A recent study indicated that patients with chronic heart failure benefited from having high levels of cholesterol rather than low.

In every study with rodents to date, statins have caused cancer. Why have we not seen such a dramatic correlation in human studies? Because cancer takes a long time to develop and most of the statin trials do not go longer than two or three years. Still, in one trial, the CARE trial, breast cancer rates of those taking a statin went up 1,500 percent. In the Heart Protection Study, non-melanoma skin cancer occurred in 243 patients treated with Simvastatin (Statin drug) compared with 202 cases in the control group. Manufacturers of statin drugs have recognized the fact that statins depress the immune system, an effect that can lead to cancer and infectious disease, recommending statin use for inflammatory arthritis and as an immune suppressor for transplant patients.

High cholesterol is the health issue of the 21st century. It is actually an invented disease, a "problem" that emerged when health professionals learned how to measure cholesterol levels in the blood. High cholesterol exhibits no outward signs, unlike other conditions of the blood, such as diabetes or anemia, diseases that manifest tell-tale symptoms like thirst or weakness, high cholesterol requires the services of a physician to detect its presence. Many people who feel perfectly healthy suffer from high cholesterol-in fact, feeling good is actually a symptom of high cholesterol.

We conclude that a deficiency of nutrients particularly, Vitamin C and Co-Q10, combined with the consumption of hydrogenated oils and statin drugs are the main causes of cardiovascular disease. In order to combat this epidemic, we have developed a dietary protocol in the solutions section (#36) of the book.

21. WHAT DO HEART DISEASE & DIABETES HAVE IN COMMON?

In order to understand heart disease, one must first understand the heart, its function and its purpose. The heart is considered the "King" of all organs. Classical internal medicine states that 'the heart commands all organs, houses the spirit, and controls emotion.' According to ancient Chinese wisdom, "when the heart is vibrant and balanced, emotions are under control; when weak and out of balance, emotions will rebel and prey upon the heart/mind, thus compromising command over the body."

From a physiological perspective, the heart governs the circulation path of the blood throughout the body. Therefore, all the organs of the body rely on sustenance and activity of the heart. Believe it or not, our thoughts and emotions influence the functions of various organs via the pulse and blood pressure, which are mastered by the heart. One fact that is absent from the young medical student's education by the time he/she enters the incomplete world of western medicine is the intimate connection between the internal organs of the human body. Instead of analyzing the body as a whole, western medicine teaches the young student to isolate a symptom and treat it by prescribing a drug, which has no harmonious or vibrational connection with the mind, body or spirit.

Internally, the heart function is even associated with the thymus gland. The thymus gland is located in the same cavity as the heart and plays an intricate role in immune system activity. Compromising emotions such as grief, anger and hatred can weaken the heart, which can create an instantaneous effect on the immune system by inhibiting thymus function. This phenomenon has been observed by eastern practitioners but barely understood by western medicine. Another connection that is overlooked is the heart muscle connection between the tongue and the heart. The color and texture of your tongue actually reflects the condition of your heart. This is what is called tongue diagnosis. The color, shape, and surface of the tongue show the different conditions of your circulatory system. This diagnosis is used widely throughout Asia and India. Changes in facial complexion are a direct reflection of blood circulation, indicting either stagnant blood flow or the presence of toxicity within the blood. The heart is considered the "fire energy, yin organ" which makes it the superior organ of the summer, because it increases circulation to the body's surface in order to expel excess body heat.

The body has its own time clock where each organ performs its activity at a higher level. The heart function has its maximum activity between 11 am and 1 p.m.. One needs to be mindful of the amount of food consumed during this time. Since the heart requires maximum blood to circulate, consuming a large meal will interrupt the energy flow because the food will cause the energy and blood flow to travel to the stomach area rather than to the heart. This can lead to an imbalance of the cardiovascular system.

Heart disease is still the number one killer of people in America, 50% of the men die from it and it is the number one killer of women. However, this health condition is one of the most preventable degenerative diseases. There are an estimated 1,500,000 new and recurrent cases of heart attacks every year, and most will bite the dust without warning. This common fatality is the end result of dietary and lifestyle neglect. Our hearts go out to the many people who had dedicated 20 to 40 years of hard work, then after only a few years into retirement they collapse and die.

About 16 million more people endure the many episodes of this thing called heart disease due to lack of equilibrium and harmony. The causes of this disharmony and degeneration are dietary neglect. We have become a fast food nation, far, far away from the "grass roots" of domestic eating. Every food product that you consume is more than likely to contain MediSins or by-products that create cell and artery wall deterioration. The white flour, white sugar, hydrogenated oils, along with tap water, causes long term decay in the human body. Not to mention the lack of Vitamin C and other micro nutrients that can reduce the risk of a cardiovascular breakdown, starting from the cellular level.

Every 33 seconds an American falls to the mercy of CVD, or around 954, 000 annually, with nearly 50% resulting in mortality. According to institutional research, 52.3% of women and 47.7% of men are a statistic of heart disease telling, us that one out of every 2.5 deaths in America is a result of heart disease. The American Heart Association estimated that heart disease cost the American public more than $151 billion and was expected to climb to nearly $352 billion in 2003 and of course the episode continues. Don't blame this statistic on anything else but your own dietary neglect.

If we break the divine laws of eating, there is a penalty that will be paid. Hippocrates said "Let thy food be thy medicine and thy medicine be thy food". Obviously, the masses have taken the law of health for granted. Remember, your diet is just like Karma, you know what goes around comes around or you reap what you sow. It's the same principle with dietary neglect. If you live by the extreme of consuming so much commercial meat, hydrogenated oils, white sugar, tap water, commercial snacks and commercial dairy you will experience extreme health complications of the heart.

A few years back, former President Bill "Slick" Clinton went under the knife to receive his by-pass surgery. If Clinton does not change his diet he'll be dead in less than a decade. By-pass surgery is a temporary fix that has drastic results. Running (exercise) may seem very impressive, but dietary neglect will always take its toll on the body (athletes are a prime example).

We don't know what the standard meal was for the great celebrities, like singer Robert Palmer, comedian Robin Harris, singer Johnny Taylor or any other average person that has experienced a heart attack but we can be sure it was due to some form of dietary neglect. What we also know is that heart disease is not some hereditary sin that you acquire, because your forefathers bit the apple. Hereditary theories are a great way for the doctor to tell his/her patients not to have responsibility for their health. The only thing hereditary is the fact that what your mother ate and what her mother ate and what her mother ate, if it was all the same diet, will have the same result you will get each time. For example, if your grandmother had arthritis and she ate whatever, and then your mother gets arthritis because she ate whatever, and then you eat like your mother, then you'll get arthritis also. It's that simple. By reintroducing more organic whole grains, yams, organic grass-fed beef, lamb, or clean ocean fish, the heart would respond only in an optimum way. This diet should include mineral rich organic vegetables, fruits and natural cold pressed oils like flax, hemp, or olive.

It would be wise to comprehend and decipher the composition of processed food, which represents premature disease and death. Most of what you carry to the check-out lane is not food, but a substitute to fill the void of hunger. Practically every type of food ranging from ramen noodles to frozen meals is comprised of hydrogenated oils, preservatives and a high sodium content that will eventually cause blood energy flow stagnation. So, after years of this modern dietary neglect your arteries will eventually clog, your tissues will weaken, your breath will shorten, your blood will coagulate, and a short life span will be certain. Until we learn to reform ourselves through the dietary and holistic laws of fasting, detoxification and exercise, the medications that we depend on will slowly walk us to our grave.

HIGH BLOOD PRESSURE

High blood pressure literally means the pressure of blood in your arteries, which is measured by two numbers. The first number (top) is always higher than the second (bottom) one. This is because the first number given is always the measurement of the pressure of blood in the arteries when blood is pumped out of the heart. The arteries transport the blood from the heart to the organs and tissues throughout your body. Your arteries need the elasticity to handle the extra blood temporarily exiting out of the heart until the heart fills up again, of course this is a very rapid response. As a result there is temporary elevation of pressure. This exists only until the heart refills itself from the blood supply brought back to it by the body's main vein. The arteries have to have enough elasticity to handle the rise in pressure during every heart beat. The first number is called the systolic pressure.

The second number is basically the lowest pressure of blood in the arteries when the heart refilling, releasing the extra pressure, allows blood to move through the arteries and veins back into the other side of the heart before it is pushed out again. It is known as the diastolic pressure.

Normal blood pressure can vary. The younger you are the lower your blood pressure is due to several factors (elasticity, mineral supply, stress, etc.) Average adult blood pressure measured in mm/hg (millimeters of mercury) is about 120/70 mm/hg. The systolic blood pressure as the heart contracts and pumps blood out into the arteries is 120 mm/hg, the diastolic blood pressure as the heart refills from blood circulated back to it by the vein is 70 mm/hg. However, this can vary on how fit you are or how well you are: people with kidney disease often have high blood pressure, no matter how old or young they may be.

The subject of high blood pressure is no mysterious health concern to most people since it is so common among the older adults and the seniors. However, on the flip side there are several indications or forms of hypertension starting with:

I. Benign Hypertension: runs a long and relatively symptom free course.
II. Borderline Hypertension: the zone between the highest acceptable "normal" blood pressure and "true" hypertension, i.e. pressures between 140 and 160 mm/Hg systolic and 90-95 diastolic blood pressure.
III. Essential Hypertension (also known as: EHT; hyperpiesia; idiopathic hypertension, primary hypertension) is hypertension of unknown cause. This form of hypertension is diagnosed in over 90% of hypertension patients.
IV. Goldblatt Hypertension: caused by obstruction of blood circulation to the kidneys.
V. Intracranial Hypertension: localized in the skull's chamber
VI. Postpartum Hypertension: follows the completion of labor after pregnancy.
VII. Pulmonary Hypertension: occurs within the pulmonary circuit.
VIII. Renal Hypertension results from narrowing of the renal artery.
IX. Symptomatic Hypertension (also known as Secondary Hypertension): from disease of the arteries.

The kidneys and high blood pressure have an intricate relationship. When you incur high blood pressure or hypertension chances are your kidneys will also be affected. The vessels in your kidneys become damaged which will prevent them from removing waste and extra fluid from the blood. The extra fluid retained may cause your blood pressure to elevate. You may also experience heart damage if there is not enough blood flow through your kidneys. So if balance is not maintained in your once healthy kidneys, you could incur the end-stage renal disease (ESRD) or potential kidney failure, one of the end results of hypertension.

High blood pressure appears to be the leading cause of kidney failure next to diabetes. Every year high blood pressure contributes to over 15,000 new cases of ESRD in America. Patients with ESRD have two choices from the medical establishment. It's either dialysis or receive a new kidney transplant. Do you ever wonder why so many dialysis centers are popping up around the country? I guess maybe the conventional and corporate establishments want you to feel a little prestigious to have a machine filter your blood and waste fluids instead of the old fashion way!

WHY HEART DISEASE EFFECTS MORE AFRICAN-AMERICANS MORE THAN OTHER RACES

Recently it was found that African descendants in America have larger hearts and thicker heart muscle walls than people in America of European decent. This apparently contributes to higher degrees of hypertension according to a report from the New York Presbyterian Hospital. African-American communities around the nation are experiencing an enormous increase in hypertension, heart attacks and congestive heart failure. Cardiovascular disease among African-American men is approaching 55%, while African-American females are around 70%. This is not a result of a "soul food" diet, but from lack of exercise, stress, poor food choices, and mental exhaustion.

Although African-Americans have lost the true connection with their ancestral diet (due to slavery), for the most part, some foods like greens and yams are still present in the diet. Cassava, sorghum, millet, citrus and other wholesome foods are absent from today's diet. Though the fast food restaurant is practically everywhere, it has predominately infiltrated the African-American community, leaving in its path a trail of obesity, diabetes and heart disease.

Although hypertension appears to be a hereditary issue among the masses of the African-American lineage, it most certainly is due to the large consumption of commercial dairy, hydrogenated oils, and swine saturated soul food and anti-hypertensive drugs. There are lengthy studies recorded about American-Americans indicating that they have a higher percentage of high blood pressure, heart attacks, strokes, and congestive heart failure than African descendants from Africa or the Caribbean according to lead study author Dr. Jorge Kizer. Dr. Kizer is an assistant professor of Medicine and Public Health at Weil Cornell Medical College. Studies have found that the left ventricular has hypertrophy – an increased muscle weight of the heart's main pumping chamber, which could be the determining factor of the illness. Dr. Kizer says "The problem has been that a whole host of other factors, including body mass index (a measure of obesity), duration of hypertension and even socio-economic status can influence left ventricular mass." So there is a connection between high blood pressure and heart enlargement. Maybe the FDA should require better supplementation, and definitely a better diet and a greater reduction of stress.

Another major research activity on the black people of Africa was conducted by world renowned Dr. Weston Price, a Doctor of Dentistry who began his interior journey in Mombassa, Kenya on the east coast of Africa. He worked inland through Kenya to the Belgian Congo, then northward through Uganda and the Sudan. Dr. Price conducted studies in isolated populations on native diets. He was repeatedly astonished by the contrast of native sturdiness and optimum health. The Native African tribes he studied were the Masai of Tankanika, Chewya of Kenya, Muhima of Uganda, and the Neurs tribes on the western side of the Nile in the Sudan who were all cattle keeping people. These tribes had a similar dietary lifestyle, which consisted of animal meats that contained fat-soluble vitamins, unprocessed milk, fish, grains, fruits and vegetables. Dr. Price discovered that these fat-soluble vitamins produced excellent development and disease free bodies. These tribes were noted for their physiques and fine well arched teeth. In some tribes women averaged over 6 feet tall and men reach almost seven feet in height. Examinations of their teeth revealed very few dental caries usually less than 0.5%, some tribes were found to have no dental decay at all!

More than 40 years after Dr. Price's great research, doctors Edward and Peter Williams wrote on their experience in Africa. They discovered that by the late 1970's, the nomadic cattle herding tribes of the Sudan had vanished. The whole food diet of millet, cassava flour, whole grains and green foods were replaced by processed millet and soon other foods. Commercial tea had become a favorite drink and sugar was very popular, with the average daily adult intake reported to be at that time at least 100 grams. Peanut and cottonseed oil was soon added to the diet, just like how both the commercial food and health food industry infiltrated our diet with canola or "rapeseed oil." And of course you know cigarettes and alcohol had to make their MediSin debut to get their share of the pie. It is very apparent that when processed foods enter the equation of any diet, the results are always the same: destruction and death.

Like any other people in this country, the only way that high blood pressure, heart attacks and congestive heart failure can be avoided is through a whole food (practically organic) chemical free diet with exercise and natural supplementation. According to numerous studies, just by taking economical supplements like Vitamin C, selenium, folic acid, B-6, B-12, and Coenzyme-Q10 along with a whole food diet and a little cardiovascular exercise the risk of heart disease will be greatly eliminated.

DIABETES and DIETARY NEGLECT

Diabetes or "Sugar", the nickname for diabetes, was once considered a disease of "old age" since it was more common in people over the age of 60. However, with the advent of adulterated foods along with fast food, diabetes has infiltrated over 17 million Americans followed by a potential 12 million developing the disease. Diabetes has become a serious MediSin among the people of all ages in America. It has become as American as apple pie! In fact, American teens and younger children are increasingly developing adult-onset-diabetes. Apparently Americans have their head anywhere but the underlying cause of this relatively curable disease.

There are several major contributors to diabetes:

I. Food poisoning (when food has been stripped of its natural resources and then replaced with synthetic vitamins and minerals).

II. Refined sugars and carbohydrates and overeating.

III. Severe chromium, vanadium, zinc, omega 3 fatty acid and enzyme deficiency.

IV. Excessive environmental, physical and emotional stress.

Diabetes, like most diseases in America, is self inflicted through dietary neglect. By disobeying the laws of natural health, the body experiences episodes of imbalance. Americans now grow up on refined and dead carbohydrates (cereals) along with enzyme depletion, which causes the pancreas to shut down.

The masses in America do not have a dietary principle that is parallel to their ancestry or their blood type. People in America follow a standard western type diet of hot dogs, frozen foods, canned foods, micro-waved foods, soda beverages, refined candy and cakes and other toxic foods of commerce.

The ancestral diet proves to be a more wholesome diet because it meets the essential needs of that certain group of people. Most of the Asian-American, Hispanic-American, and Native-American and some African and European-Americans may follow a traditional or ancestral diet based on what dietary principles have been passed down. We do find very low statistics of diabetes in Asian-Americans because their diet pyramid is totally different than the Standard American Diet. They thrive on whole grains and a balance of meat, vegetables, fruits and they often use medicinal herbs, roots or leaves in the meal preparations. On the other hand, most African and European-Americans have a high statistic of diabetes, which is based on a more commercialized diet: white flour, white sugar, refined table salt, fried meals and improperly slaughtered meats and other adulterated foods that create a foundation for degenerative disease. Obesity in America is at an all time high and is still on the rise throughout the entire world. Foods of commerce have infiltrated every corner of the earth by corporate, commercial and political persuasion. As a result, diabetes, followed by other degenerating diseases, is taking the world by storm. It's a shame that we have the most powerful medical institutions in the world, but yet cannot eradicate something as simple as diabetes.

Diabetes is commonly regarded by some western doctors as incurable and all efforts are directed at controlling or managing the symptoms. However, not only is diabetes preventable but is reversible by first replacing the standard American food chain with wholesome unrefined, organic foods which you will find at a reputable health food store. Secondly, seek qualified alternative practitioners like clinical nutritionists, naturopaths, doctors of oriental medicine or a Medical Doctor who has some integrity and some knowledge of natural medicine. The diabetic has to be willing to make dietary sacrifices in order for the alternative applications to be effective. In other words, a person would really need to surrender pork fried rice, white flour, fried chicken, frozen food dinners, service station meals, and other life taxing foods that contain MediSins. The present corporate medical treatment for diabetes is either a pill for a non-insulin dependent diabetic or an insulin injection for someone who is an insulin dependent diabetic. Either way, both will eventually lead to a major side effect, because the conventional applications will only address the symptoms, not the underlying cause.

For mothers who are thinking of having children, bottle feeding with commercialized milk is not an option. Bottle-fed infants have a great chance of becoming type I diabetics compared to the children that grow on breast milk. According to researchers, it is believed that the cow's milk protein, albumin, triggers an autoimmune reaction against the pancreas setting it up for future cell destruction. A study involving several hundred diabetic children revealed an immune or allergic response to a fragment of cows' milk protein in the entire group. The study also showed that the milk protein element has the same composition as the P69 beta cell of the pancreas. This P69 cell is usually protected inside the pancreatic beta cells and comes to surface only during a sign of microbial or viral infection. The immune system can mistake the P69 for milk protein and attack and destroy the pancreatic beta cell in the process. This is why "bottle-fed" infants are very susceptible to colds, respiratory and gastrointestinal infections.

People have naively assumed that chances of dying from diabetes was greatly reduced after the discovery of insulin, unfortunately that's not the case. Formerly, diabetics were treated with a reasonably effective diet high in proteins and low in sugars. With the advent of insulin, this effective diet has been ignored by patients, and they assume that they can chow down on anything because the insulin is appearing as a safety net. This unfortunately, will create long term consequences.

Another factor regarding insulin is the toxicity effect. All diabetics develop immune reactions against injected insulin and may become more or less allergic against the application. Life-threatening reactions are now rare but were common with the impure products used initially. Through corporate greed of course, the more effective animal-based insulin is being phased out by synthetic human insulin, which now presents a questionable danger to the patient. For the insulin- sensitive patient, this new synthetic application can be more of a MediSin than their medicine.

The commercial foods that children are being fed are fattening them up for a miserable and extremely unhealthy life. Parents do not even put any forethought into a child's dietary lifestyle. The food that we feed our children has been only in the best interest of the manufacturer not our children. Heart disease and diabetes have one thing in common: dietary neglect.

Diabetes Type I Protocol: 300 mcg. GTF Chromium
(Mega Foods, Inc.)

1 tablespoon Cod Liver Oil
(Carlson or Nordic Naturals)

Diabetes Type II Protocol: 300 mcg. GTF Chromium
(Mega Foods, Inc.)

1 tablespoon Cod Liver Oil (Carlson or Nordic Naturals)
Bitter Melon, Gymnema Sylvestre

Heart Protocol: 400 mcg. Selenium (Mega Foods, Inc.)
1 tablespoon cod liver oil (Carlson or Nordic naturals)
600 mg. of Magnesium Citrate
Hawthorne Berries

Protocols are daily dosages.

22. HOMOCYSTEINE: THE OVERLOOKED VILLAIN

In section twenty of the book, we gave you a fair overview about the alleged evils of cholesterol and its role in cardiovascular disease. It was proven without doubt that cholesterol is an absolute essential body compound, comprising a high concentration of normal brain tissue and serving as a basic building material for the manufacture of cortisone, sex hormones, Vitamin D and other essential body substances. The real villain that determines your condition in regards to atherosclerosis and heart disease, besides the standard American diet, is homocysteine. Thanks to heart researcher Kilmer S. McCully, M.D., for publishing a 1969 unorthodox conclusion in the American Journal of Pathology stating that a substance called homocysteine could reach high levels in the body causing degenerative arteries and heart disease. This article would soon cost him his job at Harvard University!

If the amino acid methionine is not properly converted into cytokine, homocysteine levels will increase in the body. Due to deficiencies in vitamin B6, folic acid, and vitamin B12 the conversion of methionine cannot take place. As a result free radicals are generated thus allowing the oxidation of cholesterol to proliferate. Studies show that a moderate intake of methionine found in quality grass-fed red meats, raw milk and its by-products do not create this problem. However, without proper conversion, it has been found that men with high homocysteine levels have three times more heart attacks than men with low levels. The same institution that removed Dr. McCully from his position at Harvard proved that men with homocysteine levels of only 12% higher than the average had three times the risk of a heart attack of those with normal levels also. Also that same year, the

European Journal of Clinical Investigation showed that 40% of the stroke victims had elevated homocysteine levels compared to only 6% of the controlled studies.

In 1995, the Journal of the American Medical Association reviewed 209 studies that linked homocysteine with heart disease. For the most part, homocysteine is considered a manifestation of the abnormal processing of protein in a persons body due to a deficiency of B-vitamins. Dr. McCully discovered that a person's homocysteine levels are more controlled when they supplement their diet with vitamin B12 combined with folic acid and vitamin B6. Dr. McCully suggested that the intake of 350 to 400 mcg of folic acid, 3-3.5 mg of B-6 and at least 3 mcg daily of vitamin B-12 would solve the problem. Dr. McCully additionally suggested that taking betaine hydrochloride, which is the stomach's primary digestive acid and vitamin C, would lower homocysteine levels in the person's blood. In most health food stores you can find actual homocysteine formulas featuring vitamin B6, B12, and folic acid. Also, have your homocysteine levels measured when you visit your favorite HMO representative for your yearly check-up.

23. WHY ARE THE RELIGIOUS FAITHFUL NOT DISEASE FREE?

People of many religious persuasions experience many forms of ill health and disease in America and the world due to a lack of knowledge. Many of the religious faithful have lost faith in the Creator, and rely on man-made science to solve all the problems. The statistics of ill-health obviously show that there is no harmonious connection between The Creator and our health. The masses of various religious sects in American may give their mind and spirit to "God" but they surely give their bodies to science and MediSin.

The genuine scriptures and the spoken words of the great prophets of the Creator were delivered to mankind as guidance against sorcery. This sorcery has come to mankind in the form of processed foods, drugs, and vaccines that are developed by tenacious men and women who serve a dark entity of evil and arrogance. These men and women orchestrate the foundation of deception to make it appear that their products of commerce are superior to the Creator's. They perpetrate, infiltrate and influence a nation's state of mind to the point of compromise and destruction.

The destiny of mankind has allowed his trust to unconsciously fall into the hands of mortal serpents that have achieved enlightenment over the masses with the knowledge of the seen and the unseen. Though the knowledge they contain is only a particle of dust compared to the Creator's galaxy of universal existence, they still arrogantly advance the practice of mortal medical, and mathematical and commercial trickery.

The Book of Hosea (4:6) mentions; "My people are destroyed for lack of knowledge." There is a great deal of divine knowledge that has been intentionally suppressed and as long as the masses continue not to seek that knowledge, they will surely die in vain. Desire for knowledge is the essence of wisdom and life. Those who pacify their minds with fantasy, soap operas, and music videos are only a corpse. It is knowledge and wisdom that sets us free from the dogma and institutional deception so that we may heal ourselves physically, mentally and spiritually. It is paramount to understand that disease is not the will of the Creator but from man's ignorance and misunderstanding, truth is only a thin line away from deception. Over the centuries, the masses of the world have been influenced by many vehicles of trickery to obtain power over education, government, and the industries of medicine, food, and health. In order for this domination of evil to exist, there must be a division between man and his creator.

One of the foundations of disease in the human body is the illness of the heart. The heart is where emotions are directed and where good and evil manifest. One of the greatest books of guidance speaks of two types of illnesses, the illness of the heart and illness of the body. In regards to the heart, it comprises of two types. The first is suspicion and doubt, and the second is desire, allurement and sin. In that regard, the Creator says: "Their hearts are sick, and the Creator has caused their sickness to intensify" (Qur'an 2:10). It is the mission of Satan and his disciples to influence one's heart so that an ill body and spirit will become crippled. The hearts of men and women have become the flesh of granite governed by arrogance. The words of revelation and truth become so dull that they are unable to pierce the spirit. This is the origin of destruction. Unless the religious faithful heed with piety, they will be destroyed because of their disobedience, arrogance and lack of knowledge.

The Holy Scriptures of the Torah, Psalms, and Qur'an provide us with medical and holistic guidance, which was instituted by the messengers of God (peace be upon all of them). Surely, there is no better way to apply such knowledge than through the guidance of Noah, Abraham, Moses, Jesus, Muhammad, and the other messengers of the almighty God. As for the medicine of the heart, it can only be acquired through humility and sacrifice. Many of the religious faithful have experienced chronic disease and illnesses of the body and yet they still gravitate to the medical deities (MD) of MediSin. Whether you are a Christian, Muslim, Jew or Buddhist and believe that human creation is perfect, then why do you run away from the Creator's food and settle for soda pops, Suzy-Qs, fruit loops, and super sizes? Why would you pray for recovery from chemotherapy when you were warned about the deception of sorcery (Rev. 18:23)? Statistics have shown that the average survival time from chemo treatment is only five years because of the devastating effects on the bone marrow and other components of the immune system. Besides, why would you indulge in any medication that contains a molecular structure that is nowhere to be found in natural creation and that carries a skull and cross bones on the label?

Biblical readings confirmed that the Creator used a balance of universal materials in the making of man: "In the sweat of thy face shall thou eat, till thou return unto the ground; for out of it were thou taken; for dust thou art, and unto dust shall thou return." (Genesis 3:19) You may also refer to Psalms 103:14 and Ecclesiastics 12:7. So why are the religious faithful sick as Hell? Surely, the masses are not cursed with cancer or born in a diabetic or a hypertensive state. There has to be a manifestation of dietary neglect and an alienated lifestyle.

Common diseases are a result of your lifestyle not a curse from God. Diabetes is the end result of a refined carbohydrate diet which exhausts the pancreas and the adrenal glands. Cardiovascular disease is the end result of hydrogenated oils, tap water, refined foods, and mineral deficiencies. Cancer is the end result of carcinogenic chemicals like nitrates, nitrites, sulfur dioxide, radiation exposure, fluoride and other cell manipulating chemicals. All these diseases are a manifestation of over-industrialization and technological perversion.

Man has replaced natural raw sugar with white refined sugar, whole grain brown bread with white bread, and naturally dense brown rice with white rice. Foods in their natural food state are replaced with synthetic and genetically engineered by-products. Our commercial herbs and meats are irradiated, our commercial breads don't even mold any more! This demonstrates the arrogance of mankind and his disrespect for creation. The scientists of modern technology think they can outsmart the Creator with their genetic and nuclear technology. However, they are destroying the world because they cannot co-exist with the natural laws of the Creator. Mankind would rather risk thousand of lives for the sake of modern medicine instead of understanding the underlying cause of disease. One of the Messenger's of God (Prophet Muhammad of Arabia) said: "For every disease, God has created a cure." So for every malady there is a modality. So, when you hear allopathic medicine saying there are no cures for this or that, WHO DO YOU BELIEVE? Prophet Muhammad also said: "The stomach is the house of every disease, and abstinence (fasting) is the head of every remedy, so make this your custom." Folks were talking about fasting here, something as simple as not eating for a certain amount of time.

It is common for the religious faithful to reject this knowledge and freely indulge in their perverted appetite and behavior on their way to a diseased body, soul and a premature death. The masses have the audacity to pray in vain when the scripture clearly states what is good and not good for the temple: "Be not deceived; God is not mocked: Whatsoever a man soweth, that shall he also reap." (Galatians 6:7) This is why the religious faithful are as sick as Hell!

Because of commercial, corporate and medical trickery, people of all sects of religious faith tend to be very fatalistic in their view of sickness, often attributing it to or even blaming God for their illness. These are several reasons sickness and disease rule a nation:

1. Denial is one of the main reasons for one's experience with disease, a carefree attitude, lack of consciousness and an unholy lifestyle practice is what accelerates an untimely death to the mind, body and spirit. Repentance and atonement will assist in the recovery of ill health and spirit.

2. With lack of humility and the character of arrogance, people of all parts of the world feel that they no longer need spiritual guidance. This carefree attitude has left the world in the hands of provocateurs while they arrogantly wander blindly.

3. The violations of the Natural Laws of God is the cause of over 90% of all sickness and physical suffering being experienced today. Consider the several hundred thousand deaths and permanent adverse effects from prescription drugs, surgery and misdiagnosis.

4. Our poor eating habits, chemical based foods, lifestyle along with lack of exercise are the underlining factors of our health conditions.

Let's review a synopsis of various religious teachings:

Seventh Day Adventist, founded by Ellen G. White, advocates that their followers refrain from coffee, tea, tobacco and alcoholic beverages. They also refrain from swine just as the Muslims and those who follow the Torah. Though the followers of Seventh Day Adventist do not follow all of the teachings, statistics show that the Adventist has less occurrence of cancer. They also appear to be healthier and live, on the average six years longer than the average American.

The Mormons founded by Joseph Smith practice certain dietary restrictions. These restrictions included alcohol, coffee, tobacco, tea, cola and other drug potentials.

Islam specifically prohibits the flesh of swine due to its parasitic nature. The consumption of carrion is also prohibited in Islamic law for the same reason; that is to say, it adversely affects the moral qualities of the human and also increases physical disease. If the blood of an animal remains inside the body of the animal from abuse such strangulation or brutal beating they are called carrion because of the poison adrenaline settled in the flesh.

Pentecostals teach that the healing of the body is included in the atonement and they use Healing services and prayer lines via telephone and in some cases they may apply some oil along with the prayer. Pentecostals will demand healing in the "name of Jesus," but prayer without consciousness and mindfulness only equates sickness and ignorance.

Baptists are often extremely fatalistic when it comes to sickness, they pray very sincerely and they accept treatment with drugs, radiation and surgery by the allopathic medical profession as a means that God uses to heal Christians who are sick. If prayers and the efforts of the medical profession don't bring healing, then it is accepted as the "Will of God." In spite of the repeated medical failures in treating many diseases especially cancer, the religious faithful still refuse to massively choose or at least research a natural alternative. There is nothing in any scripture that endorses chemo, radiation, surgery or chemical prescription!

The Bible gives valid reasons for sickness or physical problems among the religious faithful:

I. In the Gospel of John, Chapter 9 verse 1-3, we read of a man who was blind from birth. Neither he nor his parents had sinned. The Bible asks: Who did sin, this man or his parents that he was born blind?" Jesus answered, "Neither hath this man sinned, nor his parents, but that the works of God should be made manifest in him."

II. Corinthians 11:28-32 elaborates on weakness, sickness and early death coming upon believers when they would not confess their sins, and God had to judge them. "For this cause many are weak and sickly among you, and many sleep. For, if we would judge ourselves we should not be judged. But when we are judged, we are chastened of the Lord, that we should not be condemned with the world."

One thing that needs to be politically corrected is the acronym MD. This does not really stand for Medical Doctor, but Medical Deity. Though the Medical Doctor appears to be an authoritative profession and is the medium between health and disease, this profession is the third leading cause of death in America with the approach for #1 around the corner. Just observe their pattern: wrong prescription, misdiagnosis, surgery negligence, and over prescribing. The religious faithful need to understand that without divine guidance, medical professionals are lost.

BLESSING THY FOODS

Traditionally, before eating we bless our food, but blessing a food that has already been manufactured with MediSin is like praying over crack cocaine before you snort or inject it. We often see people bless their foods (ham, catfish, chitterlings, etc.) when the food has already been cursed.

The commercialized meat industry represses the unpleasant reality that we are devouring an improperly slaughtered cow, lamb, chicken or "just dead meat." They have fine tuned the names of foods to limit our curiosity and intelligence. As children, when we heard the names of food like "sweetbreads" our mouths would water. But as we got older we realized "sweetbreads", meant innards the (intestines) of baby lambs and calves, or not to mention the famous "Rocky Mountain Oysters" which really are the pig's testicles.

Our very language has become an instrument of denial. When we consume the meat of a cow we have designated names for the part we are eating, rib-eye, brisket, T-bone, and quarter house steak. We have been systematically trained not to see beyond what's on the plate or how that cow was raised, how it was fed and how it was slaughtered. Then we say our grace over a meal that has been fed irradiated grains, injected with hormones, antibiotics and has saturated itself with poisonous adrenaline because of the abused death it had anticipated.

All animals should be properly nourished, properly raised and properly slaughtered before selling them to the public. We must refrain from the life-taxing products masquerading as food. The only way to nourish the Holy Temple within yourself is by not just praying over your meal, but making sure it meets guidelines of wholesomeness. Remember "...I have set before you life and death, blessing and cursing: therefore choose life that both thou and thy seed may live." (Deuteronomy 30:19)

There needs to be a clear understanding between sickness and obedience. The religious faithful need to understand that when you consume white flour, chemically bombarded grains, toxic dyes, irradiated food, improperly slaughtered and fed cattle, you are choosing death. And the end result will be heart disease, cancer, diabetes, stroke, and accelerating aging. Choose life by growing some of your own fruits and vegetables, if you choose to eat the cleaner of meats and chemical free foods, you and your future offspring may be blessed with the eradication of disease.

24. The Green Monkey: Medical Terrorism

"If you want to know what to do to be healthy, go to a physician. Whatever he advises, do just the opposite and you'll be just fine."
– Dr. Herbert Shelton

People of the world especially Americans are among the most brainwashed people on this planet. And we always thought it was in Russia and in other countries that this dastardly practice was perpetrated.

For instance, Americans are taught a phony nutrition. The basic four food group diet is a fraudulent imposition that has nothing to do with nutrition. The stipulations to eat so many servings from each food group amounts to a division of the marketplace. The basic four is a pathogenic arrangement that is responsible for along list of diseases including acne, diabetes, arthritis, asthma, cardiovascular and heart problems, cancer, lupus, and psoriasis. This is evident when a mere change in diet enables sufferers to become free of their problems and live healthful lives.

Toxins, especially drugs, are deadly to all cells including the first line of defense, the white blood cells. It is these cells which actively apprehend poisons and get them out of the system. But, when they are killed by the poisons they apprehend, they do, indeed, become reduced in numbers that the body must redirect body faculties to extraordinary elimination which manifest as some illness or disease or in AIDS parlance, opportunistic infections. The white blood cell complement would normally have handled the situation with ease. But chemicals and harsh drugs are by no means normal and all cases of AIDS with rare exception are caused by poisons from drugs, food or other sources.
The cartel goals in promoting the AIDS farce is enlarging the market for drugs from which it derives enormous profits.

America is a drug culture, and the drug culture keeps enlarging. The modus operandi by which drugs are promoted in the case of AIDS is strictly supplier directed. For instance, from the beginning, chemotherapy was the treatment of choice without any tests whatsoever for efficacy. As a result almost every AIDS sufferer died. They still do if they submit to the medical system, whereas those who do not submit are surviving!

We are told there is no cure for AIDS. Yet the system does not hesitate to administer drugs massively as if they were curative. Further, test kits are developed and sold to "detect" "AIDS virus carriers." Not only are the tests fraudulent in themselves but, if followed up as the "system" insists, hundreds of thousands will die martyr's deaths being treated for a nonexistent disease which the "system" declares to be inevitable and which it insists on treating "to protect the population at large."

For instance the tests are to detect "antibodies" that supposedly is evidence that the presence of the AIDS virus which somehow they do not find and which, of course, does not and cannot cause what is called AIDS. All that these tests detect are specialized proteins called opsonins which are recognition factors for special types of food. In imposing this upon us, they have undermined their rationale for immunizations! Antibodies created by virtue of vaccinations are supposed to confer immunity to disease. But here, the antibodies are supposed to make one liable to the disease they have called AIDS. That reversal alone constitutes fraud!

So those who test positive for the AIDS virus (because they have antibodies the tests would detect) would be subjected to a course of drugs which are in themselves immunosuppressive and cause the very conditions they are supposed to prevent or overcome, that is, AIDS. Millions might well test positive by these tests and, undoubtedly, thousands upon thousands will be subjected to "virus eradicating" treatments which they would not survive. Thousands more will die and their deaths, instead of being attributed to drugs, will become additional AIDS statistics deaths. However, the ghoulish objectives of the cartel will have been served nonetheless-increased drug sales and profits.

The major perpetrator of the scam, Dr. Robert Gallo, has been found guilty of "scientific misconduct," an interesting euphemism for scheming, lying thievery. When finally brought to trial for his real crime, his defense will undoubtedly be that the AIDS hypothesis has never been anything but a hypothesis, and thus he will try to escape responsibility.

Let's look at the real facts:

1) AIDS is simply a new name for 25 diseases that have always existed.
2) The causes of acquired immune deficiency have been listed in medical texts (Merck manual) for over 70 years. They are, in order of importance: malnutrition (starvation), drugs, radiation, and chemotherapy.
3) It appeared to be an epidemic at first, because the drug addicted segment of the gay population began to suffer the effects from years of drug use. They became an identifiable group when they came out of the closet just prior to the "epidemic."
4) AIDS in Africa is what it has always been-slow starvation and malnutrition-and it hasn't changed at all, except for the name. Simply compare any AIDS patient with the appearance of a crack cocaine baby or the horrible tel-lie-vision pictures of starving Iraqis, or prisoners in Concentration camps (Guatameno Bay). The epidemic in Africa simply does not exist. It has been an invention based on completely false information provided by indigent families seeking funds from charitable agencies and also by AIDS workers seeking to protect lucrative jobs. The statistics released are all unverified estimates that have proven to be 100% wrong.
5) Hemophiliacs get AIDS in small numbers because of additives and contaminants in their frequent blood transfusions.
6) AZT, a drug so toxic that it was discarded as a treatment for cancer, and which causes AIDS, is being given to individuals because they tested positive for antibodies to an innocent "virus." They will die of an acquired deficiency caused by AZT-and many of them are perfectly healthy!

"WARNING: Retrovir (AZT)… has been associated with symptomatic myopathy, similar to that produced by Human Immunodeficiency Virus…"

Glaxo Wellcome literature!!

7) Not one single reference paper (scientific proof) exists proving that HIV is the cause or even a co-factor of AIDS.
8) Condoms cannot stop a disease that is caused by starvation and drugs.

Saga of AIDS

1952: meeting behind closed doors in Ottawa, Canada, of Canadian, American, and British researchers studying retroviruses.

1961: Vaccination by living viruses begins.

1963: It is reported that the number of cases of leukemia has increased in States where the anti-polio vaccine containing SV 40 was administered.

1963: A biological research program is launched under the auspices of the CIA and the US Army at Fort Detrick, in Maryland. It is attached to the national Cancer Institute.

1968: American virologists set up their sophisticated equipment in Zaire.

1973: Berg and other leaders in biochemistry reveal the general principles of a new science. Genetic engineering is born.

1975: Gallo, an American researcher, announces the discovery of HTLV and states that this virus gives leukemia to certain population groups.

1977: First case of immuno-deficiency. (Acquired by a young African woman doctor).

1978: Vaccination against hepatitis B of homosexuals in New York.

1980: Vaccinations against hepatitis B of homosexuals in San Francisco, St. Louis, Denver, Chicago, and Atlanta.

1981: The official debut of the AIDS epidemic.

"I have known so many people who have died of AIDS...and all of them-all of them-took the drugs they were told to by their doctors...I have never taken any of them and I haven't gotten sick. Not even a cold. The doctors told me I had five years left to live...these drug companies that produce the medication are getting very rich...everyone I knew who has been HIV positive-and that's a lot of people-has died after taking these drugs."
Goldie Glitters-30 years old "living with the virus."

The Great "HIV" Hoax

The multi-billion dollar AIDS/HIV fraud is based on two fabrications: that AIDS is a single disease and that it is caused by the HI virus or the "HIV virus" as some medical/media masterminds call it. Perhaps they think the V in HIV stands for victory. In Japan "AIDS" is virtually unknown: yet, in random tests 25% of people were found to be "HIV-positive."

HIV-positive response means nothing of any relevance to health: it can be triggered by vaccination, malnutrition, influenza, leprosy, hepatitis...: over sixty different conditions. By grouping together 25-plus different diseases and other allied factors-pneumonia, herpes, Candida, salmonella, vaccine and antibiotic damage, amyl nitrate, malnutrition etc. and particularly in Africa, TB, malaria, dysentery and "slim disease" and calling the whole thing an "AIDS epidemic", a multi-billion scam has been created.

"If you think a virus is the cause of AIDS, do a control without... it hasn't been done. The epidemiology of AIDS is a pile of anecdotal stories, selected to fit the virus/AIDS hypothesis....
Peter Duesberg Member, National Academy of Sciences.

"...AIDS is not a disease at all- it is a government program."
Tom Bethel, Hoover Institute researcher.

The mythical "HIV-induced AIDS plague" in the Third World generates huge sums of cash from Western relief organizations whilst smoke screening the vaccine/drug boys, responsible for the carnage. Pregnant women who are HIV-positive have been told to stop breast-feeding, dosed with AZT, have had abortions or have been sterilized. HIV-positive babies who become ill from vaccination or whatever are automatically diagnosed as "suffering from AIDS". None of which stops the medical trade from pushing it on every trusting sap who is not ill to start with but is labeled with the "HIV-positive" nonsense and then destroyed by AZT; with "AIDS" getting the blame-and more billions pouring in for the drug boys, vivisectors, animal breeders and the rest. A particularly good scam is to haul into court someone "guilty of deliberately infecting the victim with the HI-Virus which supposedly causes AIDS' "which then develops into "full-blown AIDS"- no mention of vaccine, antibiotic damage, etc. or full-blown AZT. Over 2000 and rising, of the world's scientists are now disputing the HIV hoax, their efforts being continually suppressed by the AIDS establishment, the pharmaceutical/vivisection syndicate and their political and media lackeys.

Taking the "HIV test" is of no use whatsoever to anyone other than drug companies and governments ever eager to increase their control. Those who have had their immune system damaged by vaccines, antibiotics, antipyretics, analgesics, amyl nitrates etc. need to detoxify and to build up immune strength with raw, organic, non-GMO foods, homeopathic and herbal remedies which include Selenium, Cysteine, Tryptophan and Glutamine: and above all else, to stop swallowing the " 'HIV' causes 'AIDS' " rubbish and the lethal AZT "medication."

"Roche Diagnostics...likewise say of their genetic 'HIV testing kits': The Amplicor HIV monitor test is not intended to be used as a screening test for HIV or as a diagnostic test to confirm the presence of HIV infection"
Continuum Magazine leaflet Dec 1998

"Positive tests do not prove AIDS or pre-AIDS disease status."
Manufacturers of Western Blot (HIV) test kit.

DEADLY DECEPTION (The Most Important Lies)

1) AIDS is caused by the HIV virus
2) AIDS is contagious

3) A positive HIV test means death by AIDS
4) AZT is a treatment for AIDS
5) AIDS has no CURE

25. MSG: the Hidden Poison

A chemist by the name of Dr. Kikunae Ikeda was attempting to isolate a chemical that was responsible for the taste enhancing properties of the seaweed known as Kombu or "sea tangle." The Japanese had used this seaweed based flavor-enhancer in their recipes for thousands of years. Dr. Kikunae had received training in Germany under the auspices of a famous chemist, Dr. Wolf, who had perfected the technique of isolating glutamate from proteins. It was discovered that the mysterious flavor enhancing ingredient of the seaweed was glutamate. In 1909, Professor Ikeda partnered up with Dr. Saburosuke Suzukie and established a company under the name of Ajinomoto, which would manufacture the unique so- called flavor enhancer in the form of monosodium glutamate (MSG). Ajinomoto translates into 'the essence of taste" in English.

By 1933, Japanese cooks were using over 10 million pounds of the new flavor enhancer in their meals. Now, MSG is one of the most common food MediSins in the commercial food and restaurant industry. This toxic food additive can cause abnormal fetal development, ADHD and autism in children. MSG was slowly incorporated in the American diet in 1948 and has now risen to epidemic proportions. The use of this product was minimal in America until after WWII, when it was introduced to the United States food industry as a flavoring agent that the US military discovered made Japanese army rations more palatable than our own. Do you remember when pure monosodium glutamate became available in American stores in a product called "Accent?"

In 1968, a Chinese physician, Dr. Robert Ho Man Kwok, wrote a letter to the editor of the New England Journal of Medicine to ask for help in determining why he and his friends suffered numbness, weakness, and palpitations when they dined in certain Chinese restaurants. He reported that the condition occurred 15 to 20 minutes following the meal and lasted about two hours.

The letter was published under the heading "Chinese Restaurant Syndrome." Published responses that followed indicated that Dr. Kwok's problem was a reaction to MSG.

Monosodium Glutamate (MSG) is a neuron toxin that causes headaches, joint pain, feverish flush, disorientation, heart throbbing, seizures, and brain damage. Just one teaspoon could cause a heart attack and it has won FDA approval for 40 years. MSG has no flavor of its own, but it brings out the flavor in foods while causing an addiction to them at the same time. MSG also triples the amount of insulin the pancreas creates causing humans to gain weight. MSG depletes serotonin levels, which trigger headaches, depression, fatigue, and leads to more food cravings. In fact, scientists feed glutamate to young laboratory animals as a reliable way of inducing obesity. Is this the cause of America's obese situation? MSG is found in most processed foods: Campbell's soups, the Hostess cakes, Doritos corn chips, the Lays flavored potato chips, Top Ramen, Betty Crocker, Hamburger Helper, Heinz canned gravy, Swanson frozen prepared meals, Kraft salad dressings, especially the 'healthy' low-fat ones (FDA allows MSG to be labeled by other names including "natural flavors"). Do not forget that practically all commercial restaurants use MSG in abundance, some just use more or less than others. Commercial fried chicken restaurants may be the worst of all, that's why people love that coating on the skin, the secret spice is MSG!

In 1998, the US Environmental Protection Agency (the only protecting they do is corporate pockets) granted the unconditional registration of AuxiGro containing two new active ingredients "gamma amino butyric acid (GABA) and glutei acid for use as a growth enhancer for certain food crops and ornamentals. Between, 1999-2001 spraying of AuxiGro on wine grapes (calling the spray a fertilizer) was approved by the California Department of Food and Agriculture. Since that time AuxiGro has been approved for use on ALMONDS, APRICOTS, CANTALOUPES, CHERRIES, GRAPES (ALL OR UNSPECIFIED), MELONS, NECTARINES, ONION, PEACHES, PLUMS, PRUNES, TOMATOES, and WATERMELONS. And in July, 2004, California proposed to allow cole crops to be sprayed with AuxiGro. Cole crops include BROCCOLI, BRUSSEL SPROUTS, CABBAGE, CAULIFLOWER, KALE, COLLARDS, TURNIPS, RUTABAGA, MUSTARD,

WATERCRESS, and KOHLRABI. The exemptions and registration were granted to Auxein Corporation, Lansing, Michigan. According to John Erb, a developmental disorder researcher and author of the book "The Slow Poisoning of America", the cause of ADHD and autism is no longer a mystery.

MSG is added not to enhance the flavor of the foods, but to create addiction to the foods. It is the nicotine of our food supply. It is highly reactive in the human brain and other organs. According to Erb, "when a women becomes pregnant, the placenta barrier is not fully formed in the first month of fetal development. The chemical the mother eats can go directly to the developing child. MSG stimulates rapid growth in the brain, creating ADHD symptoms, and it over-stimulates areas of the brain, resulting in neuron cell death. This destruction of neurons results in the symptoms categorized as Autism."

Here are some of the collected reports of adverse reactions to MSG:

Cardiac	**Neurological**	**Gastrointestinal**
arrythmia,	depression,	diarrhea,
lowers blood	sciatica,	nausea,
pressure,	dizziness,	spleen disorders,
rapid heartbeat,	light-headedness	stomach cramps,
angina	loss of balance,	irritable bowel
	mental confusion,	
	anxiety,	
	panic attacks,	
	hyperactivity,	
	behavioral problems,	
	lethargy,	
	sleepiness,	
	insomnia,	
	migraine headaches,	
	seizures	

Circulatory	**Respiratory**	**Muscular**
Swelling/Edema	flu-like aches	

Visual	Skin	Urological
	shortness of breath	joint pain
	runny nose / asthma	stiffness
Blurred vision	hive / rash	swelling of prostate
	flushing	
	extreme dryness of the mouth	

In 1969, just as the dangers of MSG were being discovered, the glutamate industry formed a non-profit organization, the International Glutamate Technical Committee (IGTC), and in 1977 formed a subsidiary, The Glutamate Association (TGA), to defend the safety of its product, MSG. This is very similar to the dairy industry when it formed a National Dairy Council to support the bogus facts of pasteurized milk. To this day IGTC serves as a research organization for the MSG industry, interacting with scientists and providing research grants for studies on the subject of MSG. Until several years ago, the TGA served as the MSG industry's connection to consumers, acting somewhat like a public relations firm. This is how the games are played, the corporations have the finance to develop PR firms, third party research and doctors on contract to sugar coat the dirt they sell to the public. And since you, the consumer, have limited resources and access to information, you trust what their media delivers to you.

MSG is being added to mass produce food to increase its palatability. Women are being exposed to this toxic chemical, which can cause irreparable damage to their unborn child. They say that it is a flavor enhancer, but why do you need a flavor enhancer when the Creator blessed us with thousands of herbs and spices to enhance our foods. The problem is that we are dealing with intellectual, upscale psychopaths that "want to corrupt you while making a buck."

MSG: THE MISSING LINK BEHIND OBESITY

It is reported that obesity is responsible for $90 billion in medical cost and over 300,000 premature deaths in America. Since people are not genetically born to be obese, this condition has to be chemically driven. There are people with larger body frames, but prior to the 1950's there were few overweight people in America. It was relatively rare to find an individual that was grotesquely obese.

In 1968, John W. Olney, M.D., a respected researcher at Washington University Medical School, St. Louis, Missouri, and member of the National Academy of Science, found that mice in his laboratory that were being used to replicate a 1957 study by Luca and New house, in which the administration of MSG had resulted in retinal damage, had become grotesquely obese. Dr. Olney decided to sacrifice some of the mice and found lesions in the hypothalamus portion of the brain, the portion of the brain, as defined in Stedman's Online Medical Dictionary, that is "... prominently involved in the functions of the autonomic (visceral motor) nervous system and, through its vascular link with the interior lobe of the hypothesis, in endocrine mechanisms: it also appears to play a role in neural mechanisms underlying moods and motivational states."

Dr. Olney published a paper on his research in 1969, in which he described the hypothalamic lesion, stunted skeletal development, and obesity in maturing mice which had been given the food ingredient MSG. Olney also commented on the pathological changes found in several brain regions associated with endocrine function in maturing mice. Until 1978, research showed that baby food was a main supplier of MSG to developing infants. After 10 years of pressure from concerned parents and scientists, MSG was "voluntarily" removed from "baby food" by its manufacturers. However, in January of 1998, the EPA approved using processed free glutei acid (MSG) in pesticide products and plant growth enhancers—and fruits, grains, nut seeds and vegetables. Since "baby food" is made from processed vegetables/fruits that are made from products that were sprayed with pesticides, the baby food has once again become re-poisoned.

MSG: THE SCIENTIFIC CONFIRMATION

Many scientists have confirmed Dr. Olney's discovery of damage to the hypothalamus from MSG resulting in obesity. Take the time and retrieve the information from the web site, www.publmed.gov, you will also find 151 studies that correspond to

Dr. Olney's study. Initial experiments showed that the hypothalamus was damaged by MSG on small laboratory animals like mice and rats. Although research designed to produce brain lesions could not be executed in human subjects, studies revealed positive results of MSG damage when it was tested on primates such as the Rhesus monkeys. Neuroscientists have determined that humans are 5 times more sensitive to MSG than the mouse, and 20 times more sensitive to MSG than monkeys, based on blood plasma levels of glutamate following an oral dose of 150 mg/kg of glutei acid. Furthermore, individual variability in plasma response to glutamate loading is more extreme in humans than in the mice or monkeys. It should put a bitter taste in your mouth to find that neuroscientists have known about this MediSin (MSG) and its lesion producing chemical effect on the hypothalamus ever since 1969.

The glutamate industry along with the denying food corporations would of course like us to believe that MSG is not a problem for human consumption because the human brain is protected from MSG by the blood-brain barrier. However, scientific research proves different. The blood-brain barrier is underdeveloped in newborns, and there is some evidence that it is not fully developed in some children until puberty. Furthermore throughout life, certain regions of the brain, known as the circumventricular organs, lack a blood-brain barrier, and the blood-brain barrier can be damaged from high fever, stroke, trauma to the head, seizures, repeated ingestion of MSG, and the normal aging process. The developing fetus is at particular risk since the placental barrier is not impervious to MSG and it is assumed that the same is true for aspartic acid contained in aspartame, which you will find in part 26 of this book. Since most of the processed foods consumed today contain MSG, along with many other products, supplements and pharmaceuticals, it is almost impossible for a vulnerable mother to avoid this toxin during prenatal stages.

At this point, there is no question that MSG is a neurotoxin, potentially dangerous to everyone, even those that do not respond with adverse reactions such as migraine headaches, asthma, nausea, fatigue, disorientation and depression. There is scientific proof that MSG kills brain cells and causes lesions of the hypothalamus. Therefore, there is a strong link with neurological functions and obesity. MSG induced brain lesions in the area of the hypothalamus and/or accumulations of glutei acid have been shown to cause each of the following: retinal degeneration, neuroendocrine disorders, obesity, reproductive disorders, stunted growth, behavioral disorders, learning complications, memory disorders and hyperglycemia. In addition to this toxic escapade, addiction, stroke, epilepsy, Alzheimer's, Parkinson's, brain trauma, naturopathic pain, schizophrenia, anxiety, and diverse disease processes of the central nervous system were discovered.

THE SOLUTION TO MSG SYNDROME

In a testimony before FASEB on April 7, 1993, neuroscientist Richard C. Henneberry, Ph.D. summed up his presentation by saying: "I consider it ironic that the pharmaceutical industry is investing vast resources in the development of glutamate receptor blockers to protect CNS neurons against glutamate neurotoxicity in common neurological disorders, while at the same time the food industry, with the blessing of the FDA, continues to add great quantities of glutamate to the food supply. Although MSG sensitive individuals must stay away from MSG, I feel that MSG is not good for anyone." A growing number of neuroscientists believe that MSG may be a "slow neurotoxin," resulting in neurodegenerative diseases such as Alzheimer's and Parkinson's later in life." So why aren't the scientists, physicians, politicians, and health care administrators stepping up to the plate to summarize the true cause of the adverse effects of monosodium glutamate? We can now see that this MediSin is causing obesity, cardiac, respiratory, muscular and other physical and neurological complications. Once again the love for money and control has precedence over integrity. So therefore, the solution to eradicating the problems caused by MSG is to stop purchasing anything that contains a MSG by-product and purchase more foods that are close to a natural state.

It's amazing that a toxic substance like MSG is allowed to run rampant in the food supply and be protected by government agencies. At this present moment, that current low-life President George W. Bush and his corporate lackeys are pushing a bill through Congress called the "Personal Responsibility in Food Consumption Act", also known as the "Cheeseburger Bill." This sweeping law bars anyone from suing food manufacturers, sellers, and distributors, even if it turns out that they purposely added addictive chemicals to their foods. The Bill has already been rushed through the House of Representatives, and is due for the same rubber stamp at the Senate level.

THE HIDDEN SOURCES BEHIND MSG

The sooner you take a careful inventory of your groceries, the safer you and your family will be. MSG has been a hidden food additive under the following ingredients:

Hydrolyzed vegetable protein,
Autolyzed yeast extract,
Soy protein isolate
Sodium caseinate
Calcium caseinate
Hydrolyzed protein
Malt extract
Malt flavoring
Bouillon
So-called natural flavors
Whey protein concentrate
Carrageenan

26. WHY IS AMERICA AFRAID OF A WEED CALLED HEMP?

The world's view of the hemp plant is related to derogatory connotations similar to narcotics or cocaine with the status of an illegal drug by state and federal standards. In fact, hemp is the world's premier renewable resource of food, fiber and energy. The global hemp market is a thriving commercial success. Unfortunately, due to the outdated attitudes and drug war paranoia in the District of Columbia, America is the only major industrialized nation to prohibit the growing and processing of hemp. Since Jamestown and up to 1937, American farmers cultivated industrial hemp without restrictions. Today, a large, cross-section of citizens is demanding that right to be restored.

For a government to falsely charge hemp with a crime of this magnitude, it had to be something else about this extraordinary plant besides getting a high and having a sexual appetite. Could it be that hemp is the standard fiber of the world, which has great tensile strength and durability? Over 5,000 safe textile products can be produced from hemp ranging from rope to fine string. The woody "pulp" remaining after the fiber has been removed contains over 77% cellulose, which can be converted to more than 25,000 products, ranging from dynamite to cellophane.

Henry Ford even built his Ford Model-T using hemp to line the side panels. The impact strength was measured to be ten times stronger than steel alone! This could reduce many vehicle fatalities today. The Model-T was also designed to run on hemp fuel, which Henry Ford grew from his own yard. This was illustrated in the Popular Mechanics Magazine in the February 1938 edition. Concentrated extract of cannabis from the flowers was the second most used medicines in American for over 150 years, for over 100 separate medical illnesses.

Hemp contains several medicinal benefits and can be considered a natural medicine for glaucoma, stress, nausea, arthritis, asthma and even epilepsy. It is estimated that hemp would have at least 50,000 commercial uses if it were legal in America today.

The Cannabis/Hemp plant has been used throughout the world since the beginning of time for just about everything that mankind needed. The paper produced from hemp was used for books, bibles, maps, and even money. You can produce 4 times as much paper from an acre of hemp as you can from an acre of trees at 1⁄4 the cost and 1/5 the pollution. It is 26 times stronger than cotton and can last up to 1,000 years instead of only 50 for cotton. Hemp can be recycled at four times the amount of paper from wood pulp, which could save the destruction of the rain forest from the Americans and the Japanese. The American Constitution was originally written on hemp paper as well as the drafts of the Declaration of Independence.

Hemp is one of the strongest natural fibers on the planet, not to mention among the fastest growing plants, growing four times faster than corn. According to studies, the seed of hemp contains a very high source of vegetable protein. It also contains essential fatty acids that are not matched by any other plant. Hemp can be produced into machine-grade lubricants for engines, which can actually replace petroleum oil. It seems as though when any herb, weed, perennial, or any viable resource is available with little cost, it becomes practically banned. Just as corn can be converted into clean-burning ethanol fuel so can hemp. In 1794, President George Washington quoted, "make the most you can of the Indian hemp seed and sow it everywhere."

Another reason that hemp is so intimidating is that it threatened the cotton industry. On an annual basis, one acre of hemp will produce as much fiber as two to three acres of cotton. It is much stronger and softer than cotton, lasts twice as long, and it will not mildew. Fortunately, many textile products like jackets, pants, backpacks, paper and even houses are available from 100% hemp. Hemp is also an easy crop to grow and will yield from three to six tons per acre on any land that will grow corn, wheat, or oats. It can also be grown in any state in America. Due to its short growing season, it can be planted after other crops are planted. The long roots will penetrate the soil without harm, leaving it in perfect condition for the following year's crops.

Today, we are told that hemp is bad, but for the first 162 years of American existence, hemp was totally legal and was a common crop. However by the 1930s, American citizens were receiving derogatory press about this amazingly resourceful plant, which led to its prohibition. Some of the headlines made about hemp in the 1930s were: *"Marijuana: The assassin of youth"*, *"Marijuana: The devils weed with roots in hell."* In 1936, the liquor industry funded the infamous movie titled Reefer Madness. This movie depicts a man going insane from smoking marijuana, and then murdering his entire family with an ax. It was campaigns and media press like this that created such an illegal stigma on hemp. Let it be noted that prior to 1935, the word marijuana was NEVER used to identify hemp. This connotation was started by William Randolph Hearst (who owned all newspapers at that time) and DuPont (chemicals) to make sure it carried a negative idea in the minds of the masses, because it supposedly was being used by Mexicans to get high. While DuPont was protecting his empire (chemicals in which hemp would have eliminated the use of), Hearst was being paid to write the falsehood!

Thanks to the Marijuana Tax Act of 1937, hemp was declared illegal. New technologies were being developed that made hemp a potential competitor. The newly founded synthetic fiber (nylon, polyester, etc.) and plastic industries joined forces to get rid of it. Hemp's potential for producing paper also posed a threat to the timber industry. There is much evidence that commercial interest had a great deal to lose from hemp resource competition, so there had to be propaganda created to foster hysteria. Corporations used their heavyweight influence to lobby for Marijuana Prohibition.

In 1937, Harry J. Anslinger, the director of Furniture Brands International (FBN), was the leading advocate of Marijuana Prohibition. Anslinger testified before congress in favor of banning marijuana stating that, *"Marijuana is the most violent causing drug in the history of mankind." Most marijuana smokers are Negroes,*

Hispanics, Filipinos and entertainers. Their satanic music, jazz, and swing, result from marijuana usage. This marijuana causes white women to seek sexual relations with Negroes." This is how desperate corporations can get when it comes to a natural product potentially compromising their corruption.

The main reason that hemp is illegal in America today is because the families of wealth like the Harrimans, the Rockefellers (Standard Oil), the Whitneys (Eli Whitney-Cotton Gin), DuPont (chemicals in wood pulp processing and cotton pesticides), and Hearst (newspapers, media) find it more profitable to sell the masses cheap unnecessary chemicals, petroleum products (from gasoline to cosmetic ingredients) that are immune system-destroying pharmaceuticals. Not to mention the destruction of trees, all at inflated prices and at the expense of our health and life sustaining environment. Almost everything that is considered a commodity in America is exported across the globe. The estimated value of oil, petrochemicals, and pharmaceutical sales has reached the trillion dollar mark. However, if America was humble enough to see the 50,000 commercial products and the potential for the production of farm raised hemp, America would become a richer nation. By the way, man made alcohol and God made hemp. Whom do you trust?

27. PLASTIC IN MY VEINS: THE REAL CAUSE of CARDIOVASCULAR DISEASE

At the turn of the century a criminal process was discovered that uses heat in the presence of hydrogen and certain metal catalysts to convert natural liquid vegetable oils into solid fats. This physical change occurs because unsaturated bonds become saturated (fully hydrogenated) and others are converted from their natural origin (fatty acids) to an unnatural (trans fatty acids) position, creating straight molecules that pack together more solidly. None of these molecules have ever been encountered in nature. This process called hydrogenation was rapidly commercialized to create vegetable shortening, containing 30% to 40% trans fatty acids at a cost lower than that of palm, coconut or animal fats. Even by 1910, per capita production of margarine and vegetable shortening was above 4,000 grams per year. Production rose steadily over the course of the century, further augmented by the substitution of margarine for butter for both economic and alleged health benefits. Much of the success of refined hydrogenated oils is due to the economic appeal of their longer shelf life and decreased expense, compared with other fats. However, products containing hydrogenating oils, especially margarine, have been heavily promoted on the basis of health claims. Such claims have never been substantiated and concerns have been expressed regarding possible adverse health effects of hydrogenated oils.

I. OIL USAGE

Fresh seed oils are noticeable by their seed-specific characteristics, odor, and flavor. They are light, easy to digest, sustain health, and have therapeutic benefits. Have you ever wondered why that clear plastic bottle of oil sitting on most grocery store shelves has no smell or color at all? In Europe, during the early 1900s, seed oils such as flax, walnut, and olive were made in small glass bottles (12 oz.) and delivered to homes for their therapeutic value.

By the end of WWII, flaxseed oil, one of the more nutritious oils, had virtually disappeared from the market. Flax oil spoils quickly due to its high content of both essential fatty acids (EFA): Linoleic Acid (LA) and Alpha-Linolenic Acid (LNA). These fatty acids are needed everyday because our bodies cannot produce them. We must obtain them from the foods we eat. The usefulness of LA and LNA in our body results from their chemical properties. EFA attracts oxygen and absorbs sunlight while carrying slight negative charges. They keep membranes fluid, a property that is important in membrane functions. Their tendency to disperse surface activity gives biological systems the power to carry substances, such as toxins, to the surface of the skin, intestinal tract, kidneys or lungs, where these substances can be eliminated. EFA allows the one-way movement of electrons and energy to take place between molecules. The chemical reactions, on which life depends, require this one-way movement.

Overall, EFA are involved with producing life energy in our body from food substances, and moving that energy throughout our systems. LA and LNA appear to hold oxygen in our cell membranes where the oxygen acts as a barrier to viruses, fungi, bacteria and other foreign organisms that cannot thrive in its presence. LNA produces smooth, silky skin, increases stamina, speeds healing, increases vitality and brings a feeling of calmness. LNA reduces inflammation, water retention, platelet stickiness and blood pressure. It also inhibits the growth of tumors. LNA enhances some immune functions, reduces pain and swelling of arthritis, and completely reverses premenstrual syndrome in some cases. LNA kills malaria (in animal studies) and has been used successfully to treat bacterial infections. In short, EFA governs every life process in our body. Life without them is impossible. When our foods are EFA-deficient, we can expect a range of health problems.

The symptoms of LA deficiency include:

- Eczema
- Loss of hair
- Liver degeneration
- Excessive water loss through the skin
- Drying up of glands
- Susceptibility of infection
- Failure of wound healing
- Sterility in males
- Miscarriage in females
- Arthritis-like conditions
- Heart and circulatory problems
- Growth retardation
- Kidney degeneration
- Behavioral problems

The symptoms of LNA deficiency include:

- Weakness
- Impairment of vision and learning disability
- Motor coordination
- Tingling sensation in arms and legs
- High triglycerides
- Low metabolic rate
- High blood pressure
- Sticky platelets
- Tissue inflammation
- Edema
- Dry skin
- Mental deterioration
- Immune dysfunction

Over the years, natural, unrefined oils were replaced by bland or tasteless oils. People have come to accept that oils should be tasteless. These tasteless, low-quality oils have had molecules with health benefits removed, altered or destroyed. On the contrary, fresh natural seed oils have the delicate aromas and flavors of the seeds from which they are pressed. Due to ignorance and improper usage of modern technology, the majority of the oils in supermarkets have lost the complex, natural substances that oils contain, which help to digest and metabolize the oils. These substances include lecithin, phyto-sterols (plant chemicals), Vitamin E, and chlorophyll. Lecithin is the balancing factor for cholesterol. Where lecithin and cholesterol appear in food (i.e. eggs) they are counter-balanced and no harm results in the user. However, lecithin is heat-unstable or readily destroyed by high temperatures. So, when you consume hydrogenated fats you get the full blast of the cholesterol without the balancing lecithin phyto-sterols which block cholesterol absorption from our intestine.

Fat-soluble Vitamin E complex protects the oil against spoilage during storage and acts as an anti-oxidant in our bodies. Anti-oxidants prevent toxic reactions in the body called "free radicals." Free radicals are electrons that move about the body creating unstable chemical reactions resulting in degenerative diseases. The anti-oxidants neutralize these "free radicals" with nutrients such as vitamin C, B, selenium, bioflavonoids, zinc, coenzyme Q10, and copper. Chlorophyll, which is the essence of life, rich in magnesium, aromatic volatile compounds, and minerals are also present in the oils. Chlorophyll acts as an internal cleanser for the body, eliminating heavy metals, toxins, and dead cells.

Edible, refined oils have become the oil of choice here in America and across most of the "so-called" industrialized world. These oils are contaminated with pesticide residues that interfere with nerve functions and oxidation processes, therefore lowering our vitality. The invention of chemical extraction introduced gasoline-like chemical hexane in our oils. The chemicals are lung irritants and nerve depressants. Small amounts can have a detrimental effect on our well being. The use of non-natural anti-oxidants was added to these edible oils to improve shelf life, but their ingestion interferes with energy production, metabolism, and respiration. Since our bodies are made from natural substances, these unrelated substances do not fit precisely into the molecular architecture of our enzyme and membrane systems. Over time, they contribute to degenerative diseases and chronic fatigue.

II. HYDROGENATION

Hydrogenation, a process introduced on a large scale in the 1930's for making margarine and shortening, produces many toxic substances in our food supply. Just one of them called trans (short for transformed)-fatty acids bring twice as many food additives from all the food sources combined. Hydrogenation is the most common way of drastically changing natural oils to an unnatural substance. The process has major effects on our health. Industry's reason for using this process is to provide cheap spreadable products to unconscious consumers, and to provide shelf stability (100 years) at the expense of nutritional value. Imagine a processed food product remaining on the shelf for 100 years and never spoiling? It is important to know the effects of hydrogenated oil molecules because they destroy our health. Individuals should make well informed choices about whether or not to consume such a deadly product.

Hydrogenation changes the unsaturated and EFA present in natural oil to an un-natural product. In the process, oils are reacted under pressure with hydrogen gas at high temperatures of 450-500 degrees Fahrenheit in the presence of a metal catalyst (usually Nickel) for 6-8 hours. A nickel catalyst often used in hydrogenation is actually 50 percent nickel and 50 percent aluminum. Remnants of both metals remain in the products containing hydrogenated oils and are eaten by people and domesticated animals. Nickel destroys the vitamin pyridoxine (vitamin B6). Parkinson's disease is associated with the absence of Vitamin B6 in the body. The presence of aluminum is particularly dangerous; because its presence in the human body is linked to Alzheimer's disease (mental senility), osteoporosis, and will facilitate the development of cancer.

After the oil has been under pressure for the time allowed, the hydrogenation is complete and it contains no life (no nutrients, enzymes, etc.) at all. Such an oil is "safe" because it does not spoil, resulting in a longer shelf "life" (if that term can be applied to a dead substance). Complete hydrogenated oil which is now a solid "fat" can be heated without further damage: fried, baked, roasted, and boiled. Since the hydrogenation process has transformed these fats they are no longer accepted by the body, and act as toxins in our cell membranes. In recent years, measurements of trans-fatty acids in membranes of human red blood cells have been 20 percent, when the figure should be zero. Trans-fatty acids in cell membranes weaken the membrane's protective structure and function. This alters normal transport of minerals and other nutrients across the membrane allowing deceased membranes and toxic chemicals into our cells more easily. The result: sick, weakened cells, poor organ function and an exhausted immune system, which lowers our resistance and increases the risk of disease.

Trans-fatty acids can also derail the body's normal mechanisms for eliminating cholesterol. The liver normally puts excess cholesterol in the bile and sends it to the gall bladder, which empties into the small intestine just below the stomach. Trans-fatty acids block the normal conversion of cholesterol in the liver and contribute to elevated cholesterol levels in the blood. Trans-fatty acids also cause an increase in the amount of low-density lipoproteins (LDL'S) considered to be one of the main instigators of arterial disease (hardening of the arteries). Meanwhile, Trans-fatty acids lower the amount of high-density lipoproteins (HDL'S) which help protect the cardiovascular system from the adverse affects of the (LDLS). Trans-fatty acids also increase the level of Apolipoprotein A, a substance in the blood; which is another risk factor for heart disease. Another adverse effect of trans-fatty acids in the diet is an enhancement of the body's pro-inflammatory hormones (prostaglandin 2), and an inhibition of the anti-inflammatory types (prostaglandin 1 and 3).

Prostaglandins are short-lived, hormone-like chemicals that regulate cellular activities on a moment-to-moment basis. Healthy human beings make the prostaglandins they need from EFA, but trans-fatty acids and metabolic conditions can block the ability to convert EFA into prostaglandins. This undesirable influence executed by trans-fatty acids on prostaglandin balance may render you more vulnerable to inflammatory conditions that do not want to heal! Prostaglandins also regulate many metabolic functions. Tiny amounts of trans-fatty acids cause significant changes in allergic reactions, blood pressure, clotting, cholesterol levels, hormone activity and immune function.

A report by the Danish Nutrition Counsel said that the consumption of trans-fatty acids from margarine is equally, or perhaps more responsible for the development of arteriosclerosis than saturated (animal fatty acids). Another report by the Harvard School of Public Health analyzed the diets of 239 patients admitted to the Boston Hospital for their first heart attack, and compared them with the diets of 282 healthy control subjects. After adjusting for several lifestyle variables, they found that margarine intake was significantly the number one reason for their first heart attack.

The American Journal of Clinical Nutrition published a study 50 years ago between the heart disease rates of populations in Northern and Southern India. The Northerners were meat eaters and had high cholesterol levels. Their main source of dietary fat was ghee (clarified butter). The Southerners were vegetarians and had a much lower cholesterol level. Present day "wisdom" would predict the vegetarians to have the lower rate of heart disease, but in fact, the opposite was true. The vegetarians had 15 times the rate of heart disease when compared to their Northern counterparts! What was the reason for the surprising difference? Aside from meat versus vegetables, the major dietary difference was that the Southerners had replaced their traditional ghee (a real food) with margarine and refined oils (medisins). Twenty years later, the British medical journal "The Lancet" did a follow-up to the American Journal and noted an increase in heart attack deaths amongst the Northern Indians. The Northerners had largely replaced the ghee in their diets with margarine and refined oils.

Many of these problems with trans-fatty acids have been known or suspected for 20 years, but have been largely ignored in the U.S. In Europe, trans-fatty acids are restricted in food products, and some countries allow no more than 0.1% trans-fatty acid content. In contrast, margarine in the U.S. may contain up to 50 percent trans-fatty acids. Margarine contains no cholesterol, but lacks the minerals and vitamins for its metabolism. Margarine contains fewer pesticides than butter and no antibiotics. However, margarine contains trans-fatty acids in substantial amounts, and is a major source of unwanted aluminum and nickel in our body. In making the oils used in margarines, manufacturers remove all proteins, all fiber, about 95 to 99 percent of all minerals, 65 to 100 percent of all vitamins, almost all of the lecithin, phytosterols, and other minor components. The consumer ends up with a product that has had almost all of its essential nutrients deliberately removed or destroyed. The 60 grams (2 ounces) of margarine consumed each day contains more than twice as many toxic food additives that are found in the many other grams of food that people consume each day.

Trans-fatty acids increase blood cholesterol levels by 150 percent and blood fat levels by up to 55 percent. When hydrogenated oils containing 38 percent trans-fatty acids are ingested, the result is high TG levels. Triglycerides play a big role in developing cardiovascular disease. High blood TG levels increase our risk of heart disease. They are produced by overeating and by high dietary intake of refined sugars, refined carbohydrates, and too few antioxidants. Under these conditions, TG fatty acids oxidize and damage the insides of our arteries. High blood TG levels may also increase the tendency of blood cells to clump together. Excess stored triglyceride fats (in overweight or obese people) correlate with high blood cholesterol and triglyceride levels. All increase our risk of cardiovascular disease, high blood pressure, kidney failure, and cancer.

Many kinds of cancer are associated with diets high in refined fats. When the information is analyzed and compared to the increase in the incidence of deaths from cancer over the last 80 years (from 1 in 30 people to 1 in 4 people in 1999), cancer increase parallels the increase in the consumption of hydrogenated oils. The fact that trans-fatty acids interfere with vital metabolic functions, which cause the body to retain toxins and alter cellular structure makes their involvement in cancer frightening!

One hundred years ago, cardiovascular disease was virtually unknown. Today, two thirds of the U.S. citizens develop heart disease. Remember that the process of hydrogenation in regard to its use in food is comparatively new. It was only during the past thirty years, that it has become widely used. In these thirty years, we have seen the incidence of heart disease grow rapidly. There is no doubt in our minds that the incidence of heart disease can be charted almost accurately with the incidence of the increased use of hydrogenated oils in our food supply.

One other such oil that is being promoted as healthy is canola oil. First of all, there is no seed called canola. This oil is produced from the rapeseed, which is a monounsaturated oil that had been used extensively in many parts of the world, notably in China, Japan and India. It contains almost 60 percent monounsaturated fatty acids (compared to about 70 percent in olive oil). Unfortunately, about two-thirds of the monounsaturated fatty acids in rapeseed oil are erucic acid, a 22-carbon monounsaturated fatty acid that had been associated with Keshan's disease, characterized by fibrotic lesions of the heart. In the late 1970s, using a technique of genetic manipulation involving seed splitting, Canadian plant breeders came up with a variety of rapeseed that produced a monounsaturated oil low in 22-carbon erucic and high in 18-carbon oleic acid.

The new oil referred to as LEAR oil, for Low Erucic Acid Rapeseed, was slow to catch on in the U.S. In 1986, Cargill announced the sale of LEAR oil seed to U.S. farmers and provided LEAR oil processing at its Riverside, North Dakota plant but prices dropped and farmers took a hit. Before LEAR oil could be promoted as a healthy alternative, it needed a new name. Neither "rape" nor "leer" could be expected to invoke a healthy image for the "wonder" crop. In 1988, the industry settled on "Canola," for "Canadian oil," since most of the new rapeseed at that time was grown in Canada.

By the late 1990s, canola use had soared and not just in the US. Today China, Japan, Europe, Mexico, Bangladesh and Pakistan all buy significant amounts. It is the oil of choice in gourmet and health food markets like Fresh Fields (Whole Foods) markets and shows up in many supermarket items as well. With all this fanfare it would seem like a godsend for those looking for the ultimate oil. But hold on to your horses! Canola was the first seed oil to be CREATED THROUGH GENETIC MANIPULATION; canola is also the focus of a variety of genetic engineering projects in which genetic material from other species is inserted into the seeds in order to magnify certain traits in the resultant plant. Herbicide-resistant genetic canola now comprises a large portion of the total canola crop.

By ingesting this hydrogenated oil, people are subjecting their bodies to fibrotic lesions of the heart, decreased vitamin E output, undesirable changes in blood platelets and a shortened lifespan in stroke victims. Furthermore, it retards growth, which is why the FDA (of all people) does not allow the use of canola oil in infant formula. When fed to animals in Europe in the early 1990s, canola oil caused them to go blind and crazy from scrapie, cows attacked people and had to be shot. So much for the great wonder oil out of Canada!

It is now recognized that the United States is one of the unhealthiest countries in the world for men 25 years of age and older with respect to heart disease. Most middle-age American men have severe coronary arteriosclerosis and young children are close behind. Young children are now found to have the beginning stages of heart disease in their blood vessels. We predict that the incidence of heart attacks will reach epidemic proportions and those men and perhaps women will be dropping dead on the streets, in their automobiles, in buses, streetcars, in subway trains and anywhere human beings congregate. Also, we predict that heart attacks will strike people of young ages. From 55 that it used to be, it will go down to 45 and from 45 it will go down to 30 and from 30 it will drop to the 20's and eventually into the teens where some of that is now scratching the surface. You hear about many high school athletes dropping dead during athletic events and that will only increase with time.

The problem is that 95% of the American population use foods containing hydrogenated oils (margarine) with particularly every meal. The continued pileup of these dangerous plastics in your body can have in our sincere opinion, but one result: ill health, sickness and untimely death. We suggest you call hydrogenated oils what they really are, a synthetic chemical compound: plastic. There is no justification, rhyme or reason for calling it an oil or fat. It is no more an oil suited for human consumption than is motor oil. Please use organic butter, extra-virgin olive oil, and unrefined coconut oil as your choice of fats in your diet.

28. ASPARTAME: A SWEET MISERY

It all began in 1964, when an international pharmaceutical company, G.D. Searle and Company was working on an ulcer drug looking for an inhibitor of the gastrointestinal secretory hormone gastric (Stegink 1984). In 1965, while creating a bioassay, an intermediate chemical was synthesized, aspartylphenylalanine-methylester (aspartame). James Schlatter (member of G.D Searle) was recrystalling aspartame from ethanol when the mixture spilled onto the outside of the flask. Some of the liquid got onto his fingers. Schlatter unconsciously licked his fingers to pick up a piece of paper. History was about to begin as he noticed an extremely sweet taste. He figured that taste must have come from the chemical aspartame. Apparently, he convinced himself that the dipeptide aspartame was non-toxic so he indulged in tasting more of the chemical. The first report on the discovery was revealed in the Journal of the American Chemical Society stating (Mazur 1969):

"We wish to report another accidental discovery of an organic compound with a profound sucrose (table sugar) like taste ... Preliminary tasting showed this compound to have a potency of 100-200 times sucrose depending on concentration and on what other flavors are present and to be devoid of unpleasant aftertaste."

In August of 1970, G.D. Searle conducted two 78-week toxicity studies on rats for what was to become a best selling heart medication Aldactone. In March 1972, the rats that were studied were then autopsied and pathologically analyzed. Pathologist Dr. Jacqueline Mauro discovered that the drug aspartame appeared to induce tumors in the liver, testes and thyroid of the rats. The report submitted to G.D. Searle by Dr. Mauro was known as the MBR report. On March 5, 1973, G.D. Searle's petition to the FDA for approval to market aspartame as a sweetening agent was published in the Federal Register (1973). These statistically significant findings were confirmed by G.D. Searle's Mathematic-Statistics Department. Instead of submitting these findings of toxicity to the FDA, G.D. Searle contracted another pathologist, Dr. Donald A Willigan. Dr. Willigan was given 1,000 slides to examine this report and concluded that there were no liver tumors caused by aspartame. Dr. Willigan's report revealed a significant increase in thyroid and testes tumors, but not in liver tumors, which are of more concern to the FDA. The Willigan report was immediately submitted to the FDA. G.D. Searle did not disclose the MBR Report to the FDA until August 18, 1975, 27 months after it had been given to G.D. Searle.

At first, G.D. Searle claimed that they did not submit the MBR Report to the FDA because of an "oversight." Alexander Schmidt, M.D., the FDA Commissioner from 1972 to 1976 felt that *"Superficially, it seemed like, if there would ever be a safe kind of product that would be it. The idea that two naturally-occurring amino acids could harm someone in relatively small amounts....."*

In a FDA memorandum dated September 12, 1973, Martha M. Freeman, M.D. of the FDA Division of Metabolic and Endocrine Drug Products addressed the adequacy of the information submitted by G.D. Searle in their petition to approve aspartame (Freeman 1973):

"Although it was stated that studies were also performed with dikatopiperazine [DKP] an impurity which results from acid hydrolysis of Aspartame, no data was provided on this product."

Commenting on one particular single dose study:
"It is not feasible to extrapolate results of a single dose testing to the likely condition of use of Aspartame as an "artificial sweetener."

It is important to note that Dr. Freeman pointed out the inadequacy of single-dose tests of aspartame as early as 1973. The approval of aspartame is a great example of political progress at work. In 1977, Donald Rumsfeld, who was a member of Congress and the Chief of Staff in the Gerald Ford Administration, was recruited as G.D. Searle's president. Attorney James Turner alleged that G.D. Searle hired Rumsfeld to handle the aspartame approval difficulty as a "legal problem rather than a scientific problem." (US Senate 1987) In January of 1977, FDA Chief Counsel, Richard Merrill recommended to U.S. Attorney, Sam Skinner, in a 33-page letter emphasizing violations of the law, that a grand jury be set up to investigate G.D. Searle. In the letter Merrill stated:

"We request that your office convene a Grand Jury investigation into apparent violation of the Federal Food, Drug and Cosmetic Act, 21 U.S.C. 331(e), and the False Reports to the Government Act, 18 U.S.S. 1001, by reports to the Food and Drug Administration required by Act, 21 U.S.C. 355(i), and for concealing material facts and making false statements in reports of animal studies conducted to establish the safety of the drug Aldactone and the food additive Aspartame."

There were other studies where the violations of the law appeared to be especially flagrant. Studies cited by Merrill included the 52 week toxicity study on infant monkeys performed by Dr. Waisman which G.D. Searle withheld key information from the FDA, and the 46-week toxicity study of hamsters where G.D. Searle had taken blood from healthy animals at the 26th week and claimed that the test had actually been performed at the 38th week. Many of the animals from which G.D. Searle claimed to have drawn blood were actually dead at the 38th week. So why would anyone consume anything that has to be taken through so many trial studies? This product is detrimental to the human body, so why in the hell is this MediSin in the American food chain? Due to politics, greed and demonic nature, that's why!

Another chemical poisoning that is derived from aspartame is methanol, which causes blindness. In aspartame, methanol alcohol poisoning and poisoning from methanol's breakdown components (formaldehyde and formic acid) can have widespread and devastating effects. This occurs in even small amounts and can cause a great deal of damage when introduced with toxic, free form amino acids, called excitotoxins. Methanol is quickly absorbed through the intestinal lining called the mucosa and the small intestines. The methanol is converted into formaldehyde (a known carcinogen). Then, via aldehyde hydrogenase, the formaldehyde is converted to formic acid. These two metabolites of methanol are toxic and cumulative.

Since there is mass consumption of aspartame, there is the belief that it has been contributing to Sudden Cardiac Death (SCD). According to Betty Martini of Mission Possible, an Aspartame Awareness group; Sudden Cardiac Death is not a clogged artery fatality like heart attack or myocardial infarction, it is an electrical problem in which the cardiac conduction system that generates the impulses regulating the heart suddenly outputs rapid or chaotic electrical impulses or both. The heart ceases its rhythmic contractions, the brain is starved of oxygen and the victim loses consciousness in seconds.

It appears that aspartame not only has no bias but it also doesn't spare any structure or system in the body, so it wouldn't be logical to try to mentally isolate it to a few structures or a few systems in the body. In fact, the FDA identified 92 documented symptoms triggered by aspartame, including death. A comment made by Dr. James Bowen appeared in the Atlanta Journal Constitution (AJC) stated:

"Sudden death in high school athletes is a topic that has received a lot of attention recently." In many cases aspartame victims may have had pre-existent or congenital undiagnosed cardiac problems. The fatal abnormalities induced by NutraSweet would have quicker and greater effect on these unfortunate individuals."

The article in the AJC discussed accidents that may have been caused by sudden cardiac arrest. It brings to mind the death of Sonny Bono who had an accident while skiing and hit a tree. The new paper reported Bono was not drinking alcohol, only a "Diet Coke." Another interesting case is that of Charles Fleming, who drank ten diet drinks a day and other aspartame products. He became ill after playing basketball and died. His autopsy revealed a classic death by aspartame. It showed pulmonary edema that is often evident. According to Dr. H.J. Roberts who wrote an article in the Townsend Letter for Doctors, the report stated that Mr. Fleming had chronic methanol poisoning which was shown by a fatty liver. Methanol is classified as a narcotic, and is one of the three components of aspartame. The police did not know that aspartame causes chronic methanol poisoning (one of the reasons that it mimics MS – destroys the CNS (Central Nervous System) and thought that Mr. Fleming's wife murdered him even though she passed the polygraph test. She was sentenced to 50 years in prison where she remains in Troy, Virginia. Mrs. Fleming was a Sunday school teacher and helped the homeless. Aspartame caused her to lose everything.

So, just how toxic is aspartame (NutraSweet, Spoonful, or Equal)? Aspartame (C14H18N205) is a compound of three components. These components are methanol, aspartic acid and phenylalanine (the latter being free-form amino acids). Methanol (methyl alcohol or wood alcohol) is a colorless, poisonous, flammable liquid. It is used for making formaldehyde (used in making embalming fluid), acetic acid, methyl-t-butyl ether (a gasoline additive), paint strippers, carburetor cleaners for your car's engine, and chloromethane. This poison can be inhaled from vapors, absorbed through the skin, and digested.

Today, there are hundreds of millions of Americans, and millions more worldwide, that are consuming foods and soft drinks laced with NutraSweet or Equal in their cakes, pies, coffee, puddings, cereals, juices and over 9,000 other consumer foods and products. In late 1982, Searle petitioned the FDA approval to use the sweetener in diet soft drinks and even in children's vitamins. It is these chemical MediSins like aspartame, MSG, Splenda, NutraSweet, Saccharin and any other laboratory chemical that is portrayed as a food or additive that is killing not only America but also the world. This stuff will not only cause mental disarray but will compromise your soul. This is why they are called excitotoxins, because the chemicals excite your cells to death! Remember all excitotoxins play a key role in degenerative diseases, such as Parkinson's, Alzheimer's, Huntington's and other new age diseases that are ruining your career, your health and your family. Stop it before it's too late! Read the book, "Excitotoxins" the Taste that Kills, by Russell L. Blaylock, M.D., for more on chemicals called excitotoxins.

29. SPLENDA: IT REALLY ISN'T SPLENDID

When the masses of Americans began to replace the sugar substitutes with Splenda they chose a far worse MediSin than white refined sugar. They might as well go back to saccharin, because Splenda is sucralose and sucralose is a chlorocarbon. Chlorocarbons have long been known to cause organ, genetic and reproductive damage. The FDA even reveals that it has been shown to cause up to 40% shrinkage of the thymus gland (the gland that has a major responsibility of producing T-Cells and maintaining a strong immune system). Not to mention that Splenda also causes swelling of both the liver and kidneys particularly calcification of the kidney.

Sucralose is (sold under the name Splenda) a non-caloric artificial sweetener that is 600 times sweeter than sucrose (white sugar). It was discovered in 1976 by researchers employed under Tate & Lyle Ltd, a British sugar refiner. Four years later, Tate & Lyle arranged with Johnson & Johnson to develop sucralose. Johnson & Johnson quickly formed McNeil Specialty Products Company in the 1980s to commercialize sucralose. It was in 1998 that the US Food and Drug Administration granted approval for sucralose to be used in a variety of food products, and diet RC cola was the first U.S. product to contain sucralose, in that same year.

Sucralose is made by chlorinating white sugar (sucrose). The chemical structure of sugar is manipulated by substituting three chlorine atoms for three hydroxyl groups. The anti-life process of this MediSin will alarm most people, understanding that chloride is an extremely poisonous agent. According to Mosby's Medical, Nursing and Allied Health Dictionary, chlorine is a yellowish-green, gaseous element of the halogen group. Its atomic number is 17; its atomic weight is 35.453. It gives off a strong, distinctive odor, is irritating to the respiratory tract, removes all Vitamin E from the body, and is poisonous if ingested or inhaled.... Chlorine compounds in general use include many solvents, cleaning fluids and chloroform (formed when taking showers without a shower filter). Most of the solvents and cleaning fluid containing chlorine are toxic when inhaled or ingested. Despite the facts that sucralose contains such well-known poisons, its manufactures adamantly assure us that Splenda is not only safe but has a great taste.

If you go to the Splenda website, (www.splenda.com), you will find out what type of political and corporate beast the world is challenged with. Review the myriad of information concerning this MediSin! It states: "Splenda Brand Sweetener is made from sugar, so it tastes like sugar, with no unpleasant aftertaste. It can be used virtually anywhere sugar is used. In cooking and baking, Splenda No Calorie Sweetener, or sucralose, is made from sugar through a patented, multi-step process that selectively replaces three hydrogen-oxygen groups on the sugar molecule with three chlorine atoms. The website further states that after consumption, sucralose passes through the body without being broken down. Splenda manufacturers claim that the sweetener is safe to use and does not break down after consumption. They claim that this is the most extensive studied food additives today; it is also one of the most toxic studied food additives today.

The manufacturers of the MediSin Splenda feel that replacing sugar with a toxic chemical is no big deal. But anything that passes right through the spleen (which is the master of digestion) and does not break down is a major problem. Since sucralose is a chlorocarbon, it should belong on the same shelf as DDT. The company heinously denied that sucralose was a chlorocarbaon. They stated that is was merely a salt, like sodium chloride! They were also very covert in hiding the fact the sucralose is absorbed from the digestive tract, chlorocarbons are significantly absorbed from the digestive tract.

Here are the side effects that come with Splenda:

Shrunken thymus
Enlarged kidney and liver
Reduced growth rate
Decreased red blood cell count
Aborted pregnancy
Diarrhea
Spiritual death

People, you are not making progress with something as toxic and synthetic as sucralose. Any sugar substitute is detrimental to your health and you cannot expect anything wholesome from a lab and a patent. If it's calories you are watching, then you are going by it totally wrong! First of all, all food should be consumed from its natural state or as close to it as possible. Try other health benefiting natural sugar alternatives like stevia, raw honey, grade B or C maple syrup or xylitol.

30. CRIME AND THE REFINED DIET

Whoever said that there is no connection between a person's behavior and the food they ate is not only wrong but also crazy! Just in the last 15 years America and other parts of the world have witnessed more child violence, child murders, more hyperactivity, more irrational behavior, more drop outs, more apathy, and less balance than ever in the history of man's civilization. Child violence and behavioral disorders are a new societal epidemic, the main vector of this modern day crisis of psycho-revolutionary violence or "looking for love in the wrong damn place" is a combination of subliminal music, violent television and most of all chronic malnutrition. If body chemistry plays a definitive role in causing abnormal physical behavior, psychological thinking and irrational responding are not only a theory but a true hypothesis, it is pointless to treat hyperactive children with Ritalin, Prozac or to increase the prison population when the combination of dietary neglect and the media projections of violence is the critical factor during the persons growth process.

Up to the decade of the 70's, parental guidance and domestic nutrition was much more wholesome, even though some families were at the poverty borderline, the home and the food it provided was much more simplistic and less toxic. Less television, more physical activity and "on-the-spot" family and neighborly support was much more essential for rational thinking and productivity. Now fast food, unsupervised, unregulated television programming, fashionable clothing trends have manifested into youth gang violence, drug abuse, youth depression, suicide and mass murder. This American system of political and demonic design has intentionally eradicated youth and nutrition programs by the multitudes. While countries like Cuba and Japan place nutrition and education at an unprecedented level, the United States of George Bush focuses on only what his administration thinks is important, "the war on terrorism" instead of nutritional reform. Besides the terrorist are right here on the home front and they don't were turbans.

By using the science of hair analysis it is much easier to observe the mineral profiles of individuals and how the patterns of violent and non-violet criminals differ. Researchers suggest that murder can result from anger "with volume turned up" with the body's terrain of abnormal chemistry manifested by an undernourished lifestyle and environmental influence. It is almost apparent that a child surrounded by a violent environment whether it be the inter-urban, low-income community or a prestigious wealth estate, the outcome of a child's development can be progressive or destructive. Just compare various crime episodes between the black youth in the "hood" to an episode of mass murder committed by an upper-middle class white youth at Columbine high school in Colorado. Though many aspects of media, parental guidance or societal corruption could off-set the psyche of the developing mind, what secures and protects the infrastructure of rationale and critical thinking is an essential diet.

There have been numerous studies conducted on the incarcerated population and it has been found that nutritional deficiencies and imbalances can impair one's brain function especially in young adults that set the stage for delinquent and criminal behavior. Experts have also found that when subjects are given supplements supported by a wholesome non-toxic diet the results are nothing short of dramatic!

In the early 70's Bill Walsh a Ph.D. and analytical chemist was working as a scientist at Argonne National Laboratory and involved in some volunteer work at Illinois' State Prison decided to conduct a study with Carl Pfeiffer a M.D., Ph.D., a nutritionally oriented physician. Pfeiffer understood that low levels of essential nutrients and high levels of toxic metals could affect one's behavior. By inviting other Argonne scientists and using state-of-the-art analytical equipment, Walsh studied mineral levels by conducting a hair analysis on 24 pairs of brothers. In each case, one brother appeared to be balanced and progressive and the other was violent, aggressive and irrational.

The results were obviously surprising, the positive group of boys had normal mineral levels, but the delinquents had two distinctive mineral patterns: One pattern consisted of very high copper and very low zinc, sodium, and potassium; the other consisted of very low zinc and copper and very high sodium and potassium. Most of the violent subjects systems contained lead and cadmium levels three times higher than the more progressive, balanced brothers. Walsh extended his study on mineral patterns in a group of 192 adults, half incarcerated criminal and half "law-abiding adults," the results were similar, some of the subjects appeared to be normal while others would have be described as a sociopath.

According to Walsh, children that were born with a metal metabolism disorder had the inability to properly regulate trace minerals. This disorder is related to poor metallothionein activity in the gut. Metallothionein, a protein needed for absorption of zinc, also plays a key role in removing hazardous metals such as lead and cadmium. According to clinical and nutritional research, metalloionein levels can be boosted with supplemental zinc and other minerals.

In 1981, Dr. Walsh established a non-for-profit corporation called the Health Research Institute in Naperville, IL which consists of the research institute, the Pfeiffer treatment center, and a pharmacy for patients. Since the establishment of the Institute, Dr. Walsh has conducted mineral analysis of 28 serial killers and mass murders, including Charles Manson. All subjects fell into the two abnormal mineral patterns with lead and cadmium levels typically being elevated. It was discovered that Manson had one of the most extreme mineral patterns among the 14,000 patients in the center's database. According to Dr. Walsh, Manson always blamed his behavior on how he grew up. But based on the mineral analysis, he would have been criminal minded regardless of his childhood social environment.

The overall purpose of the Health Research Institute and Pfeiffer Treatment Center is to address unfortunately the common behavioral and psychological disorders in everyday America like: autisms, depression, bipolar disorder, schizophrenia and ADD (attention-deficit-disorder) which really is nothing but a label. Dr. Walsh has analyzed and observed over 200 consecutive (i.e. random) patients diagnosed with behavioral disorders, which include destructive behavior, uncontrollable mood swings and tempers, all of whom were treated with nutritional applications at the Pfeiffer Treatment Center. In fact 92% of the aggressive subjects who followed their nutritional and dietary protocol improved, and 58% completely eliminated this type of behavior. Eighty percent of the destructive patients progressed, 53% completely eliminated and 92% of the subjects that had conditions of temper outburst improved, 11% completely eliminated.

There was another observation made by Stephen J. Schoenthler, Ph.D., a sociology professor at the Stanislaus campus of California State University that discovered a powerful connection between nutrition and behavior. Like most pediatricians and psychologist (psy-quakery) in America, Schoenthaler was a skeptic but after 20 years of studies and broad-minded research he became an advocate in the health benefits of dietary balance and nutritional supplementation.

During Schoenthler's numerous observations he and his colleagues found sometimes startling results. For example, one study of juvenile delinquents and adult felons of five different states found that the offenders with the most aggressive behavior had very limited vitamin and mineral intake. It was also found that among the prison population in California Institutions inmates that reveal up to four nutritional deficiencies were 50% more likely to incur violent episodes, and those with five to nine essential deficiencies were 90% more likely to experience violent or uncontrollable incidents.

An experiment involving 8,000 teenagers in 9 different correctional facilities who consume a diet of high sugar and refined carbohydrates receive a replacement diet high in vegetable, fruits and other wholesome foods. The study ended with a near fifty-percent decrease in violence and anti-social incidents. In the 1980's Schoenthaler was involved in a study that altered the nutritional content of school lunches for 1.1 million New York public school students. Within one year this more wholesome, less refined food program contributed to a 16% increase in academic performance and a 41 percent decrease in learning disabled children.

In another investigation, people receiving a multivitamin/mineral supplement incurred less anti-social or violent behavior, compared with those receiving a placebo. Schoenthaler stated that "The most common vitamins to be low among children whose conduct and academic performance improved after nutritional intervention are pyridoxine, folic acid, thiamine, niacin and vitamin C."

Since many of the newly commercialized foods have been completely stripped of all essential nutrients and replaced with synthetic chemicals, including aspartame, dyes, canola oil, etc. that not only tax the body of stored nutrients, but encourage neurological disharmony. It is now absolutely clear that nutritional components have a profound effect on the brain's activity. For example, thiamine (vitamin B1) deficiency can result in irritability and unregulated behavior. By supplementing thiamine, a person can go from rude and stupefied to rational and reasonable. Studies have shown that mineral deficiencies causing abnormal chemistry can result in violent anger.

Refined sugar was known to have physiological and psychological affects even though it is still sold to the masses around the world. Refined sugar causes children and young adults to become hyper, lethargic, and irritable. Next time you are at your grocery market, take a look at the children who cry out when mommy does not give them their candy! Hormone contaminated meats stimulate character and mood imbalance, while fluoride calcifies the secret pineal gland and blocks intuitive thought. Foods that are created with by-products of a synthetic nature will create severe molecular and physiological changes because of the foreign activity that goes on in the process of metabolism. For example, give a person alcohol and their psychological functions change. Some that indulge become passive, while others may become violent, depending on the mental, physical or spiritual constitution.

In 1979, Frank Kern, assistant director at Tidewater Detention Center in Chesapeake, Virginia conducted a dietary reform using macrobiotics as a base. He arranged an experiment among twenty-four inmates. The inmates would have sugar completely taken out of their diet. The subjects were between 12 and 18 years of age with offenses ranging from disorderly conduct, to larceny and burglary, to alcohol and narcotics violations. Soda beverage machines were also removed from premises and substituted with fruit juice. The refined sugar was replaced with honey and other unrefined sweeteners.

The three-month trial was designed as a double-blind case-control study. Neither the detention center personnel nor the inmates were aware that the tests were being conducted. At the end of the trial period, the regular staff records on the inmate's behavior were checked against a control group of 34 youngsters who had been institutionalized previously. Researchers found that the youngsters on the modified diet exhibited a 45 percent lower incident of formal disciplinary actions and antisocial behavior than the control group. Over the following years the absence of sugar resulted in a 82% reduction in assaults, 77% reduction in thefts, 65% reduction in misconduct and 55% reduction in insubordination.

There are many case studies that prove that refined carbohydrates are the underlying cause of violent and irrational behavior. But still the quacks of authority are exercising the application of Ritalin on children instead of themselves. Plain and simple the chemical structure in Ritalin, Zoloft, Prozac or any mind altering drug is causing maximum disharmony with the psyche of any healthy individual. The administration of these drugs is a medical sin and is manufactured not for the good, but for the financial gain and evil intent. So, modify and be more mindful of what you and your children consume. If it is refined, enriched, adulterated or chemically created, avoid it. Find a health food store or grow it yourself!

Youth Violence

The diet of youths today is a disaster. It usually begins with a high-carbohydrate breakfast cereal (the box that the cereal is in is more nutritious than the cereal itself) then the child is inundated at school with soft drinks (soften your bones) and junk food from vending machines throughout the day. In many families, dinner consists of carryout or convenience foods. No wonder our young people are subject to depression, psychological problems and, in a number of cases, senseless violence.

Constant parental guidance was available fifty years ago, with the mother at home cooking good wholesome meals and providing on-the-spot emotional support. Ever since higher taxes forced both parents to work outside the home, purchase factory foods and allow unsupervised television programming that breeds rampant materialism latch-key kids have been killing for fashionable clothes, and joining gangs as a substitute for the caring intimacy no longer provided by their family. All these contribute to our sick society, but the major culprit is processed food.

What specific nutrients are missing from their diets? The four primary nutrients missing are zinc, iron, B vitamins, and protein. Zinc is perhaps the single most common nutritional deficiency in the American population. Estimates are that more than 80% of the population is deficient in zinc. As a result of that deficiency, people's immune systems are impaired, they're not able to resist infectious diseases and it impairs neurological function.

So many young children are raised with nutritional imbalances which then distort their mental function, their mood, their response to stress and their ability to be successful in modern society. At the same time we have B-vitamin deficiencies, which is interesting because so many of the popular food products sold in grocery stores all over the country and around the world actually deplete the body of B vitamins. For example, when a person eats a donut, that donut contains both white flour and added sugars, which deplete the body of B vitamins, causing deficiencies. And it is these deficiencies that lead to antisocial behavior, aggressive behavior and ultimately criminal behavior-especially among males.

Instead of spending a few dollars a month on nutritional supplements that would prevent these chronic diseases and aggressive behaviors, we end up spending hundreds of billions of dollars a year on building new prisons and treating people with expensive prescriptions and mind-altering drugs. When it comes to children, for example, instead of giving them the food they need to be healthy, which prevents these disorders, we dose them on Ritalin, antidepressants and mind-altering drugs. This is good for the drug pushers (pharmaceutical companies), but it impairs the child's learning capability while at the same time increasing the child's risk of violent behavior and suicide.

Another point worth mentioning here is that the national food supply doesn't offer consumers sufficient quantities of these vitamins and minerals. There's a great myth out there that is frequently promoted by conventionally trained medical doctors that says you get all the nutrition you need from eating three balanced meals a day. But this is nothing more than a myth. "Three balanced meals a day" is meaningless because a lot of people think that one breakfast at Denny's, lunch at McDonalds and dinner at home with macaroni and cheese (mucous pie) is "balanced." It is neither balanced nor a meal. It's simply junk food that promotes chronic disease, obesity, and depression to name a few.

As anyone can plainly see that the majority of youth in America and across most of the so-called "civilized nations" of the world are drowning in the cesspools of moral bankruptcy, irresponsibility, and sexual promiscuity that a solution is needed like yesterday. Essentially, we are raising tomorrow's criminals. Right now in America, we have a system that literally gives rise to a population of emotionally imbalanced, mentally deranged criminals. And they are that way because, in part, they don't have good nutrition. They simply don't get the vitamins and minerals that their nervous systems need to fully develop and function in a healthy way.

The following are modern processed foods that contribute to violence:

Soy Infant Formula: Very high in inorganic manganese against which a baby's brain has no protection. High levels of manganese in the brain have been linked to violent criminal tendencies.

Refined Sugar and White Flour: Empty carbohydrates = same effect as cocaine.

Cold Breakfast Cereals: The process of making cereals creates chaotic protein fragments which can have neurotoxic effects; processed grain extruded products block assimilation of zinc in the body.

MSG and artificial flavors: Consumption of MSG has been associated with violent behavior.

Infant feeding: Crucial for the development of tomorrow's youth

The chief aim of corporations is to maximize profits by expanding markets, increasing the use of products, inventing new products and extending the length of their use. Their greed appears insatiable as more and more babies suck rubber in vain searching for the juice of life. Their main concern is profit, not public health. It's clear that breastfeeding is not good for the baby food industry. The baby food industry (which includes the production of bottles and nipples) is an eight-billion-dollar a year industry with an enormous profit margin and vicious intercompany competition. Corporations invest only to maximize their returns. Formula companies give money to doctors, nurses, medical students and department of pediatrics for research, equipment, gifts, payments, conferences, travel and publications, with the goal of enlisting their endorsement and promotion of their products.

Money spent on promotion and lobbying means less for quality control, research and basic ingredients. WHO (Wicked Health Organization) has recommended that docosahexaenoic acid (DHA), essential to infant brain development, be added to infant formula. Europe and Asia have done this but formula makers in the US have resisted. We're sure profits are the underlining cause for this resistance. Infant food companies influence government health policies and have made the medical profession their handmaiden. They use "science" to scare mothers, exploit women's working rights and men's desires to adapt to family realities. Aggressive formula marketing has deceived mothers into believing that formula is equivalent to breast milk. Good lactating breasts have been removed from the mouths of infants and promoted only as sexual organs.

With restrictions to formula distribution, the corporations become more devious, lobbying governments, challenging the law and establishing clinics and hospitals as marketing agents and centers. When other promotion avenues fail, companies go directly to governments to meet their needs. The formula industry was able to persuade the FDA to classify formula as a food, not a drug, so that they would be subject to less stringent review. The FDA allows the use of soy protein isolate even though it does not have Generally Recognized as Safe (GRAS) status.

There are financial incentives for governments to import infant foods. Governments get extra income through sales taxes and import duties. In Zimbabwe, income is generated for governments through the 17.5 percent sales tax on imported formula and a 10 percent import duty. Thus, the government shares in the profits when mothers abandon breastfeeding.

WHAT'S IN INFANT FORMULA?

Water: Tap water which contains fluoride & chlorine.

Corn Syrup: Contains glucose. Mother's milk contains lactose as the main carbohydrate. It destroys the pancreas setting the stage for infantile diabetes.

Soy Oil: Genetic, chemically laced with aluminum, rancid.

Soy Protein Isolate: Highly processed, contains estrogens that adversely affect baby's hormonal development and depress thyroid function.

Carrageenan: Extremely hard to digest. Main cause of digestive disorders in formula-fed infants. Caused liver problems and retarded growth in rats.

Soy Lecithin: Waste product of the soy industry. High in pesticides.

Synthetic Vitamins: Opposite effect of natural vitamins naturally occurring in real food.

Free Glutamic Acid (MSG) and Aspartic Acid: Neurotoxins that destroy the development of the nervous system.

US INFANT FORMULA RECALLS 1982-1994

1985 Cow & Gate Improved Modified Infant: Deficient in copper & linoleic acid
1986 SMA Ready to Feed (Wyeth Labs): Curdling, discoloration
1993 Nutramigen (Mead Johnson): Glass Contamination
1994 Soyalac (Nutricia Inc.): Salmonella contamination

Myth of ADHD

The vast majority of Ritalin and Adderall are given to school children to treat an alleged disease called ADHD (Attention Deficient Hyperactivity Disorder). Children suffer from ADHD are said to be in attentive, impulsive, and hyperactive. They often get bored easily in class squirm in their seats, are always on the go, or don't get along with other students or the teacher. In other words, many children diagnosed with ADHD may simply be normal kids, full of energy, and bored out of their minds sitting in mind-numbing, public or private-school classrooms.

Boredom is not the only reason children can exhibit symptoms of ADHD. Perfectly normal children who are over-active (have a lot of energy), rebellious, impulsive, day-dreamers, sensitive, undisciplined, bored easily (because they are bright), slow in learning, immature, troubled (for any number of reasons), learning disabled (dyslexia, for example), can also be inattentive, impulsive, or hyperactive.

Many factors outside the classroom can stress or emotionally affect children, causing some children to exhibit ADHD-like symptoms." Some of these factors are: not getting love, closeness, or attention from their parents; if a parent, friend, or sibling is sick or dies; if the parents are divorcing and there is anger, shouting, or conflict at home; domestic violence at home; sexual, physical, or emotional abuse by parents or siblings; inattention and neglect at home; personality clashes with parents or siblings; envy or cruelty directed at a child by classmates or by siblings at home, and many other factors.

Also, many other medical conditions can cause children to mimic some or all of ADHD's symptoms. Some of these conditions are: hypoglycemic (low blood sugar), allergies, learning disabilities, hyper or hypothyroidism, hearing and vision problems, mild to high lead levels, toxin exposures, sleeping disorders, high mercury levels, iron deficiency, worms, parasites, and malnutrition to name a few.

Since these medical conditions can cause some or all of ADHD's symptoms, it becomes next to impossible for any teacher, principal, or family doctor to claim with any certainty that a child has ADHD. To be certain, a doctor would have to test the child for all these other possible medical conditions. Since parents or doctors don't do this, every diagnosis of ADHD is one big fat LIE!

Many reputable authorities deny that ADHD, the disorder for which Ritalin (kiddy crack) is most commonly prescribed, even exists. According to Breggin in "Talking Back to Ritalin,"

"There are no objective diagnostic criteria for ADHD… no physical symptoms, no neurological signs, and no blood tests. ADHD and Ritalin are American and Canadian medical fads. The U.S. uses 90% of the world's Ritalin…there is no solid evidence that ADHD is a genuine disorder or disease of any kind… there is NO PROOF of any physical abnormalities in the brains or bodies of children who are routinely labeled ADHD. They do not have known biochemical imbalances or 'crossed wires'…ADHD is a controversial diagnosis with little or no scientific basis…. A parent, teacher, or doctor can feel in good company when utterly dismissing the diagnosis and refusing to apply it to children."

In other words, by labeling these normal personality traits of children a "disease," public school authorities in many states can now pressure parents to give their children mind-altering drugs to make the kids "behave" in class. This is a classic case of blaming the victim, the children, for public or private schools' education disorder.

Parents do not fall for the ADHD arguments that some public or private school authorities are now attempting to foist on you and your children. Although a few children do exhibit extreme "symptoms" ADHD, for most normal kids ADDHD turns out to be a questionable 'disease' at best, and a bogus disease at worst. Parents do not succumb to the temptation to drug your children with mind-altering drugs because a public-school teacher or school nurse tells you that your child is not "behaving properly" or "paying attention" in class. There are many other ways to deal with children's "behavior" problems in school besides drugging your children. One of the best ways is to take your children out of public school so they aren't bored to death sitting in public school classrooms. When children get engrossed in learning in a stimulating home school environment, they are far less likely to misbehave.

Healthy School Lunches

School lunches can be healthy and can serve as a model for healthy eating of other meals. A dietary experiment producing dramatic success in teenage athletics, academics and morale over a ten year period in the 1960s at Helix High School in San Diego County, California, has been preserved on video(1). This documentary gives specific recommendations by improving cafeteria lunches, and suggests that the money saved reducing athletic injuries and insurance costs was significant. Also shown in the documentary is the Georgia school system of over 70 schools that successfully modeled their program after Helix High School. Another example of a holistic lunch program was also done in Appleton, Wisconsin in 2003 and it is still being used today.

Recommendations for child health (mental & physical):

1 teaspoon: Cod Liver Oil/daily-seek out companies such as Carlson, Nordic Naturals, or Quantum Nutrition.

B-Complex: 50 mg/daily-seek out companies such as New Chapter or Mega Foods.

Heavy Metal Detox: use Metal Flush by Chi Enterprises (714) 777-1542

1. The video is available from the Price-Pottenger Nutrition Foundation (619) 462-7600, info@price-pottenger.org

31. FRANKENFOODS: THE GENETICALLY MODIFIED FOOD CHAIN

"The CDC (Center for Disease Control) now says that food is responsible for twice the number of illnesses in the United States as scientists thought just seven years ago.... At least 80 percent of the food-related illnesses are caused by toxins or other pathogens that scientists cannot even identify." New York Times, March 18, 2001

Since the above quote was mentioned over three years ago there have been 35,000 deaths, over 2 million hospitalizations, and 500 million illnesses related to food. And, these are only the REPORTED CASES. This increase roughly corresponds to the eating period since Americans have been eating GM (Genetic Modified) foods. During this time, obesity has become a national concern. Back in 1990, not one state reported 15 percent or more of its population as obese. By 2001, only one state remained in this lower obesity category. Diabetes has risen by a phenomenal 52 percent in just 14 years (1990-2004). Lymphatic cancers are increasing, and many other illnesses are on the rise.

All living things have been wondrously and marvelously made by the Creator and are unique and distinct unto their kind. Consequently, all living organisms, both plants and animals, have unique gene codes written into their DNA. These codes are the blueprints that make each God-created species distinct. Each gene represents a specific trait for that particular species. DNA is the primary genetic material that contains and transmits this biological information from generation to generation. Through genetic alteration, scientists and researchers are now able to artificially modify the DNA code within a species and, worse yet, transfer genes from one species to another. This is what creates genetically modified organisms.

More worrisome than the unpredictable nutrition in GM foods are the effects of introducing proteins previously unknown to humans. Current biotech foods carry genes from bacteria, viruses, and other organisms. Without testing, we do not know what the allergy-causing potential of each of these foods might be. What we do know is that people went into anaphylactic shock and some died from eating Starlink GM corn. This product from Aventis (a Swiss company) was not approved for human consumption. Eventually, it was found in tacos, tortillas, and other corn products (remember Taco Bell). Over 300 items were recalled and Aventis paid out an estimated $1 billion for the contamination. Even though very little acreage was dedicated to raising corn from these bad seeds, Aventis admitted that due to cross pollination and other factors, Starlink would remain in the food supply FOREVER.

On the other hand, Roundup Ready soybeans are still on the market. In fact, 90 percent of the U.S. soybean crop is GMOs (Genetic Modified Organisms). In March 1999, scientists at the UK's York Laboratory (Europe's leading food sensitivity specialists) discovered that soy allergy had jumped 50 percent from the previous year. People reacted with a range of chronic illnesses, including irritable bowel syndrome, digestion problems, and skin complaints. They also suffered neurological conditions with chronic fatigue syndrome, headaches, and lethargy. Scientists confirmed the link with soy by detecting increased levels of antibodies in the blood of the patients. At the time, most of the soy in the UK was imported from the U.S. and contained a significant amount of the Roundup Ready variety.

A public health disaster was narrowly averted in 1996 when a group of researchers tried to improve soybeans by giving them a gene from the Brazil nut. The goal was to improve the nutritional value of soybeans by forcing them to produce more methionine, an essential amino acid. The gene from the Brazil nut was successfully transferred to soybeans. Many people are allergic to nuts, particularly Brazil nuts. In some people, allergic reaction to Brazil nuts is swift and fatal (Dr. Whitaker can verify with the previous sentence, although the outcome was not fatal, the allergic reaction was brutal). This is just one example of how these deadly Franken foods can have a devastating effect upon the human population.

Roundup Ready crops share gene sequences identical to those found in a shrimp allergen and in a house dust mite allergen. In 2002, Dutch scientists discovered the sequences in the two herbicide resistant proteins, which occur in the Monsanto-owned GMOs. In this country, soy and soy derivatives are ingredients in more than 60 percent of all processed foods. GM soy is mixed with natural soy and the foods are not labeled. Once again, the FDA relies entirely on each company's own safety assessments, as it does for all GM crops. This is critical in regards to the risk to children. Children are three to four times more susceptible to allergies than adults. Infants (less than two years) have the highest incidence of reactions. They are especially sensitive to new allergens in their diets. The corporate controlled mass media have largely maintained silence about the genetic engineering revolution in agriculture, and government regulators have imposed no labeling requirements, so the public has little or no knowledge that genetically altered foods are already being sold in grocery stores everywhere, and that soon few traditional foods will remain on the shelves.

Three federal agencies regulate genetically-engineered crops and foods: the U.S Department of Agriculture (USDA), the U.S. Food and Drug Administration (FDA), and the U.S. Environmental Protection Agency (EPA). The heads of all three agencies are on record with speeches that make them sound remarkably like cheerleaders for genetic engineering, rather than impartial judges of a novel and powerful new technology, and all three agencies have set policies that:

1) No public records need be kept of which farms are using genetically-engineered seeds.

2) Companies that buy from farmers and sell to food manufacturers and grocery chains do not need to keep genetically-engineered crops separate from traditional crops, so purchasers have no way to avoid purchasing genetically engineered foods.

3) No one needs to label any crops, or any food products, with information about their genetically engineered origins, so consumers have no way to exercise informed choice in the grocery store. In the U.S., every food carries a label listing its important ingredients, with the remarkable exception of genetically engineered foods.

These policies have two main effects:
1) They have kept the public in the dark about the rapid spread of genetically engineered foods onto the family dinner table, and

2) They will prevent epidemiologists from being able to trace health effects, should any appear, because no one will know who has been exposed to novel gene products and who has not.

Today Pillsbury food products are made from genetically-engineered crops. Other foods that are now genetically engineered include Crisco; Kraft salad dressings; Nestlé's chocolate; Green Giant harvest burgers; Parkay margarine; Isomil and Prosobee infant formulas; and Wesson vegetable oils. Fritos, Doritos, Tostitos and Ruffles Chips and French fried potatoes sold by McDonalds are genetically engineered.

It is safe to say that never before in the history of the world has such a rapid and large-scale revolution occurred in a nation's food supply. And not just the U.S. is target for change. The genetic engineering companies (all of whom used to be chemical companies)-Dow, DuPont, Novartis, and preeminently, Monsanto, are aggressively promoting their genetically engineered seeds in Europe, Brazil, Argentina, Mexico, India, China, Africa, and elsewhere. Huge opposition has developed to Monsanto's technology everywhere it has been introduced outside the United States. Only in the U.S. has the "a biotech" revolution been greeted with a dazed silence.

Monsanto, the clear leader in genetically engineered crops argues that genetic engineering is necessary if the world's food supply is to keep up with human population growth. Monsanto says. that without genetic engineering, billions will starve. However, neither Monsanto nor any other genetic engineering company appears to be developing genetically engineered crops that might solve global food shortages. Quite the opposite! Monsanto is America's most dangerous criminal. History will judge them to be murderers. Since their creation of Agent Orange, Monsanto has introduced many horrible chemicals into our food supply and environment. History will reveal that George Bush was elected by a key vote from one Supreme Court Justice who also served as Monsanto's attorney (Clarence Thomas). History will also expose that the George Bush cabinet was filled with employees and friends of Monsanto, from Cheney to Ashcroft to Rumsfeld. Two others from our Monsanto's "hall of shame" include Secretary of Agriculture Ann Veneman (who was on the board of directors of Biogen), and FDA's boss Tommy Thomson, Secretary of the Department of Health and Human Services. Thompson was Monsanto's bed partner as governor of Wisconsin, investing over $300 million of state funds to promote GMO's. We also would like to mention that Bill "Slick" Clinton praised Monsanto in his state-of-the union address while in office.

If genetically engineered crops were aimed at feeding the hungry, then Monsanto and the others would be developing seeds with certain predictable characteristics: (a) ability to grow on substandard or marginal soil; (b) plants able to produce more high-quality protein, with increased per-acre yield, without increasing the need for expensive machinery, chemicals, fertilizers, or water; (c) they would aim to favor small farms over larger farms; (d) the seeds would be cheap and freely available without restrictive licensing; and (e) they would be for crops that feed people, not animals.

None of the genetically engineered crops now available or in development (to the extent that these have been announced) has any of these desirable characteristics. The new genetically engineered seeds require high-quality soils, enormous investment in machinery, and increased use of chemicals. There is evidence that their per-acre yields are about 10% lower than traditional varieties (at least in the case of soybeans), and they produce crops largely intended as feed for animals, not to provide protein for people. The genetic revolution has nothing to do with feeding the world's hungry.

Crops are genetically modified chiefly as a way to sell more pesticides. In some cases, the modified crops change the pesticides themselves, giving them new toxicity. The herbicide bromoxynil falls into this category. Bromoxynil is already recognized by the U.S. EPA as a carcinogen and as a teratogen (causes birth defects). Calgene (now owned by Monsanto) developed a strain of cotton plants called BXN Cotton that can withstand direct spraying with bromoxynil. Unfortunately, the bromoxynil–resistant gene in cotton modifies the bromoxynil, turning it into a chemical byproduct called DBHA, which is at least as toxic as bromoxynil itself. Although humans do not eat cotton, traditional silage for cattle contains up to 50% cotton slash, gin mill leavings, and cotton debris. Both bromoxynil and DBHA are fat-soluble, so they accumulate in the fat of animals. Therefore, DBHA will make its way into the human food chain through meat. Furthermore, cottonseed oil is widely used as a direct human food and as a cooking additive.

In rats and rabbits, bromoxynil causes serious birth defects, including changes in the bones of the spine and skull, and hydrocephaly (water on the brain). These birth defects appear in offspring at doses of bromoxynil that are not toxic to the mother. Despite these findings and despite a law (the Food Quality Protection Act of 1996) that explicitly gives the EPA the power to reduce exposure standards to protect infants, the EPA in 1997 declined to require a special safety factor to protect children from bromoxynil. Lastly, when the EPA added up the cancer-causing potential of bromoxynil, they found bromoxynil to be 2.7 per million, and they promptly declared this to be "well within" the one-in-a-million regulatory limit. Is 2.7 less than one? Somebody help us!

Most fundamentally, GMO crops substitute human wisdom for the wisdom of nature. As GMO crops are planted on tens of millions of acres, the diversity of our agricultural systems is being further diminished. Genetic engineering is by far the most powerful technology humans have ever discovered, and it is being deployed by the same corporations that, historically, have produced one large-scale calamity after another. In sum, Monsanto is achieving a complete monopoly of the soy crop and progressing very quickly to monopolize every major food crop here and abroad. If something does not change soon, it is safe to predict that a small number of "life science" corporations (they like calling themselves) will have a monopoly on the seed needed to raise all of the world's major food crops. Then the hungry, like the well-fed, will have to pay the owners of this new technology for permission to eat.

Genetically Modified Foods in American Crops:

Soy (90%), cotton (75%), canola (70%), corn (50%), Hawaiian papaya (over 60%), a small amount of zucchini and yellow squash, and Quest brand tobacco.

Dairy products from cows injected with rBST & cloned animals which were recently approved by your FDA for human consumption.

Food additives, enzymes, flavorings, and processing agents, including aspartame, and the rennet used to make hard cheeses; meat, eggs, and dairy products from animals that have eaten GM feed; honey and bee pollen that may have GM sources of pollen.

URGENT SPECIAL NOTE:
To avoid GMO food products check your produce tag number. There will be four or five numbers on a sticker on the produce you pick. If the sticker has four numbers it was grown conventionally, if the sticker has five numbers and the first one begins with an 8 then it's genetic, if the sticker has five numbers and begins with a 9 then it is organic.

30. THE REAL PROBLEM WITH COMMERCIAL MEATS

"He caused the grass to grow for the cattle, and herb for the service of man: that he may bring forth food out of the earth" Psalms 104:14

America is the land of meat, meat and more meat. Beef, poultry, farm-raised fish, factory eggs, milk, and other meat by-products are the backbone of the standard American diet and most of the so-called civilized world. Physiologically, meat gives the human organism an immediate burst of energy and strength. It was this raw power that allowed nomadic tribes of Indo-Europeans to over run traditional grain and vegetable consuming cultures in ancient Greece, Italy, the Near East, and India. In the Americas, heavy meat-centered diets enabled pioneers to level whole regions of the continent quickly and efficiently, though at high cost to the native peoples and their environment.

While meats and processed meat by-products are a part of the traditional American diet, it is massively commercialized. Though America over consumes commercial meat, which leads to a variety of health complications, the other major problem is how the meat is slaughtered, processed and packaged. The first problem is that America's commercial cattle are improperly fed. The grain supply contains many toxic by-products, non foods, meat scraps, hormones and antibiotics. As this feed fattens the cattle at an enormous rate, the chemicals and other by-products build toxicity within the cattle's body and by the time it arrives to your kitchen table, the chemical and hormone toxicity is consumed right along with the meat, making it a MediSin.

The next problem is that the cattle are improperly slaughtered. Since the commercial cow is in a state of fear and is anticipating death, adrenalin rushes throughout the flesh creating more toxicity. This unholy toxic slaughtering procedure also arrives at your dinner table making it a MediSin. John Robbin's video, "Diet for a New America" captures a very good example of how nasty the meat processing is really achieved.

HEY MOMS, HOT DOGS DO BITE!

So what's wrong with hot dogs? Well, according to several different studies it has been concluded that this standard America picnic, ballpark and birthday party treat is actually a MediSin, because it is a risk factor for childhood cancer. Peters et al studied the relationship between the intake of certain foods and the risk of leukemia in children from birth to age ten in Los Angeles between 1980 and 1987. The study found that children eating more than 12 hot dogs per month have nine times the normal risk of developing childhood leukemia. A strong risk for childhood leukemia also existed for those children whose fathers' intake of hot dogs was 12 or more per month, according to one study conducted at the University of Southern California (USC) School of Medicine. The USC study tested other possible links to childhood cancer such as the consumption of other "danger" foods (among them bacon, sausage and corned beef).

How do hotdogs cause cancer?
The same preservatives in commercial meats are in hotdogs: sodium nitrates and nitrites which are a cancer causing preservative, used primarily to fight botulism. During the cooking process, nitrites combine with amines naturally present in meat to form carcinogenic nitrosamines, which have been shown to cause cancer in laboratory animals by forming tight chemical bonds to DNA.

Is there an alternative to commercial hotdogs?
Yes there is. It is only the commercial hotdog that appears to be a risk. Many health food stores now offer brands that understand the danger of nitrites and nitrates, so they manufacture nitrate free hotdogs made from properly slaughtered meats. So you don't have to give up your favorite past time social food. Just

be more selective and don't over consume. When you consume commercially processed meat, you also consume all of the commercial crap that comes along with it. What we have found to be a much healthier selection is "grass fed, halal or kosher beef, lamb, goat, buffalo or venison. These selections of meat are properly slaughtered (allowed to fully bleed the initial blood from the body before processing) and processed. Grass fed beef and lamb even have a natural chemical called CLA (conjugated linoleic acid) which has been shown to encourage weight loss, lean muscle mass and can stimulate the immune system, even against cancer.

THE OTHER WHITE MEAT, SCIENTIFIC VIEW OF THE HOG

We have reason to believe that God made the pig for a unique purpose other than for eating. Make no mistake about it, the Creator declared the *"other white meat"* that is loved so much by the masses as unclean for food for logical reasons (see Leviticus chapter 11 or the Quran chapter 5).

One major observation of the swine is its sty. When you straighten out its forelegs you will see an open sore a few inches above the pig's foot on the inner side. If you would grasp the leg high up and press downward, you would witness a discharge. This discharge is waste matter that has to be conveyed through this unique system of drainage. The liver of the pig is full of abscesses which develop millions of embryonic worms consisting of a pair of hook worms. The shape of these worms forms a twisting motion which will cause them to penetrate the tissue in the fashion of a corkscrew. Countless number of these worms may be taken into the system since a single tapeworm is capable of producing more than two million eggs. According to the Chicago Academy of Medicine the "other white meat' also contains the deadly Trichinae parasite. This parasite is enclosed in a little cyst or sac, which, when taken into the stomach is dissolved by the gastric juice. The parasite eventually penetrates the walls of your stomach and gradually works its way throughout the whole muscular system then on to the bone tissue. It has been scientifically proven that pork consumption proliferates arthritis, heart disease, diabetes and other life-taxing illnesses.

Dr. Glen Shephered wrote an article on the dangers of eating pork in the 31st May, 1952 issue of the Washington Post, and the following extracts are taken from that article:

"One in six people in the United States of America and Canada have worms in their muscles-Trichinosis-from eating pork infested with Trichnis. Many people so infected have no symptoms. Most of those who do have, recover slowly. Some die. Some are reduced to permanent invalids. All were careless pork eaters." He continues: *"No one is immune from this disease and there is no cure. Neither antibiotics nor drugs nor vaccines affect these tiny deadly worms."* After reading these statements of Dr. Shephered, we can presume that there is no guarantee of immunity when eating pork which is affected by Trichinosis worm.

Another parasite that was discovered in the pig by Tom Cobbold (1875) and Mark Looss (1907) was the Clonorchis Sinesis. The Clonorchis Sinesis is a sucking worm, a kind of parasite which inhibits the bile passage of a pig's liver, which is a source of these parasites infecting people in close contact with pigs. The occurrence of the disease in China, Formosa, Japan, Korea and Southern India again points to the close association with pigs. This parasite created many serious diseases of the liver and the chest in human beings. If this parasite is present in the lungs, it may cause pneumonia, if it is in the air tubes it causes suffocation and if in the intestines, it causes intestinal obstruction, or acute pancreatitis. Then there is Clonorchiasis, a peculiar liver disease. The liver becomes enlarged accompanied with severe jaundice, diarrhea and emaciation. This disease could be fatal. Medical science, in spite of its strenuous efforts, has not yet been able to produce any specific treatment for it. Complications caused by this disease are stone formation in the liver and cancer. To eat pork, then, is an extremely risky gamble with one's health.

In directing the dietary principles of the children of Israel and thereafter of the Muslims, God meant these rules to be a source of continued benefit to mankind. The transfer of disease, as modern medical research has substantiated, would be adequate justification for this divine law.

33. SOY: THE MEATLESS DECEPTION

"Doctors give drugs of which they know little into bodies, of which they know less, for diseases of which they know nothing at all
-Voltaire

For the past decade, an unfermented and genetic bean has swept America like Hurricane Ivan. This inexpensive plant has been touted as America's new health food by newspapers, magazines, and best selling health writers proclaiming the "joy of soy" as the key to disease prevention and maximum longevity.

Americans rarely hear anything negative about soy. Thanks to the unethical public relations campaign waged by Archer Daniels Midland (ADM), Protein Technologies International (PTI), the American Soybean Association, Monsanto, and the Food and Drug Administration's (FDA) 1999 approval of the health claim that soy protein lowers cholesterol, soy maintains a "healthy" image. The truth unfortunately is far more complex. Unfermented soy foods come in a variety of forms, including many heavily processed modern products such as soy burgers and soy cheese. Most important, many respected scientists have issued warnings stating that the possible benefits of eating unfermented soy should be weighed against the proven risks. Indeed, thousands of studies link unfermented soy to malnutrition, digestive distress, immune-system breakdown, thyroid dysfunction, cognitive decline, reproductive disorders, infertility, cancer and heart disease.

Those who dare speak about this over-exaggerated bean get stares and one stock answers: Soy foods could not possibly have a downside because Asians eat large quantities of soy every day and consequently remain free of most western diseases. In fact, the people of China, Japan, and other countries in Asia eat very little or if any unfermented soy. Having lived in South Korea for two years myself (Dr. Whitaker), I never saw soy in any Korean Restaurants as the main course. The soy industry's own figures show that soy consumption in China, Indonesia, Korea, Japan, and Taiwan ranges from 9.3 to 36 grams per day.(1) That's grams of soy food, not grams of soy protein alone. Compare this with a cup of tofu (252 grams) or soy milk (240 grams). (2) Many gullible Americans today think nothing of consuming a cup of tofu, a couple glasses of soy milk, handfuls of soy nuts, soy "energy bars, " and veggie burgers. Infants on soy formula receive loads of estrogen in quantity and in proportion to body weight. Infants' consuming an eight ounce glass of soy milk is equivalent of five birth control pills in a single setting due to the high estrogen levels of the unfermented soy bean.

In short, there is no historical precedent for eating the large amounts of unfermented soy food now being consumed by infants fed soy formula, and vegetarians who favor soy as their main source of protein, or for the large amounts of soy being recommended by Dr. Andrew Weil, Dr. Christiane Northrup, and many other popular so-called health experts.

What's more, the rural poor in China have never seen–let alone feasted on-soy sausages, chili made with Textured Vegetable Protein (TVP), tofu cheesecake, packaged soy milk, soy "energy bars," or other newfangled soy products that have infiltrated the American marketplace. The ancient Chinese honored the soybean with the name "the yellow jewel" but used it as "green manure" –a cover crop plowed under to enrich soil. Soy did not become human food until late in the Chou Dynasty (1134-246 B.C), when the Chinese developed a fermentation process to make soybean paste, best known today by it's Japanese name, miso. (3) Soy sauce–the natural type sold under the Japanese name Shoyu-began as a liquid poured off during the production of miso. Two other popular fermented soy foods, natto and tempeh entered the food supply around 1,000 A.D. or later in Japan and Indonesia, respectively. The Chinese never ate boiled or baked unfermented soybeans or cooked with soy flour except in times of famine. Modern soy products such as soy protein isolate, TVP, soy-protein concentrate, and other soy-protein products made using high-tech industrial processes, were UNKNOWN in Asia until after WW II.(4)

Contrary to popular belief, neither soymilk nor soy infant formula is traditional in Asia. Soy milk originated as a waste product through the process of making tofu, the earliest reference to it as a beverage appeared in 1866. (5) By the 1920s and 1930s, it was popular in Asia as an occasional drink served to the elderly. (6-8) The first person to manufacture soy milk in China was an American-Henry Miller, a Seventh Day Adventist physician and missionary. (9)

Unfermented soy protein isolate lurks in nearly 65 percent of the foods sold in supermarkets and natural food stores. Much of this is hidden in products where it would not ordinarily be expected, such as fast-food burgers and Bumblebee canned tuna. There's nothing natural about modern unfermented soy protein products. The process of making soy protein isolate (SPI) begins with defatted soybean meal, which is mixed with a caustic alkaline solution to remove the fiber, then washed in an acid solution to precipitate out the protein. The protein curds are then dipped into another alkaline solution and spray-dried at extremely high temperatures. These refining processes remove the nasty smell and flavor, but vitamin, mineral, and protein quality are sacrificed and levels of carcinogens such as nitrosamines are increased. (17-22) SPIs appear in so many products that consumers would never guess that the Federation of American Societies for Experimental Biology (FASEB) decreed in 1979 that the only safe use for SPIs was for sealers for CARDBOARD PACKAGES. (23)

Scientists who have studied the use of unfermented soy protein in animal feeds over the years have discovered a number of components in soy that cause poor growth, digestive distress, malnutrition and infertility. The best known case concerns the cheetahs at the Cincinnati Zoo. In the 1980s, Kenneth D.R. Setchell, Ph.D. discovered one reason the big cats were not reproducing. The female cheetahs were suffering from liver disease and reproductive failure caused by the high concentrations of unfermented soy in their feed. The phytic acid in unfermented soy blocks mineral absorption, causing zinc, iron, and calcium deficiencies. (29-34) Lectins and saponins have caused leaky gut syndrome and immune dysfunction. (35-36) Oxalates surprisingly high in unfermented soy may cause problems for people prone to kidney stones and women suffering from vulvodyna, a painful condition marked by burning, stinging, and itching of the external genitalia. (37) Finally, oligosaccharides give soy its notorious reputation as a gas producer. Although these are present in all beans, soy is such a powerful "musical fruit" that the soy industry has identified "the flatulence factor" as a major obstacle that must be overcome for soy to achieve full consumer acceptance (39, 40)

Unfermented soy is one of the top eight allergens that cause immediate hypersensitivity reactions such as coughing, sneezing, runny nose, hives, diarrhea, difficultly swallowing, and anaphylactic shock. Delayed allergic responses are even more common and occur anywhere from several hours to several days after the food is eaten. This MediSin has been linked to sleep disturbances, bedwetting, sinus and ear infections, crankiness, joint paint, chronic fatigue, gastrointestinal woes, and other mysterious symptoms. (52, 53)

Soy allergies are on the rise for three reasons: the growing use of soy infant formula (now 30 percent of the formula market), the increase in soy-containing foods in grocery stores, and the possibility of the greater allergen from genetically modified soybeans. (54) Although severe reactions to unfermented soy are rare compared to reactions to peanuts, tree nuts, fish, and shellfish, soy has been underestimated as a cause of food anaphylaxis. Recently, after a young girl in Sweden suffered an asthma attack and died after eating a hamburger that contained only 2.2 percent soy protein, Swedish researchers looked into a possible soybean connection. They concluded that the soy-in-the-hamburger case was not a fluke, and that minute amounts of soy "hidden" in regular food had caused four of the total of five deaths caused by allergic reactions in Sweden between 1993 and 1996. Of the children who suffered fatal attacks, all had been able to eat soy without any adverse reactions right up until the dinner that caused their deaths. (55) According to the Swedish Ministry of Health and Social Affairs, children at highest risk are those who suffer from peanut allergies and asthma; parents of such children should make every effort to eliminate all soy from their children's diets. (56)

More than 70 years of human, animal, and laboratory studies show that unfermented soybeans put the thyroid at risk. The chief culprits are the plant hormones or isoflavones. (57-59) The United Kingdom's Committee on Toxicology has identified several populations at special risk: Infants on soy formula, vegans who use soy as their principal meat and dairy replacements, and men and women who self-medicate with soy foods and/or isoflavone supplements in an attempt to prevent or reverse menopausal symptoms, cancer, or heart disease. (60)

Infants with congenital hypothyroidism need 20 to 25 percent higher doses of thyroxin drug than usual if they are bottle-fed with soy formula (61) Likewise, adults who boost their thyroid with drugs such as Synthroid while also eating thyroid-inhibiting foods such as soy, raw broccoli, raw cabbage, and raw cauliflower put extreme stress on their thyroid. Toxicologist Michael Fitzpatrick, PhD, points out that this is the way that researchers induce thyroid cancers in laboratory animals. (62)

Scientists have known since the mid-1940s that phyto-estrogens (plant estrogens) can impair fertility. Fertility problems in cows, sheep, rabbits, guinea pigs, birds, and mice have all been reported.(63-64) Although scientists only recently stated that soy lowers testosterone levels (65) tofu has traditionally been used in Buddhist monasteries to decrease libido, and by Japanese women to punish straying husbands. Humans and animals appear to be most vulnerable to the effects of soy estrogens during infancy, puberty, pregnancy, lactation, and during the hormonal shifts of menopause. Of all these groups, infants on soy formula are the most devastated since formula is their main source of 'nutrients.' (66-67)

A crucial time for the programming of the human reproduction system is right after birth, the very time when bottles of soy formula are given to many non-breast fed babies. Normally during this period, the body surges with natural estrogens, testosterones, and other hormones that are meant to program the baby's reproductive development from infancy through puberty and into adulthood. For infants on soy formula, this programming is interrupted. (68-70)

Male infants experience a testosterone surge during the first few months of life and produce androgens in amounts equal to those of adult men. So much testosterone at such a tender age is needed to program the body for puberty, the time when a male's sex organs should develop and he should begin to express male characteristics such as facial and pubic hair and a deep voice. If receptor sites intended for the hormone testosterone are occupied by soy estrogens, however, appropriate development may never take place. (71-74) To date, most of the evidence damning soy formula can be found only in animal studies, because investigations in which humans' sex hormone levels are lowered experimentally cannot ethically be done. However, in the years since soy formula has been in the marketplace, parents and pediatricians have reported growing numbers of boys whose physical maturation are either delayed or does not occur at all. We also feel that the increased interest in homosexuality in males is linked to this MediSin. Breast enlargement, nipple discharge, underdeveloped gonads, undecided testicles (cryptorchidism), and steroid insufficiencies are increasingly common. Sperm counts are also falling. (75-79)

Soy formula is bad news for girls as well. Natural estrogen levels approximately double during the first month of life, then decline and remain at low levels until puberty. With increased estrogens in the environment and diet, an alarming number of girls are entering puberty much earlier than normal.(80-82) Ten percent of girls now show signs of puberty, such as breast development or pubic hair, before the age of three. By the age of eight, 14.7 percent of Caucasian girls and 48.3 percent of African-American girls had one or both of these characteristics. (83) The fact that African-Americans experience earlier puberties than whites is not a racial difference but a recent phenomenon.
(84-85)

Most experts blame this epidemic of "precocious puberty" on environmental estrogens from plastics, pesticides, commercial meats, etc., but some pediatric endocrinologists believe that unfermented soy is a contributor. The author's strongly believe it is the unfermented soy causing all the damage. Of all the estrogens found in the environment, unfermented soy is the likeliest explanation of why African-American girls reach puberty so quickly. Is this some type of genocide? Since its establishment in 1974, the federal government's Women, Infants and Children (WIC) program had provided free infant formula to teenage and other low-income mothers while failing to encourage breastfeeding. Due to the perceived or real lactose intolerance, African-American babies are much more likely to receive soy formula than Caucasian babies.

Early maturation in girls heralds reproductive problems later in life, including amenorrhea (failure to menstruate), anovulatory cycles (cycles in which no egg is released), impaired follicular development (follicles failing to mature and develop into healthy eggs), erratic hormonal surges, and other problems associated with infertility. Since the mammary glands depend on estrogen for their development and functioning, the presence of soy estrogens at a susceptible time predispose girls to breast cancer, another condition that is on the rise and definitively linked to early puberty.

Recently, a team of researchers headed by Brian Strom, MD, studied the use of soy formula and its long-term impact on reproductive health. They announced only one adverse finding: longer, more painful menstrual periods among women who'd been fed soy formula in infancy.(88) Dr. Strom's conclusion that the results were "reassuring" made newspaper headlines all over the world, though the data in the body of the report was misleading. Indeed, data left out of the headlines and buried in the report revealed higher incidences of allergies, asthma, higher rates of cervical cancer, polycystic ovarian syndrome, blocked fallopian tubes, and pelvic inflammatory disease. (89) Although thyroid damage from soy formula has been the principal concern of critics for decades, the researchers excluded the thyroid function as a subject for study. Not surprisingly, this study was funded in part by the corrupt infant formula industry.

Most of the fears concerning soy formula have focused on estrogens. There are other problems as well, notably much higher levels of ALUMINUM, FLUORIDE, and MANGANESE than are found neither in breast milk or dairy formulas (90-96). All

three metals have the potential to adversely affect brain development. Although trace amounts of manganese are vital to the development of the brain, toxic levels accrued from ingestion of soy formula during infancy have been found in children suffering from attention-deficit disorders, dyslexia, and other learning problems.
(97-98)

Meanwhile, the jury is still out on whether unfermented soy might help alleviate menopausal symptoms or prevent osteoporosis and breast cancer. The soy industry's top scientists, convened at the Fifth International Symposium on the Role of Soy in the Preventing and Reversing Chronic Disease (Orlando 9/03), conceded that the data are confusing and contradictory, with some studies suggesting that soy might be helpful, and others showing that soy contributes to osteoporosis and promotes breast cancer. Well, if they're unsure, then who is making all these false claims about the "joy of soy"? Why is it certain that the levels of soy estrogens that might possibly have a beneficial effect on hormonally related diseases have been proven to jeopardize the health of the thyroid? Likewise, the 25 grams of soy protein per day touted by the FDA to lower cholesterol is very likely to harm the thyroid, and thus increase one of the risk factors for heart disease.

The bottom line is that the safety of unfermented soy foods has yet to be proven, and that human beings have become guinea pigs for the corporations. All these facts should make you think twice about using this MediSin in your diets. From a nutritional standpoint, think soy in separate categories: Non-fermented and fermented. The troubles we've documented are associated with using primarily processed, non-fermented, genetically modified soy foods such as soymilk, flour, nuts, baby formula, and the many more soy products flooding the market; as well as, foods on your grocery store shelves you do not know about that may contain soy. Studies have shown traditionally fermented soy-the form that is widely popular in many Asian countries-aids in preventing and reducing a variety of diseases including certain forms of heart disease and cancers. Why? Fermentation destroys the effect phytic acid has on your system and the beans being used are not genetic. Daniel Sheehan, formerly senior toxicologist with the FDA's National Center for Toxicological Research, has called this soy ploy a "large uncontrolled and basically unmonitored human experiment." (111)

34. COMMERCIAL DAIRY AND THE TRAGEDY OF FLO JO

The source of most commercial milk is the modern Holstein cow, bred to produce large quantities of milk three times as much as the old-fashioned cow (Jersey or Guernseys). She needs special feed and antibiotics to keep her well. Her milk contains high levels of growth hormone from her pituitary gland, even when she is spared the evils of genetically engineered Bovine Growth Hormone (rBGH) to push her to the udder limits of milk production. Real feed for cows is green grass in Spring, Summer and Fall; green feed, silage, hay, and root vegetables in Winter. It is not soy meal, cottonseed meal or other commercial feeds, nor is it bakery waste or chicken manure laced with pesticides. Soy meal has the wrong protein profile for the dairy cow, resulting in a short burst of high milk production followed by premature death.

Commercial milk is pasteurized and homogenized which destroys enzymes, diminishes vitamin content, denatures fragile milk proteins, destroys vitamin B12 and B6, kills beneficial bacteria, promotes pathogens and is associated with allergies, increased tooth decay, colic in infants, osteoporosis, arthritis, heart disease and cancer. Calves fed pasteurized milk die before maturity. Pasteurization laws favor large, industrialized dairy operations and squeeze out small farmers. The homogenization of commercial milk is a process that breaks down butterfat globules so they do not rise to the top. Homogenized milk has been linked to heart disease. Powdered skim milk, a source of dangerous oxidized cholesterol and neurotoxic amino acids, is added to 1% and 2% milk. Low-fat yogurts and sour creams contain mucopolysaccharide slime to give them body. Pale butter from hay-fed cows contains colorings to make it look like vitamin-rich butter from grass-fed cows. Bioengineered enzymes are used in large-scale cheese production. Many mass produced cheeses contain additives and colorings and imitation cheese products contain hydrogenated vegetable oils.

America's Food and Drug Administration approved the use of Monsanto's genetically engineered bovine growth hormone (rBGH) for cows in February 1994. Remarkably, milk from rBGH-treated test herds was allowed into America's supply seven years before actual approval. Since 1994, most of America's milk supply has been tainted with milk produced from cows injected with genetically modified organisms. The approval process for rBGH was the most controversial drug application in the history of the FDA. In order to address that controversy, the FDA published an article in the journal SCIENCE (August 24, 1990). Data in that paper revealed that the average male rat injected with rBGH developed a spleen 39.6 percent larger than the spleen of the control animals after just 90 days of treatment. The spleens from rBGH-treated females increased in size by a factor of 46 percent. Lab animals treated with rBGH developed lymphatic abnormalities.

Cows treated with Monsanto's rBGH produce milk with increased levels of another powerful hormone, IGF-I. There are hundreds of millions of different proteins in nature, and only one hormone that is identical between any two species. That powerful growth hormone, insulin-like growth factor, or IGF-I survive digestion and has been identified as a key factor in cancer's growth. IGF-I is identical in human and cow. The Lancet (vol. 351) reported in May 1998:

"Insulin-like growth factors (IGFs), in particular IGF-I and IGF-II, strongly stimulate the proliferation of a variety of cancer cells, including those from lung cancer. High plasma levels of IGF-I were associated with an increased risk of lung cancer. Plasma levels of IGF-I are higher...in patients with lung cancer than in control subjects."

Studies have indicated that levels of IGF-I can increase as much as 70 percent during milk pasteurization, and the meat of cows treated with rBGH has been found to contain unusually high amounts of IGF-I. One aspect of pasteurized dairy that is overlooked is the casein. Casein represents eighty percent of all milk protein, which is found in cheese, milk cream, butter and other products of the dairy family. This glue-like protein cannot be assimilated easily and begins to accumulate in an undigested state in the upper intestines putrefying and producing toxins leading to a weakening of the gastric and pancreatic systems, as well as heavy deposits of mucus in the cavities of the body (chest/head). Another problem with pasteurized dairy is that most individuals are lactose intolerant with the inability to breakdown the lactose or milk sugar in pasteurized dairy.

It turns out that 50 to 90 percent of the world's population groups with the exception of those of Scandinavian and European origin and some other groups of European ancestry, have an intolerance for cow's milk. Unfortunately, pasteurized dairy foods affect all organs and systems of the body. Since dairy is a product of the mammary gland, it primarily affects the human glands, especially the reproductive organs such as the breast, uterus, ovaries, thyroid, prostate, pituitary gland, the cerebral surrounding the mid-brain and the nasal cavities. The over-consumption of commercial dairy causes the accumulation of mucus, which would eventually proliferate, cysts, tumors, and finally cancer.

The accumulation of dairy deposits does not stop at the head and nasal passages. The accumulation of fatty deposits from pasteurized dairy also ends up in the kidneys and gallbladder, which eventually leads to stones from the inorganic calcium. Other complications with the over-consumption of commercial dairy are vaginal discharges, uterine cancer, ovarian cancer, breast cyst, and prostate cancer. More studies are now linking the consumption of dairy to a wide variety of sicknesses including anti-social behavior, iron-deficiency anemia, cramps, and aggressive children. It also has been found that more oxygen is needed to carry hemoglobin to cells enveloped with mucus. Dairy food consumption interrupts this process along with docile reactions and emotional dependency.

As Americans continue to ingest genetically engineered milk and dairy products, lymphatic cancer death rates have soared. Americans have become laboratory subjects in genetic engineering's experiment, and the resulting data indicates extreme cause for concern. Here is the number, as recently published by the SEER cancer statistics review and the National Cancer Institute. Rates are per 100,000 of population.

Result:

From 1980 to 2000, lymphoma cancer death rates increased 37.3 percent in males, and increased 26.4 percent in females.

If you are going to consume milk and other dairy products you have to locate a farmer you can trust and purchase from him/her. Locate a health food store where they carry organic preferably grass-fed, non-antibiotic and rBGH free milk. You can even find un-pasteurized milk with the cream still at the top in some natural food stores.

THE TRAGEDY OF FLO JO

Florence Griffith Joyner was an admired role model to all as a result of her Olympic achievements in track and field. She crossed ethnic and racial barriers, and her life became an inspiration to male and female, black and white, young and old. "Flo Jo", as she was most commonly known, was a wife and friend to Al Joyner and loving mother to her eight-year old daughter, Mary Ruth (Mo Jo). She combined her athletic ability with great looks, personality and business acumen to build a financial empire that included her line of unique clothing. She was in great demand as a motivational speaker, and major corporations would seek her personal endorsement of their products and services by offering enormous financial inducements.

We will also remember Flo Jo by her appearance as a model and spokeswoman for the dairy industry. She posed with a milk mustache, and in doing so might very well have been betrayed and killed by a product that did NOT do her body good. The identity of Flo Jo's killer is contained in the actual autopsy but the coroner did not have the vision to identify the evildoer. When no steroids were found the conclusion was made that her death was due to heart disease. Eleven days after the initial autopsy was completed, histological examination of brain tissues resulted in the final explanation: *"Positional Asphyxia due to EPILEPTIFORM SEIZURE."* Simply stated Flo Jo had an epileptic seizure and smothered in her pillow.

Flo Jo knew her body was filled with mucous. She was producing histamines, the body's natural anti-body defense to an invading antigen. Her solution was to take an antihistamine, BENADRYL. Her tracheobronchial tree contained mucous and frothy fluid. The coroner, aware that her last meal was PIZZA (eaten 15 hours earlier) called the brick-sized lump of undigested food with flecks appearing to be cheese in her stomach: *"digested food."* One wonders if this doctor ever took a class in nutrition. After 15 hours, food still in the stomach creates duress and can no way be called digested. Flo Jo's body pumped enormous amounts of histamines, which in turn created enormous amounts of mucous, filling her lungs, body organs and cavities with a tenacious glue. Epileptic seizures often result in damage to lips or tongue or cheeks. Flo Jo had no such damage. Strangulation usually breaks the tiny hyoid bone in the neck. Flo Jo's bone was intact. The black and blue, petechial marks were caused by Flo Jo herself, struggling violently to breathe, gasping for breath, which was impossible to take in. As her body died, asphyxiating, the brain triggered an emergency wake-up call, an electrical and biochemical jolt and seizure that could not clear Flo Jo's lungs. This failed jump-start later appeared as an epilepiform seizure on the coroner's report.

The one-armed killer has killed before. This demon is a CEREAL killer and remains free to kill over and over again. His name is the COMERCIAL DAIRY INDUSTRY and his murder weapon is the MILK MUSTACHE AD. He has gotten away with his crimes and must not be permitted to kill again. In posing for her ad, FLO JO was BETRAYED by her killer. Her ad might have betrayed others for whom she was a role model.

Our sincere condolences go out to the Joyner family.

35. THE CARBOTARIANS

Carbohydrates, especially starches, if eaten in excess, cause cancer. In a study reported in the Lancet, *women who ate large amounts of pasta, white rice, white bread, and other starches had a 39 percent increased risk of breast cancer.* --Lancet, 1996, volume 347

While populations at large go through life changing events from one idea to another, there appears to be one idea (fad) that victimizes its opponents and holds itself as supreme authority over our eating habits. The myth of vegetarianism or veganism has propelled groups of people to look down on those who chose to eat animal products. The term vegetarian or vegan is a misnomer due to the fact that either group just eats vegetables. In our opinion, they are carbotarians. They tend to eat low-fat processed foods, refined grains, unfermented soy, and very few vegetables, hence the term carbotarians.

Along with the unjustified and unscientific saturated fat and cholesterol scares of the past several decades has come the notion that vegetarianism is a healthier dietary option for people. It seems as if every so-called health expert and government health agency is urging people to eat fewer animal products and consume more vegetables, grains, fruits and legumes. Although the recommendations could be more detailed, they leave the consumer to think that canned vegetables are equivalent to fresh, and that wonder bread is equivalent to whole grain sourdough bread. As we shall see, many of the carbotarian oops vegetarian claims cannot be substantiated and some are simply false and dangerous. There are benefits to vegetarian diets for certain health conditions, and some people function better on less fat and protein, but as holistic consultants who have dealt with several former vegetarians and vegans, we know full well the dangerous effects of a diet devoid of healthful animal products.

Dr. Weston Price, a dentist who traveled to over 60 countries covering Asia, Africa, and Europe studied the dietary customs of many cultures. He is the only documented human being in the last 100 years to accomplish such an incredible task. His findings were point blank-NO WHERE DID HE FIND A VEGETARIAN or VEGAN CULTURE. His research also found that when those cultures ate their native diet, they were disease free. It was only when they introduced western civilization foods that they had the diseases we see everyday in western countries. Any so-called health expert talking about diet and not mentioning Dr. Price is out of his mind and completely foolish.

While there is little argument that whole-grain cereals and breads are more nutritious and provide more fiber and aid detoxification, care must be taken to avoid consuming ill prepared or processed grains. Today's diet has deviated far from the wholesome foods of the early century. Food manufacturers have clung to public misperceptions with regard to white foods, particularly white breads, white rice, white sugar and white table salt, all of which are commonly referred to as WHITE DEATH by nutrition experts and the authors themselves, and for good reason!

White flour became popular sometime prior to 1872 (used to treat diarrhea because of its constipating effect), when the roller mill began to replace the stone mills of old. White flour, known to be better for making pastries and baking in general, was only available to the rich prior to the advent of the roller mill because its production required significant manual labor, which only the rich could afford. The baker was able to produce white bread at a cost that not most anyone could afford, all while the nutritious portions, the bran and germ of the grain were generally fed to pigs and other farm animals! Not long after white flour was accessible to all classes, cereals began to suffer the same fate, losing their nutritional value due to processing. Today, the nutritious portions of the grain are sold off to health food stores and supplement manufactures, so in essence, many of you pay for the same grain two or three times over in the form of flour, fiber supplements, and finally vitamin supplements such as vitamin E and wheat germ.

The other issue carbotarians fail to realize is that before the advent of farming, grain was partially germinated (sprouted).

The process of sprouting not only produces vitamin C; it changes the composition of the grain in numerous ways that make it more beneficial as a food. For example, sprouting increases the content of all the B vitamins, and carotene, which is converted to vitamin A. Even more important in today's climate of indigestion, is that phytic acid, which is a known mineral blocker, is broken down in the sprouting process. Phytic acid is present in the bran of ALL grains, the coat of nuts and seeds and inhibits the absorption of calcium, magnesium, iron, copper, and zinc. These inhibitors can neutralize our own digestive enzymes, resulting in the digestive disorders (IBS, diverticulitis, etc.) experienced by many people who eat unsprouted grains. There are many scientific indicators linking grain consumption to rheumatic and arthritic conditions as well.(1) Complex sugars responsible for intestinal gas are broken down during the sprouting and a portion of the starch in grain is transformed into sugar. Sprouting inactivates aflatoxins, which are toxins produced by fungus and are potent carcinogens found in grains and especially peanuts. Carbotarians praise themselves for eating tons of nuts and seeds, but they do not make the connection between phytic acid and absorption. Unfortunately, eating nuts and seeds without soaking them for at least 8-12 hours to break down the phytic acid can produce the same enzyme & mineral blocking effects as eating unsprouted grains.

Not surprisingly, America appears to be continuing another trend that began with the introduction of the steel roller mill- a declining birth rate. When bran and germ mills were extracted from flour it lowered the birth rate per 1000 people in England from 1872-1945.(2) Today, things are not much better. Artificial insemination, another MediSin is big business and, if not for advanced medical technologies, America would be losing a huge amount of babies who would not have survived even 100 years ago. Additionally, there are significant reductions in sperm counts among males, which may well be the result of both a carbotarian lifestyle and toxicity on our food supply. While our environment's chemical exposure is suspected, it is very likely that malnutrition, secondary to consuming too many processed foods, is a real possibility. Francis Marion Pottenger Jr., M.D. demonstrated that feeding cats processed foods led to numerous disease processes, infertility, and eventually EXTINCTION!

While carbotarians avoid animal products, we often ask them how they supply their bodies with a complete protein. The majority say they use those protein bars, unfermented soy, and food combining with grains. Since unfermented soy is being dealt with in another section of this book and food combining is being dealt within the solutions section of the book, we will deal with protein bars right now.

Protein bars look and taste like candy bars. They have a shelf life of a thousand years, contain protein and fiber, vitamins and some minerals. The real boost for the bar business came with the advent of cheap soy and whey proteins that could be added to make a "high protein" bar. Barry Sears' Boone "Programmed Nutrition" bars were among the first of these with copycats Balance Bars and Zone Perfect Bars. However, there is nothing natural about the protein used in these protein bars. Unfermented soy protein comes with an initial burden of aphetic acid, enzyme inhibitors and excess estrogen. More toxins are formed during the high-temperature chemical processing, including nitrates, MSG, and aluminum. Unfermented soy protein must be processed at very high temperatures to reduce levels of phytic acid and enzyme inhibitors, a process that over–denatures many of the proteins in unfermented soy, making them unavailable to the body. Whey protein is inherently fragile and must be processed at low temperatures or its qualities as a protein are destroyed. That is why casein rather than whey protein is used in animal food. When cheese, butter and cream were made on the farm, the whey and skim milk were given to the pigs and chickens. So today, industries have taken this excess waste problem called whey, and put it in protein energy drinks, high-protein bars, and body building formulas. Let's take a look at some of the ingredients in these bars of MediSin:

Power Bar: High fructose corn syrup, grape and pear juice concentrate, oat bran, malt dextrin, milk protein, brown rice, sesame butter, barley malt, and peanut butter.

BioZone Bar: Fructose syrup, soy protein isolate, honey, calcium caseinate, toasted soybeans, corn syrup, sugar, palm and palm kernel oils, peanut butter, cocoa powder, lactose, and whey protein concentrate.

Balance Bar: Protein Blend (soy protein isolate, honey calcium caseinate, toasted soybeans, corn syrup, sugar, whey protein concentrate, whey), fructose corn syrup, canola oil, and corn syrup.

With the exception of the fats, most of the ingredients used in energy bars are waste products. Soy protein isolate is from the soy industry and whey is from the cheese industry. Grape and pear fiber are left over from the process of making juice from those respective fruits. In short, most of the ingredients in energy bars are anything but natural, so why are they allowed in the health food industry? Maybe we should ask Dr. Andrew Weil or Dr. Michael Murray?

Just for the fun of it let's take a look at all the so-called claims carbotarians make against the killing and eating of animal products:

Falsehood #1: Vitamin B12 can be obtained from plant sources.

This falsehood is perhaps the most dangerous of all. While lacto and lacto-ova vegetarians have sources of vitamin B12 in their diets (from dairy products and eggs), vegans do not. Vegans who do not supplement their diets with vitamin B12 will eventually get anemia (a fatal condition) as well as severe nervous and digestive system damage. Every study of vegan groups has demonstrated low vitamin B12 concentrations in the majority of individuals. (3) Additionally, claims are made in vegetarian literature that B12 is present in certain algae, tempeh, and Brewers Yeast. All of them are FALSE, as B12 is ONLY found in animal products. Brewer's and nutritional yeasts do not contain B12 naturally; they are always fortified from outside sources.

Some vegetarian authorities claim that vitamin B12 is produced by certain fermenting bacteria in the lower intestines. In order for this process to take place the B12 requires the *"intrinsic factor"* from the stomach for proper absorption in the ileum. Herbaceous animals like cows have this factor to convert grass into protein. If an individual does have this factor, then they can support their bodies adequately on a vegetarian diet.

It is interesting to note that Webster's New World Dictionary defines the intrinsic factor as *"a substance secreted by the stomach which permits the absorption of vitamin B12 in the intestine..."* One test an individual can do for the intrinsic factor is swallowing the B-vitamin niacin. Niacin must be converted to niacin amide a proteinated form of niacin by the intrinsic factor in the stomach; otherwise a phenomenon known as "niacin flush" occurs. Such a flush causes a person's face to turn red and the back of the arms can itch from the release of histamine and the skin will feel warm. No harm is done by the niacin flush because it is simply a dilation of the blood vessels near the skin. The test is to take between 100 and 200 mg. of natural niacin but not niacin amide, which is often sold as supplemental niacin on an empty stomach. If a person flushes, the niacin was not converted by the stomach to niacin amide because the person lacked the intrinsic factor. Thus, a niacin flush at 100 mg. indicates the person's inability to prosper on a strictly vegetarian diet. Therefore, the only reliable sources of vitamin B12 are animal products. (4) This is one of strongest arguments to put the notion of veganism as a "natural" way of human eating to rest.

Falsehood # 2: Our needs for vitamin D can be met by sunlight.

For some reason it has been taught that one's vitamin D needs can be met simply by exposing one's skin to the sun's rays for 15-20 minutes a few times a week. Concerns about vitamin D deficiencies in carbotarians always exist as this nutrient, in its full-complex form, is only found in animal fats (5), which vegans do not consume. It is true that a limited number of plant foods such as alfalfa, sunflower seeds, and avocado, contain the plant form of vitamin D (ergocalciferol or D2). Although D2 can be used by humans, it is questionable, though, whether this form is as effective as animal-derived vitamin D3. Some studies have shown that D2 is not utilized as well as D3 in animals (6) and clinicians have reported disappointing results using vitamin D2 to treat vitamin D-related conditions. (7)

Although vitamin D can be created by our bodies by the action of sunlight on our skin, it is very difficult to obtain an optimal amount of vitamin D by a brief foray into the sun. There are three ultraviolet bands of radiation that come from sunlight named A, B, and C. Only the "B" form is capable of catalyzing the conversion of cholesterol to vitamin D in our bodies (8) and UV-B rays are only present at certain times of day, at certain latitudes, and at certain times of the year. (9) Furthermore, depending on one's skin color, obtaining 200-400 IUs (International Units) of vitamin D from the sun can take as long as two full hours of continual sunning. (10) A dark-skinned vegan, therefore, will find it impossible to obtain optimal vitamin D intake by sunning himself for 20 minutes a few times a week, even if sunning occurs during those limited times of the day and year when UV-B rays are available. This deficiency is also linked to the skin disease vitiligo (skin depigmentation). One of the most effective tools to use for reversing this condition is to use a UV-B lamp which emits those essential rays so badly needed to make melanin for skin pigmentation.

The current RDA for vitamin D is 400 IUs, but Dr. Weston Price's excellent research into the native diet of people he observed through his travels showed that their daily intake of vitamin D (from animal foods) was about 10 times that amount, or 4,000 IUs. (11) Accordingly, Dr. Price placed a great emphasis on vitamin D in the diet. Without vitamin D, for example, it is IMPOSSIBLE to utilize minerals like calcium, phosphorous, and magnesium. Since rickets and/or low vitamin D levels have been well-documented in many vegetarians and vegans (12), it is imperative that those individuals supplement with the following sources of vitamin D: cod liver oil, wild shrimp, wild salmon, organic butter, and free-range eggs.

Falsehood # 3: The body's needs for vitamin A can be entirely obtained from plants.

True vitamin A or retinol is only found in animal fats and organs such as liver. (13) Plants contain beta-carotene, a substance that the body can convert to vitamin A if certain conditions are present. The conversion from carotene to vitamin A in the intestines can only take place in the presence of bile salts. This means that fat must be eaten with the carotenes to stimulate bile secretion. Additionally, infants and people with hypothyroidism, gall bladder problems or diabetes (large segment of society) cannot make the conversion, or do so very poorly. Relying on plant sources solely for vitamin A is not a very wise idea. This provides yet another reason to include animal foods and fats in our diets. Butter from grass-fed cows and cod liver oil are excellent sources for vitamin A. Vitamin A is all-important in our diets, for it enables the body to use proteins and minerals, insures proper vision, enhances the immune system, enables reproduction, and fights infections.

Falsehood # 4: Meat (grass-fed lamb, cow, goat, bison, free-range poultry, and wild fish) eating causes osteoporosis, kidney disease, heart disease, and cancer.

Vegans and vegetarians like to use scare tactics to prove their weak points. One such tactic is that meat causes certain chronic diseases. Such claims are laughable and unproven with historical and anthropological facts. All the above mentioned diseases are 20th century occurrences, yet people have been eating meat and animal fat for many thousands of years. Further, as Dr. Price's research showed, there were/are several native peoples around the world (the Inuit, Maasai, Swiss, Hunzas, etc.) whose traditional diets were/are very rich in animal products, but whom nevertheless did/do not suffer from the above-mentioned maladies. (14)

Dr. Herta Spencer's research on protein intake and bone loss clearly showed that protein consumption in the form of real meat has no impact on bone density. Studies that supposedly proved that excessive protein consumption equaled more bone loss were not done with real meat but with fractionated protein powders and isolated amino acids. (15) Although protein-restricted diets are helpful for people with kidney disease, there is no proof that eating meat causes it. (16) Carbotarians try to claim that protein causes acidic conditions in the blood, which leeches calcium from the bones leading to kidney stones. Actually, meat contains complete proteins and vitamin D, both of which help maintain pH balance in the bloodstream. Furthermore, if one eats a diet that includes enough magnesium and vitamin B6, and restricts refined sugars, one has little to fear from kidney stones, whether one eats meat or not.

The study which began the meat= cancer theory was done by Dr. Ernest Wynder in the 1970s. Wynder claimed that there was a direct, casual connection between animal fat intake and incidence of colon cancer. (17) Actually, his data on animal fats were really refined vegetable oils. (18) Looking at the research even closer reveals that processed meats like cold cuts and sausages; which, are loaded with nitrates are the culprits in cancer causation (19) and not meat itself. Furthermore, cooking methods play a partial role in whether or not a meat becomes carcinogenic. (20) In other words, it is the added chemicals to the meat and the chosen cooking method that are at fault and not the meat itself. Further, it is usually claimed that a diet rich in plant foods like whole grains and legumes will reduce one's risk for cancer, but research going back to the last century demonstrates that carbohydrate-based diets are the prime dietary instigators of cancer, not diets based on minimally processed animal foods. (21)

The mainstream health and vegetarian media have done such an effective job of "animal bashing," that most people think there is nothing healthful about meat, especially red meat. In reality, animal flesh foods like grass-fed beef & lamb are excellent sources of vitamins A, D, B-complex, essential fatty acids, magnesium, zinc, phosphorus, potassium, iron, selenium, and conjugated linoleic acid (prevents cancer). Nutritional factors like coenzyme Q10, carnitine, and alpha-lipoic acid are also present. These nutrients are only found in animal foods plants do not supply them.

Falsehood # 5: The human body is not designed for meat consumption.

Some carbotarians claim that since humans possess grinding teeth like herbivorous animals and longer intestines than carnivorous animals; this proves the human body is better suited for vegetarianism. (22) This argument fails to note several human physiological features, which clearly indicate a design for animal product consumption. First and foremost is our stomach's production of hydrochloric acid (HCL), something not found in herbivores. HCL activates protein-splitting enzymes. Furthermore, the human pancreas manufactures a full range of digestive enzymes, which handle a wide variety of foods both of animal and plant origin. The carbotarian claim does not hold water on this subject.

Falsehood # 6: Animal products contain numerous, harmful toxins.

Hormones, nitrates and pesticides are present in commercially raised animal products (as well as commercially raised fruits, grains and vegetables) and are definitely things to be concerned about. However, one can avoid these chemicals by taking responsibility and consuming range-fed, organic meats, eggs and diary products, which do not contain harmful, man-made toxins.

It is often claimed by vegetarians that meat is harmful to our bodies because ammonia is released from the breakdown of its proteins. Although it is true that ammonia production does result from meat digestion, our bodies quickly convert this substance into harmless urea.

"Mad Cow Disease," or Bovine Spongiform Encephalopathy (BSE), is not caused by cows eating animal parts with their food, a feeding practice that has been done for over 100 years. British organic farmer Mark Purdey has argued convincingly that cows that get "Mad Cow Disease" are the ones that have had particular organophosphate insecticide applied to their backs or have grazed on soils that lack magnesium but contain high levels of aluminum. (23) Small outbreaks of "mad cow disease" have also occurred among people who reside near cement and chemical factories and in certain areas with volcanic soils. (24) Recently, Purdey has gained support from Dr. Donald Brown, a British biochemist who also argued for a non-infectious cause of BSE. Brown attributes BSE to environmental toxins, specifically manganese overload. (25)

In conclusion, different people require different nutrients based on their unique genetic make-up. Some vegetarians and vegans, in their zeal to get converts are blind to this biochemical fact. Further, due to peculiarities in genetics and individual biochemistry, some people simply cannot do a vegetarian diet because of such things as lectin intolerance and enzyme deficiencies. Lectins present in legumes, a prominent feature of vegetarian diets are not tolerated by many people. Others have grain sensitivities, especially to gluten, or to grain proteins in general. Again, since grains are a major feature of carbotarian diets, such people cannot thrive on them. (26)

Desaturase enzyme deficiencies are usually present in those people of Inuit, Scandinavian, Northern European, and sea coast ancestry. They lack the ability to convert alpha-linolenic acid into EPA and DHA, two omega-3 fatty acids intimately involved in the function of the immune and nervous systems. The reason for this is because these people's ancestors got an abundance of EPA and DHA from the large amounts of cold-water fish they ate. Over time, because of non-use, they lost the ability to manufacture the necessary enzymes to create EPA and DHA in their bodies. For these people, vegetarianism is simply not possible. They MUST get their EPA and DHA from animal food and EPA is only found in animal foods.

Though it may appear that some people do well on little or no meat and remain healthy as lacto-vegetarians or lacto-ovo-vegetarians, the reason for this is because these diets are healthier for those people, not because they're healthier in general. Though it may take years, problems will eventually ensue under such dietary regimes and they will certainly show in future generations.

Dr. Abrams said it well when he wrote:

Humans have always been meat-eaters. The fact that no human society is entirely vegetarian, and those that are almost entirely vegetarian suffer from debilitated conditions of health, seems unequivocally to prove that a plant diet must be supplemented with at least a minimum amount of animal protein to sustain health. Humans are meat-eaters and always have been. Humans are also vegetable eaters and always have been, but plant foods must be supplemented by an ample amount of animal protein to maintain optimal health. (27)

MediSin

36. SOLUTIONS TO MEDISIN

In the 1960's and 1970s, extensive studies were conducted by the Ford Foundation, as well as several U.S. Government agencies, concerning the health of America. The conclusions derived from these studies proved that the chronic degenerative diseases were increasing each year. Behavioral and scholastic problems in all public schools were increasing nationwide, and it seemed no matter how many millions of dollars were thrown at these problems, good health in general was deteriorating in America. No psychological or social factors studied could account for the above conclusions. However, much evidence pointed to a biological cause: perhaps a nutritional basis as a primary factor in reaching these conclusions.

In 1982, W.K. Kellogg Foundation commissioned Joseph D. Beasley, M.D. of the Institute of Health Policy and Practice at Bard College Center, to undertake a detailed study to determine why the conclusions of the Ford Foundation were happening in America. The conclusions of this study were published in 1991 and the results are startling. The study concluded that no one factor determines our health or any disease. Health is a quality, the most important quality of life. It is a state of being: of countless interrelationships in what is called "the web of life." Neither the most brilliant scientists nor the world's most sophisticated medical centers understand the "web of life" in enough detail to manage or control it.

Great biological systems make up "the web of life." Interacting in each of us continually, they yield our present state of health or illness. The existence of these systems has emerged into human awareness only in this century. Yet, we know that if these systems are healthy, we humans will be healthy. We cannot manage health directly, for it is a quality. But we can protect and support the biological systems out of which life arose and on which our health depends. We came to the same conclusions ten years ago and have tried to incorporate these principles in educating people everyday.

Of these biological systems, the above study concluded that there are five, which are absolutely essential to achieve the best health in today's society. The five systems are:

1. Our personal genetics, our genes inherited from our parents, the body's unique cellular code or blueprint that guides all its processes.
2. External events that cross our path by chance that affect our health such as a car wreck or biological terrorism or being in the wrong place at the wrong time.
3. Nutrition, the sustenance and fuel we provide our bodies and mind every day and especially the 50 essential nutrients.
4. The environment, the milieu of natural and man made elements, pollution, indoors and out, that supports or undermines human life and health.
5. Our behavior or lifestyle in that environment, stressful or relaxed, sedentary or active, with or without smoking, alcohol, drugs, exercise, and so forth.

Of course, some might argue that these first two systems are factors that you can do nothing about, but we disagree because we can practice better safety habits (seat belts, exposure to cold) and can by better nutrition, stimulate our genes to work at maximum efficiency. The last three systems and their improvement have been the basis of our research for the past ten years. Physicians in America today are not taught in medical school about nutrition and the proper diet, or about pollution and toxic substances in our environment. They are taught very little about lifestyle changes and their need to attain better health. We are very appreciative and honored that God has guided us to study and learn all about these important systems, so that we can give our clients the truth as to how to attain better health.

Diet and Nutrition

Essential nutrients are those substances necessary for growth, normal functioning and maintaining life. These nutrients must be supplied by foods, because the body cannot make them. We have concluded that there are several categories of essential nutrients that must be addressed to attain proper nutrition and better health. These include the following categories:

1. Proteins: primarily in the form of amino acids.
2. Carbohydrates: natural sugars and starches
3. Fats: primarily in the form of essential fatty acids
4. Vitamins: fat and water soluble
5. Minerals: essential and trace minerals
6. Water: the most important of all
7. Others: oxygen, fiber, specific anti-oxidants, etc.

Recommended Daily Allowances

Recommended daily allowances (RDA) are merely guidelines to the quantities of nutrients that the body needs each day. RDAs are opinions set by committees based on scientific evidence at hand. These recommendations are made on inadequate information and even differ from one country to another. Unfortunately, many doctors cite RDA as though they are the Gospel. This is far from the case and highlights the fact that the mere existence of RDA can lead to a misunderstanding of what is actually occurring with any individual. Many recent studies made in the past ten years are showing that even though many patients eat a "balanced diet", more than 90 percent suffer from lack of one or more essential nutrients. The idea behind setting RDA was to give at least some idea to the likelihood of groups of individuals being deficient in a specific nutrient when considering their dietary intake. This has severe limitations, because people not only have different and unique fingerprints, but also different and unique requirements. In our opinion the RDA are useful only as a guide as to what amount of these nutrients will prevent specific nutritional diseases like Scurvy, Beriberi, and Rickets. To use them as a guide to attain better health can be catastrophic.

Factors Influencing Nutritional Status

1. Quality of food
2. Quantity of food
3. Efficiency of digestion
4. Efficiency of absorption
5. Efficiency of utilization

I. The Quality of Food: Food grown on nutrient poor soil can be deficient in certain nutrients. The trace minerals in soils are largely governed by farming policies. Overworked soils and soils that have added chemicals such as pesticides, insecticides and herbicides can adversely influence the quality of the food. Hormones, antibiotics, and other chemicals fed to commercially grown cattle & poultry to make them grow faster, definitely influences the biochemistry in our bodies (see how fast young girls are developing breasts and menstrual cycles at age 8). Certain processes that foods undergo during manufacture and storage influence the nutrient content. Even food preparation procedures in our kitchen influence the nutrient content of our foods.

II. The Quantity of the Food. In America, under-nutrition is not a problem. However, malnutrition can occur anywhere as a result of wrong food choices and a dependence on large amounts of heavily refined foods. Processed foods (foods in boxes, cans and packages) have had many essential nutrients removed and can definitely influence nutrition. Whole grain and unprocessed (fresh) foods are always superior. In fact, "health food nuts" of the past insisted on whole grains and fresh vegetables, which have been proven by modern science.

III. The Efficiency of Digestion. A person who has an inefficient digestive system will naturally be more likely to have poorer nutritional status than a person with an efficient digestive system will. The former is often seen by physicians when certain patients do not have enough hydrochloric acid in their stomach to allow the stomach enzyme pepsin to work properly. This leads to impairment of other digestive enzyme activity.

IV. The Efficiency of Absorption. Digested foods must be absorbed properly from the intestine into the blood stream to provide the body with these essential nutrients. One example we see very often among people who do not absorb vital nutrients is an overgrowth of yeast called Candida. The yeast grows little finger-like projections that tend to "plug up" the absorption tissues called villa, and nutritional deficiencies can rapidly result.

V. The Efficiency of Utilization. A person may have proper digestion and absorption of their food and nutrients, but previous deficiencies of certain vitamins and coenzymes may prevent certain vital chemical reactions from taking place in the body. Some people with genetic defects may excrete excessive amounts of nutrients in the urine, which definitely influences one's nutrition.

Truths and Myths about Nutrition

The idea that the U.S. diet is excellent and healthy needs to be debunked. Below, we've listed some myths that are still widely believed by many doctors and nutritionists in America.

1. Nutritional deficiencies cannot exist in people on a so-called "healthy balanced" diet.
2. Sugar is an essential nutrient for energy.
3. Milk is necessary to maintain adequate calcium balance.
4. Food preservatives, colorings and additives do not affect good nutrition.

Truths

The American diet contains too:

1. Much commercially raised animal products
2. Much inorganic salt
3. Much refined sugar and refined food
4. Little fiber
5. Much non-herbal tea, coffee, alcohol and soda pop.
6. Little pure water

The American diet contains potentially harmful chemicals such as insecticides, pesticides, and herbicides, as well as coloring, flavorings, preservatives and additives.

A Lesson in Chemistry

You do not have to be a chemist to understand these basic principals regarding body chemistry. This information will be the most important of all in helping you understand why you must change your dietary habits if you ever hope to achieve better health. If you presently are sick or have any major or minor illnesses and sincerely desire to get well, you must remember that in order to make your life anew, you've got to change your point of view. You can slow down the aging process and eliminate the degenerative changes taking place in your body. There presently exists in the year 2005, effective medical knowledge that is sufficient to prevent and/or to reverse the many malfunctions of the body processes that are continually happening to our body systems. Unfortunately, most physicians do not understand these processes and are unable to advise their patients accordingly.

Proper Chemical Balance Keeps your Body Healthy

If you sincerely desire to attain the best possible health and to stay healthy, you should try to understand some basics of the chemistry of dissolved solids in your body fluids and how they work to keep you healthy and disease free. We must warn you that the explanation is quite technical and unfortunately many physicians do not understand these processes as they are not taught, in any depth, in our medical schools, because the processes involve colloid chemistry: the chemistry of dissolved solids in liquids.

Some Basic Definitions

To clearly understand the next section, you must comprehend some basic definitions of chemistry language, so try to understand the following definitions:

Atom: An atom is the smallest part of an element that can exist or that can enter into a chemical combination. Atoms have a negative or positive electrical charge.

Electrolyte: Any substance or compound or molecule that can separate into ions when dissolved in a solution, and thus becomes capable of conducting electricity. All salts, as table salt (NaCl), Epsom Salt (MgSO4) or baking soda (NaHCO3) etc., are electrolytes.

Element: The fundamental or elementary substance that cannot be broken down by chemical means to simpler substances. All matter in the universe is made up or composed of one or a combination of 108 presently known elements. Examples of elements are hydrogen and oxygen, which combine to form water. Elements may be liquids, gases or solids.

Compound: a compound is a distinct substance containing two or more elements chemically combined in definite proportions by weight. Compounds can be broken down into the elements that make them.

Molecule: a molecule is the smallest uncharged individual unit of a compound and is formed by the union of two or more atoms. Water is a typical molecular compound and a single molecule of water consists of two atoms of hydrogen and one atom of oxygen giving the chemical formula H2O. A molecule of table salt contains two elements: one atom of sodium (NA+) and one atom of chloride (Cl-) and when combined, form a single molecule of salt with the chemical formula (NaCl).

Ion: an ion is a positively or negatively charged atom or group of atoms. An ionic compound is held together by attractive forces that exist between positively (+) charged and negatively (-) charged ions. A positively charged ion is called a CATION and a negatively charged ion is called an ANION.

Colloid: particular matter (compounds usually in solution) in the size range of angstroms (a unit of small-size measure) to one micron (another unit of measure larger in size) in diameter, which fail to settle out when in a solution or in a liquid suspension. When colloids are dissolved in or dispersed in a liquid or solution, this system is called a colloidal system. All body fluids are an example of colloidal systems as blood, urine, saliva, etc. In fact, blood and urine are a mass of colloids, which include all electrolytes, protein particles, sugars, and dissolved solids.

Homeostasis: The state of equilibrium (balance) of the internal environment and relative constancy of all body fluids with their chemical and physical properties. Ideal homeostasis exists when all normal body fluid chemicals and dissolved solid substances are in perfect balance.

To summarize these definitions, We can state that one atom of sodium (Na^+, an element and a cation) can combine with one atom of chloride (Cl^-, an element an anion) to form one molecule of the chemical compound NaCl (table salt). Now, after dissolving the NaCl in water, and when hundreds or even thousand of these are dispersed (spread throughout the water) we then have a colloidal form of NaCl whose molecular particle size keeps the NaCl dissolved in the water and the NaCl doesn't settle out. If too much salt is added to the water, the solution will soon become oversaturated with NaCl and the excess NaCl molecules will clump together (aggregate or agglutinate) and settle to the bottom.

Understanding Colloid Chemistry –Vital for Good Health

We feel that not teaching colloid chemistry to all medical students in U.S. medical schools is a mistake. They are taught inorganic chemistry, which is the chemistry of all elements (dead things) other than carbon and their compounds. They are taught organic chemistry which is the chemistry of the compounds of carbon (live things) and biochemistry which is the study of the specific molecular basis of life, but very little is taught about colloid chemistry which is how body fluids function. As we've already mentioned, most physicians are so ignorant concerning colloid chemistry that they cannot even give you a clear definition of a colloid. This is tragic and should be immediately addressed! Without an understanding as to how these colloids or dissolved solids behave in our body fluids, it is impossible for any physician to understand the mechanisms of many disease states as well as how to treat them. This is one of the main reasons that medical students today are taught (brainwashed) to treat the symptoms of diseases with drugs instead of being taught to treat the cause of the disease.

Our Blood – Constantly Out of Chemical Balance

To put the aforementioned definitions to use, so you can understand what is really happening concerning poor health in America, let us simply explain about what is happening with the cations and anions in all our body fluids. When one is in good health and usually when one is born, each liter (1,000 cc or slightly more than a quart) of blood contains approximately 2/3 anions and 1/3 cations. However, due to the pollution of our water, air, food, and the excessive amounts of prescription and nonprescription drugs, most people have caused this ratio to reverse to 2/3 cations and 1/3 anions in our blood.

Your Drinking Water – Critical

Most all city water filtration systems do an excellent job of making our drinking water germ free, but they do a miserable job of removing excess cationic dissolved solids that are increasing each year due to the pollution of our environment. Unfortunately, most bottled waters (with the exception of "distilled" water) do not address this problem and the majority of home filtration systems on today's market do not remove these excessive cations. We cannot emphasize enough to you, the importance of drinking and cooking with the correct type of pure water that does not have excess cations.

The Air You Breathe – Critical

Another danger that puts excess cations in our blood is the increasing pollution of the air we breathe. All the smog, tobacco smoke, diesel and gas fumes, pesticides, herbicides, insecticides, detergents, deodorants, formaldehyde, and many other chemicals polluting our environment today are primarily cationic in nature and only serve to add to the burden of excessive cations in our blood. One should therefore make every effort to avoid exposure to these pollutants. We recommend an air purifier for home use.

Chemicals and Drugs You Take – Critical

The pharmaceutical and drug companies are making billions of dollars annually selling over the counter and prescription drugs. Most of the pain medications, antihistamines, cough medicines, antacids, indigestion drugs, diarrhea medications, laxatives, sleeping pills, not to mention tobacco, alcohol, and illegal drugs are primarily cationic in nature and when ingested, also serve to increase the excessive burden of cations in our blood and body fluid systems. It seems we are in a "Catch22" situation, because the more drugs and chemicals we take in, the sicker we become which to most people simply means more and more chemicals to treat the symptoms, and we then begin to develop even more serious illnesses requiring more drugs. One must not forget that drugs and chemicals of all kinds are foreign to our bodies. They not only add severe stress to our already stressed-out systems, but they cause an excessive burden on the organs of elimination. Chemicals suppress the immune system and severely compromise the imbalance of cations and anions in our blood, which in turn prevents maximum efficiency of all body processes throughout. No wonder the chronic degenerative diseases are increasing every year and the drug companies and many health practitioners keep getting richer and richer while unsuspecting citizens get sicker and sicker.

The Foods You Eat – Critical

Probably the worse source of polluting cations in our blood and body is from our polluted food chain. All the ingredients added to our food to make them look good, taste good, easy and convenient to prepare and all the preservatives added to give longer shelf life are cationic in nature and critically compromise the overburden of cations in our blood. In fact, at last count, there are over 60,000 colorings, flavorings, preservatives, taste enhancers, emulsifiers, texture balancers and a multitude of other types of food additives that serve to increase the cationic imbalance in our blood and body systems. The processing of these foods alone, in addition to poisoning with cationic additives only serves to make these foods deficient in vital nutrients such as vitamins, minerals, amino acids, and fatty acids. Many people today are eating only processed foods, so no wonder America is sick. If you are following this same pattern, then you are going to get sicker unless you take your health into your own hands. Unfortunately, most people do not have anywhere to turn to for advice because most physicians know very little about nutrition. They know even less about cations, anions, and colloidal chemistry, and the health of America continues to suffer, degenerative diseases increase, the pharmaceutical companies and most doctors get richer, and the cost of health care keeps skyrocketing!

Why Excess Cations Are Dangerous

The question now arises as to why these excessive cations are so dangerous in causing disease and why the depleted anions are protective and prevent the development of many diseases and conditions. Cations are sticky in nature and you can imagine sticky substances in your blood trying to flow through your arteries and capillaries. A good portion of these sticky substances are going to stick to the lining of your blood vessels and this can build up over a period of time. (Could this be the actual cause of arteriosclerosis or hardening of the arteries?) These sticky cations will stick to the formed elements (red blood cells, white blood cells, and platelets) and they, in turn, will have a tendency not only to stick together (agglomerate) but also stick to the blood vessel walls or lining. All of these sticky processes will finally terminate in a condition of electrolyte imbalance. Intravascular coagulation is where your organs and tissues cannot receive the proper nutrients (even if your diet has made them available). Neither can the cells and tissues properly rid themselves of the cell products of waste metabolism. This results in a severe deterioration of cellular function and degeneration begins.

Scientific studies show that heavy metal cations such as lead, mercury, aluminum, arsenic, cadmium, nickel, and beryllium are the absolute worst cations to initiate this intravascular coagulation. Other cation culprits include sweets and desserts, all processed foods (with additives of cations), white flour foods: macaroni, spaghetti, pizza, chips and dips, most cereals, canned fruits, and all fatty animal products, especially pork. This meat should be avoided, as it is highly cationic. There are unprocessed foods like oatmeal and fresh fruits that are sticky and they have high cations but they also have high amounts of anions to balance them.

The anionic foods are all vegetables, fruit, raw seeds, and nuts. If any vegetable is green, yellow, orange or red it is high in anions. For example, squash okra, broccoli, spinach, greens, cauliflower, cabbage, brussel sprouts, as well as all the fresh green leafy vegetables. Yellow-orange vegetables like squash, sweet potatoes, or pumpkins are also high in anions. The anions in the blood are slick and all the formed elements (red blood cells, white blood cells and platelets) have a built-in preference to have the anions coat their surfaces instead of cations, as well as the endothelial cells (lining) of our blood vessels. With adequate anions in our blood, you will find no intravascular coagulation (clumping) and the circulation is greatly enhanced. Those sticky cells slide quickly and easily through all our blood vessels and capillaries without clumping, and nutrients are effectively delivered to the cells and tissues. Waste products from cellular metabolism are quickly removed from their source and carried to the excretory organs for proper elimination.

Eleven Vital Nutritional and Health Topics

There are twelve "good health" practices and topics that need further discussion and/or clarification to give you a crystal clear understanding of why you should incorporate them into your overall lifestyle. There is considerable confusion and false information that have been given out by various individuals and self interest groups concerning these subjects. Most of the confusion and incorrect fallacies have been shoved down the throat of the general public in order for their perpetrators to make a profit on some "health product" they are selling to an unsuspecting public. Our desire and goal in this book is to bring you knowledge, so that you can decide between truth and falsehood. We just want you and your family to be healthy and avoid sickness. You may not be able to apply all of these principles to your lifestyles, but you will have the truth at your fingertips to use if you so desire.

1. Refined and Processed Foods

The food processing companies today are all in the business to make money. You must never forget this fact. This is the American way, and we're not being critical of them when we state this truth. There is tremendous competition among these companies and they are all striving to get you, the consumer, to buy their product and not their competitors. They do not want to harm you in processing their foods, but they simply want to make a profit from your purchases.

These companies know that in today's society both husband and wife have to work to maintain the same standards of living that that we are used to, and the same standards our parents maintained as we grew up. The average wife (or husband) simply does not have the time or energy to prepare the wholesome and nutritious meals they feel they should to feed their family. They must take shortcuts and look for ways to save time, energy and money to give the family the necessary meals required. The easiest way to do this is to purchase processed, refined and packaged foods. Knowing this and trying to get your dollar, all food companies make their packaged foods look good, taste good, and maintain a long shelf life. In order to accomplish this, they must remove many of the vitamins, minerals, fatty acids, all fiber, and other vital nutrients from the foods. They have to add color and taste enhancers, emulsifying agents, preservatives and many other additives to keep the foods looking good and preserve them. All these added chemicals are cations and dangerous to your health. With some foods (like white breads) the U.S. Government requires that they add back 7 of the 23 nutrients removed. Most of the companies try to capitalize even on this by advertising that their product is "enriched" with the 7 nutrients they added back, but they never mention the 16 other vital nutrients removed from the flour. This is fraud and deceit in my opinion as food companies try to make us believe they are "enriching" the product by adding back the previously removed nutrients.

Processed or refined foods are all packaged in boxes, bottles, cans or cellophane packages. This includes all sweets, pastries and desserts of all types, all white flour products including breads, crackers, biscuits, macaroni, spaghetti, pizza, most all soups, canned meats, vegetables, fruits and cereals. We jokingly tell our friends they can eat the packaging, but don't eat the foods in them. Truly, these cationic foods are very detrimental to your health and ideally should be avoided. The best safeguard to avoid the bad foods is to read all labels of any foods purchased and totally stay away from those items when food labels list the chemicals and additives that are put in the foods. Remember that fresh is the best, frozen or home canned is second and bottled or packaged foods are the worst. Also, all artificial sweeteners are cationic and are very dangerous. The best sweeteners would be unprocessed raw honey (with some honeycomb in the bottle), stevia, xylitol, and blackstrap molasses. White sugar or any ingredients ending in "ose" (glucose, fructose, maltose, etc.) as well as all white flour products create an acid medium in the colon, which is, destructive to good bacteria found in the colon. The good bacteria play a vital part in preventing yeast overgrowth, parasites and other harmful germs that try to grow in the colon.

Just remember refined foods and sugars are always depleted in fiber and this simply slows the progress of foods passing through the intestine, which makes one more susceptible to constipation, hemorrhoids, varicose veins, colon and rectal cancers. Also, with a slower transit time through the colon, more time is allowed for putrefaction (rotting) of the refined sugars to occur in the colon, which allows more toxic substances to be absorbed into your system.

And finally, please remember that all commercial wheat flour is prepared so that it can be stored for long periods of time without spoiling. To do this, the "life" is removed from the wheat in processing. Fresh whole-wheat flour spoils rapidly. Unfortunately, except for those fortunate enough to possess a household flour-mill, truly fresh flour is unavailable and this also applies to whole wheat breads found in most supermarkets. Probably your best choice under these circumstances is to purchase sour dough whole wheat bread or sprouted grain bread (usually in frozen or refrigerated section) from your local health food store. Make sure that the bread purchased from your grocery store has written on the package 100% whole wheat or 100% whole grain. Eat not food products prepared from commercially processed wheat flour.

2. Raw Fruits and Vegetables

All raw foods (except meats) are much more nourishing than cooked foods. The cooking process destroys or changes many vitamins, minerals and especially enzymes (cell produced catalysts involved in vital cell functions), which can severely compromise your digestion and the availability of these important nutrients. Raw fruits and vegetables are more cleansing and detoxifying than cooked foods, and their roughage or fiber value helps prevent hemorrhoids, varicose veins, diverticulitis and other colon diseases, as well as colon cancer. Also, the natural vitamins, minerals, amino and fatty acids in the raw foods are readily available for absorption and therefore play a major part in preventing deficiencies of these substances. The super abundance of natural enzymes in raw foods will ensure good digestion and absorption of essential nutrients.

Many people go for weeks with no more raw food in their diet than perhaps a small amount of head lettuce or an occasional glass of pasteurized fruit or vegetable juice. Ideally, 75% of our fruits and vegetables should be eaten raw and uncooked. This principle of nutrition is one that is most often overlooked and neglected in our American society.

You should understand that raw fruits and vegetables are "live" foods, and overcooking them makes them "dead" foods. Life diminishes in all fruits and vegetables in direct proportion to the time elapsed since picking. Life involves receiving live nutrients like vitamins, minerals, enzymes and amino acids and fatty acids, and overcooking makes many of these elements dead. We originally ate living food; that is right after harvesting or picking and even as recently as 30-40 years ago, most people obtained much of their food from their own gardens and livestock. Overcooked food is devitalized of most nutrients. Even though they will fill your stomach, they do not nourish your body and give good health.

Our Creator, with His omniscient wisdom, made our foods whole and placed within each type of whole food the proper and adequate nutrients that are necessary for our body to digest, absorb and nourish our bodies. This is why different foods contain different essential nutrients. Then, humankind comes along trying to make a profit, refines the food, and removes many of the nutrients and adds chemicals to enhance taste and appearance and to preserve shelf life. This refining destroys the God-intended value of the food.

Let us explain why the above is so critically important. In researching and studying why chronic degenerative diseases were increasing and what treatment methods could be applied to halt this onslaught on the health of America, we came to several conclusions. Of these conclusions, there were three certain, primary sources that greatly contribute to the epidemic of cardiovascular-renal disease we are seeing today:

These three vital contributing factors causing the kidneys to malfunction are:

1. Excessive mineral salts (strongly cationic) intake that is happening to most Americans today.

2. The reversal of the God-provided natural sodium-to-potassium ratio that is directly caused by food processing today.

3. The ingesting of anti-inflammatory drugs (Tylenol, Excedrin, etc.) is overworking, overwhelming and critically harming our kidneys, which results in colloid particle imbalance in the blood, and then intravascular coagulation begins. Degenerative diseases result.

We agree that a major factor contributing to the excessive mineral salts in our food supply lies in the basic misconception and lack of knowledge on the part of the FDA concerning the physical chemistry of food processing. Although the FDA limits certain chemical additives to the food up to 1% of the amount demonstrated to be without harm to experimental animals, they permit virtually unlimited use of hundreds of chemicals that they classify as GRAS (generally accepted as safe). We sincerely do not believe the FDA researchers fully understand the colloidal behavior of the excess salt, for example, found in our processed foods.

In measuring the specific electrical conductance (mineral salts) in 8 fresh vegetables (asparagus, beets, carrots, corn, lima beans, peas, string beans and tomatoes), it was found that measurement of these foods in a fresh state resulted in an average of 7,500 microcosm. These same foods measured from canned and processed sources gave an average reading of 17,500 microcosms. These readings show over 2 1/2 times the mineral salts found in these canned vegetables as compared to fresh forms.

Another example was taken from the Handbook of the U.S. Department of Agriculture (No.8), which shows the amounts of sodium and potassium and their ratios of these minerals in the natural God-given fresh state, and also after being processed. Eighteen fresh natural foods were listed (including those mentioned in the specific conductance test). In the fresh, raw state, these foods averaged (after measuring total sodium and potassium content) 14% sodium and 86% potassium, giving a ratio of 1:6, or one part sodium to six parts of potassium. These same food were listed after processing, and they showed 75% sodium and 25% potassium with a ratio of 3:1, three times as much sodium (added) to one part of potassium (most removed). These figures prove that the potassium was intended to be the major mineral with sodium the minor one. After processing, these ratios are totally reversed, which should give you the very best conclusion as to why you should eat as many of your fresh fruits and vegetables as you can, in the raw, uncooked, unprocessed form.

3. Meat Products and Proteins in Your Diet

Human muscle cells are composed primarily of protein and these proteins are made from chains of amino acids. Amino acids are molecules of chemicals that contain nitrogen bonds. Sources of these amino acids, of which there are 23 known to be required in human nutrition, include meats from land animals, fish and poultry, dairy products, and non-animal sources: chiefly legumes (beans and lentils, etc.) nuts, seeds and sprouts. Proteins are also derived from the germ portion of whole grains. Our human body makes fifteen of these twenty-three amino acids, and the additional eight are termed essential amino acids because they are not made by the body and must be included in adequate amounts in our bodies. These eight essential amino acids are tryptophan, phenylalanine, leucine, isoleucine, valine, methionine, lysine, threonine, and in children, histadine. Proteins are generally considered the building blocks in our body to make and repair new tissues, to make and repair certain cells and cellular parts, to make hormones, antibodies, enzymes and other necessary chemical compounds in the body. They also supply a certain amount of necessary anions in the body, although they are generally classed as amphoteric which means that they can act as an acid or an alkali, and may exhibit anionic or cationic properties.

The largest concern regarding proteins surrounds the controversy of animal versus vegetable sources. One of the chief problems with commercial animal protein intake is the excess fats, hormones, and the anti-biotic usage. Fats supply nine calories per gram; therefore, since each variety of meat varies in fat content, some proteins have more calories than others do. For example, two ounces of baked chicken without the skin yields 284 calories and two ounces of broiled sirloin steak will yield 392 calories. It becomes very important that if you choose to eat meat, choose grass-fed organic meats and free-range poultry. The highest fat content consists of pork and commercial red meats while the lowest calorie content includes chicken, fowl, and most types of fish and seafood products, as well as eggs and dairy products.

It should also be mentioned that animal products supply all eight essential amino acids; while vegetable sources do not supply all eight amino acids and thus must be combined to provide all essential amino acids together at the same meal. Prolonged consumption of protein poor diets can retard brain development, modify the chemical composition of the brain and produce long-term learning and behavioral deficits. It is imperative that pork (bacon, sausage, ham) be avoided at all costs. Pork not only contains extremely high amounts of saturated fat but it also has worms that cannot be destroyed by cooking. Pigs and hogs are scavengers, and God has mentioned in all revealed scripture (Quran and Torah) not to eat pork.

Excessive intake of proteins provides no more protein for the bodily needs than what is "enough", as the excess protein is used either as a carbohydrate or fat. The more important factor to be considered is the digestion of a normal quantity of protein, so that a reasonable amount is supplied each day. We recommend that if you depend on meats for protein, then you should limit protein intake to one meal a day, and preferably have an average serving of meat at the afternoon meal.

Contrary to some opinions, the grinding of meat into small particles (like hamburger) does not increase its digestibility; nor does the thorough chewing of meat. No protein digestion occurs in the mouth. Meat needs only to be chewed to the extent that it may be easily swallowed. On the other hand, grinding of meat can have deleterious effects. Ground meat spoils rapidly at room temperature and whole meat does not; in fact, a sort of "predigest ion" can occur. Nucleic acids are released in the grinding process and this changes the structure of the meat. Similar action may occur when ground meat is introduced to the intestinal tract. Here the temperature situation is ideal for spoilage. If there is insufficient hydrochloric acid in the stomach or a lack of proteolysis (protein digesting) enzymes, the possibility of putrefaction (rotting) of proteins is greatly enhanced with ground meat as compared with whole meat. Preserved meat such as wieners, sausages, bologna, potted meat, luncheon meats, salami and Vienna sausages do not have as much of a putrefaction tendency; however, they are absolutely loaded with chemicals and preservatives, which play a very detrimental part in causing poor health. They simply should be avoided totally.

4. Food Combinations

Poor food combining or food combinations can be a cause of toxicity in the body. The reason for this is that certain food groups do not digest well together. Some foods digest primarily in the stomach, others in the small intestine. Some foods digest in minutes while others may take hours. Some foods require an acid medium to digest in and others an alkaline medium. Therefore, certain foods eaten together do not digest properly and thus tend to become toxic. For example, starches digest primarily in the small intestine while protein digestion mostly occurs in the stomach. Eating the two together holds the starch in the stomach too long, which leads to putrefaction. This is one example how even the best food can become toxic to you. Fruits digest in a few minutes while starches require at least an hour or two to digest. When the two are combined, the fruit putrefies, as it is unable to pass through the intestine quickly enough. Fruit with protein usually causes the same problem. Fruit needs to pass right through the stomach and the protein food needs to digest in the stomach for a much longer period of time, and when eaten together, this blocks the fruits' passage. Also, sugar inhibits or retards the action of protein digesting enzymes. Therefore, sweet foods and dessert foods should not be eaten at the same time as animal foods like meats. As an example, beans (pinto or navy beans) are an excellent vegetable source of protein. In Mexico, the pinto bean is the major constituent of the diet and is eaten unsweetened. In this country, "baked beans" are served with refined sugar. Baked beans are noted for the digestive (flatulence) gas that they cause.

Most Americans are accustomed to finishing off a good protein meal (steak or other meat) with sweet desserts (like apple pie). Desserts should be eaten several hours after mealtime on an empty stomach for best absorption. There are many sugar-protein combinations, which may be avoided easily. The fact that most food contains some protein must be taken into consideration of course. Even natural sugars, such as honey and blackstrap molasses (which we usually recommend) are less harmful than any processed sugars, but they are best eaten at different times than with high protein meals. For example, orange juice that is high in natural sugars would not be an ideal combination with eggs (proteins). A better choice would be tomato juice.

1. **Proteins generally do not combine with starches.** This is probably the worst of the disease-producing habits. Of course, this really hits home with "meat and potato eaters", as well as those who excessively use sandwiches in their diet. In the digestive process, they tend to neutralize themselves and good digestion is impossible. The increased putrefaction and rotting takes place under these circumstances. Exceptions to this rule are avocados, which combine fairly well with grains.

2. **Fruits do not combine with starches.** Fruits digest immediately in the mouth and small intestine, while starches require more of their digestive time in these areas. The fruit sugars are quickly absorbed into the intestine, while the starch requires digestion in the mouth, stomach, and small

intestine. Ideally, one should eat a fruit meal by itself. Most people prefer to make breakfast their main fruit meal and this is a good idea.

3. **Fruits do not combine with proteins.** Here again, the fruits go directly into the intestine, while protein requires much more time digesting in the stomach. If sugars are held back in the stomach while trying to digest protein, you can count on the fruit putrefying.

4. **Fruits do not combine with vegetables.** A good way to remember this is that fruits are cleaners and vegetables are builders. It is very difficult to clean and build a house at the same time. One exception to this is the tomato, a fruit. You can have tomatoes with most salad vegetables.

5. **Acid fruits do not combine with sweet fruits.** These two food groups repel each other. Acid fruits include the citrus fruits like lemons, limes, oranges, pineapple, tangerines and grapefruit along with most available berries and tomatoes. The sweet fruits include bananas, dates, and dried fruits, including apples, apricots, figs, peaches, pears, prunes and raisins.

Food combining is usually recommended for patients in very critical health and especially those with a compromised immune system. If you've spent years as a "junk food junkie," ideally, you need more than withdrawal from these foods and changing to a natural foods diet. With the accumulation of chemicals, preservatives, and additives in these junk foods and other harmful substances in your body, a detoxification program should be implemented. Even natural foods, especially fruits, certain vegetables, and their juices possess a considerable detoxifying effect. Certain vitamins are very important in the detoxification process and especially Vitamin C.

5. Fasting

Fasting is the fastest way of bringing about elimination of toxins in the body and the quickest way of getting toxic materials out of the body. Fasting on just water, or perhaps, fresh-squeezed lemon, lime, or grapefruit juice greatly enhances body detoxification. During such a fast, the body can "live off itself" and burns up dead cells, waste materials and excess fat to supply energy. Since many toxins end up stored in the fatty tissues, the benefits of fasting for detoxification is simply logical. We're convinced that regular fasting one day per week produces great benefit in maintaining a clean system. We also recommend longer fasts of three days or more, to be taken 3 to 4 times each year, which induces more thorough body detoxification, and this can be compared to a quarterly "spring cleaning."

It is common knowledge that fasting has thousands of years of reputation as the ultimate form of detoxification. Let us briefly explain what fasting does and how it can help your health. When we speak of fasting, we're talking about the total abstinence from food but not from water, for a period of time. When one fasts, no food is being converted into energy and the body must live off of itself, process called autolysis. There's nothing harmful about this since the body must go for several weeks without food as it burns up dead cells and fatty tissues where most toxic chemicals are stored in the body. Fasting is really a sort of internal operation without surgery. When the digestive and elimination systems shut down in fasting, more energy is available for detoxification and repair. Therefore, when one fasts, one usually sees a greater increase in one's energy on the third day of the fast, than it would be when eating normally.

We believe personally, that short-term fasts, such as one day per week, can be an excellent benefit to your health. Islam requires the Muslim to fast for 30 days once a year in the month of Ramadan (ninth month of the lunar calendar) to learn self-restraint. This fast being spiritual in origin has the physical benefit of giving the organs of the body rest. Modern science today has stated that the human body needs thirty-days of fasting every year to obtain optimum health. Perhaps the Creator knows what's best for our body! By abstaining from two or three meals one day a week, this gives you a sort of weekly "house cleaning" inside your body. If you decide to fast, please remember that it can be very beneficial to your health. But, you should certainly exercise some care by following the guidelines listed below.

How to Fast Properly

When you begin to fast, the detoxification will often cause headaches, tiredness, fatigue, and even nausea. This is normal and it simply means that you are eliminating harmful toxins and substances from your body. When these side effects are seen, it merely shows that your body needs the fasting experience and these symptoms usually disappear after the third day.

1. If you decide to fast, you should begin your fast experience gradually. You should start with a one-day a week fast and probably skip only two meals. Later on, you can skip three meals a day on your fast, if you desire. Never begin a long fast unless your body is accustomed to fasting.

2. Once you begin your fasting program on a one-day-per-week basis, you will soon notice that there is very little to no discomfort because of the successful elimination of most of your accumulated toxins.

3. Fasting has been prescribed by God since time immortal. All the prophets fasted from Adam to Moses to Jesus and finally Muhammad (Peace be upon them all) to reach spiritual heights and cleanse their bodies and souls of toxic poison.

<u>Dick Gregory, the Guru of Modern Day Fasting</u>

If you want to really find a guru of fasting, look for Dick Gregory (Activist, Health Guru and Comedian). Mr. Gregory is the epitome of life, vitality and longevity. The man of holistic wisdom became a legend through the historical episodes of social, racial and political injustice in America. Mr. Gregory exercised his civil rights and anti-war activism through the symbol of fasting which created a cornerstone of protest in American history. Mr. Gregory has given the world several profound books that impacted America such as No More Lies: The Myth and Reality of American History (1971) and Natural Diet for Folks Who Eat: "Cooking with Mother Nature" (1973).

Mr. Gregory became the fasting guru of the western world by conducting an amazing 40 day fast as a symbol of protest during the Vietnam War with the assistance of the first African-

American female naturopath, Dr. Alvina Fulton. Dr. Fulton was the owner of the Fultonia Health Food Center in Chicago, IL. Dr. Fulton, who conducted many fasts during her lifetime, inspired Mr. Gregory toward his fasting venture. Through this representation of change Mr. Gregory perfected the art of detoxifying and holistic living that allowed him to overcome a major health obstacle. Now at the age of 74, "the icon of fasting" has maintained the vitality of a much younger man and is the perfect example of health and vigor.

Mr. Gregory also engineered one of the most effective natural weight loss and detoxification formulas in the history of dieting, "the Bahamian Diet" with his famous 4x formula. Although the formula has decreased in popularity in the health food world, it still will always be the epitome of a weight management formula because of its drug and chemical free ingredients. This super meal replacement required no doctor's prescription, only a mindful procedure to make a way for a slimmer you. Here are some of the "slim safe" meal replacement ingredients of vitality used in the formula: cellulose powder, Kelp powder, papain, bromelain, wheat germ, acerola, alfalfa, carob powder, chia seed powder, date powder, dulse, pumpkin seed powder, rice bran, sesame seed powder, sunflower seed powder, b-vitamins, and potassium iodide.

Currently, Mr. Dick Gregory and his brother Dr. Ron Gregory still spend a great deal of their lives bringing the world closer to a healthier lifestyle. It is because of these gentlemen that America still has a chance to wake up to the MediSins that our cheating them out of life. There would be a whole lot of change in America if America decided one day to start thinking. And one of the biggest and most important changes would be in the "traditional American diet." The old saying is true: "You are what you eat." It would be more accurate, perhaps to say: "You are what you assimilate." Your body is literally what you assimilate from the "foods" or more frequently "things" you eat to rebuild cells and what you eliminate as waste products of the cell-building activity, and these assimilation/elimination processes keep you revitalized each day.

6. Fermented Foods

Fermenting was one of the first methods of preservation discovered for foods. Because of the fermentation process, foods such as sauerkraut, pickles, yogurt, cheeses, buttermilk, and cottage cheese came into existence. All of these foods in their natural form have a long history of use and are highly acceptable in dietary items. We've learned from researching that there are two kinds of lactic acid produced by the body. When all body processes are functioning properly, the body produces a form of lactic acid called L-lactic acid, and when the body is overly stressed and not functioning properly, a bad form of lactic acid called D-lactic acid is produced. The fermentation process acts to produce primarily L-lactic acid; this natural acid is common to the previously named foods. This L-lactic acid seems to have a "preservative" effect on the intestinal tract as well. Such foods as yogurt and buttermilk thus have an enviable reputation for being favorable to the intestinal environment. The fermentation process also seems to act somewhat as a "predigesting factor." Tough fibers are made softer; nutrients may be released from their biological hold, such as lactose (milk sugar), which is richer in buttermilk than in sweet milk. It has also been found that lactose favorably influences and enhances the absorption of calcium.

Two Good Fermented Foods

There are two foods that are outstanding in the fermented food class: buttermilk and sauerkraut. They are easily available and both are very rich sources of L-lactic acid. Buttermilk is preferred, of course, because of its high protein and calcium content. But those who do not care for buttermilk should consider sauerkraut as a source of L-lactic acid. It would be a good health practice to try to include some fermented foods in your diet each day like buttermilk, yogurt, sauerkraut or cottage cheese. Make sure all your products are raw and organic and contain no added sugar or if possible, are not pasteurized. Pasteurization destroys the enzymes necessary to digest food properly.

7. Exercise and Physical Activity

Did you know that a fairly recent Gallop Poll reported that only 24% of the citizens of the U.S. exercise regularly? Due to the mechanization of our society over the past 100 years with machines and household appliances, a very small number of people now earn their living in jobs requiring persistent physical activity. Physical inactivity for the majority of Americans has become the rule and not the exception. We've asked many people "What is the most strenuous exercise that you have engaged in the past two weeks?" The great majority state that actually their exercise has been no greater than walking up a flight of stairs, walking from their car across a parking lot to their place of business, or maybe even just pushing a grocery cart. What we should understand is that "running around all day", whether it is at home or at our place of work is definitely not exercise and should not be considered as such.

There have been many new studies completed in the last ten years which have fairly well proven that the lack of exercise or habitual inactivity very often contributes to high blood pressure, chronic fatigue, premature aging, poor muscle tone and lack of flexibility, which in turn, aggravates low back pain, mental stress, coronary artery disease and especially obesity. Prolonged inactivity also slows bowel function, decreases male hormone production in men, as well as decreases sperm count. Without proper physical activity, there is very inefficient transfer of oxygen in the lungs, and it also has been shown to aggravate and make us more susceptible to developing softening of the bones or osteoporosis. We have seen that lack of exercise causes rapid deterioration of muscle tissue, as well as connective tissue in our ligaments and tendons. If you want to age faster, then do not exercise because when you don't use your muscles, it is true that "if you don't use it, you lose it." Exercise also increases the good cholesterol in the body and lowers the bad cholesterol and total cholesterol levels.

A person doesn't have to be a marathon runner or chop wood three hours a day in order to become more active. There are many forms of exercise that a person can perform and this range from walking to jogging, bicycling, swimming, rebounding or getting involved in some sport activity such as tennis, volleyball or possibly even playing golf. The most important decision for you, however, is to make a definite decision that you are going to exercise at least three days each week and begin some program. We're going to briefly discuss two types of exercise programs that we will recommend for the great majority of our clients, and they involve brisk walking and rebounding.

For those individuals who are entering their "golden years", a simple routine involving a brisk, daily walk is quite sufficient for the initial part of the exercise regime and may be all that a lot of clients need. The usual response to our walking prescription is that walking makes a person hungry. This is not true. When the body is walking briskly, the body's fat deposits are tapped freely for energy in order to supply fuel for the muscles so the blood comes fully loaded with these fuel materials. The net effect is that, not only does the muscle tissue have readily available fat to burn, but also the hunger mechanism is short circuited, and there is actually less hunger than if there had been no activity. A prolonged walk at a steady pace with constant stress on the circulatory system and the heart is beneficial in many ways. The primary concern in exercise is to increase your pulse rate and get your heart beating faster. This increase should be from fifty to seventy percent higher than your normal resting pulse, but do not overdo it. You would be wise to get in the habit of exercising twenty minutes every day with your heart beating faster. Morning exercise is better for you because it will give you more energy all day long.

In the beginning, the walk should be short and slow but gradually build up one's speed and distance. When asked how fast one should walk, we often use the following example: *"Imagine that you are wearing thin clothing and that the temperature outside is below freezing, the wind is blowing hard, and it is raining and you have to go to the bathroom very badly and you are a mile from home. How fast would you walk to get there?"* Now, that's a brisk walk!

Of all the types of exercise available, in the past year we have concluded that the very best form of exercise is rebounding or using a small mini-trampoline, called a Rebounder. This form of exercise is different from other physical activities because it puts gravity to work in your favor. It has many advantages over "regular" exercise because it is a cellular exercise. By subjecting each of the sixty trillion cells in your body to greater gravitation pull, waste produced is squeezed out and nutritional elements and oxygen are drawn into the cells. The cell functions more efficiently, the metabolism increases to its maximum. With this form of exercise, the membranes around each cell become stronger as they demand more protein from the body. These thicker membranes are better able to fight off foreign invaders like germs, toxins, poisons, and other pollutants more effectively. Hence, everything improves: the blood, the brain, the lungs, the muscles, all the internal organs, those of the senses and more.

Rebound exercising will increase the vital capacity (can handle more oxygen) in your lungs and more oxygen will be delivered to the body tissues and better absorption of oxygen will result. There appears to be a faster gaseous exchange within the lungs. The red blood cell count, as well as more blood, is pushed through these vessels. The heart muscles work more efficiently and collateral circulation improves. The result is that more oxygen is carried to the heart muscle. Elevated blood cholesterol and triglyceride levels tend to come down, and the good cholesterol levels increase. Rebounding also strengthens the adrenal glands so that the body may handle more severe stress. Your metabolism is enhanced and there is better absorption of nutrients from food intake. Digestion, appetite and elimination all get better. This type of exercise also tends to decrease any tendency for blood clotting or coagulation in the blood vessels. Many scientists believe that a prime cause or contributing factor of cancer is lack of oxygenation of the cells, and exercise is the main way to bring oxygen into the blood with which to bathe the cells.

We feel the most important benefit of rebounding however, is its effect on the lymph system. Most people are not really familiar with the lymph system. It is another circulatory system within the body and it is the system that drains and removes toxins, poisons and waste products from between each individual cell and delivers these waste products to the lymph nodes. In one sense, the lymph system is the metabolic garbage can of the body. It gets rid of toxins, dead cells, cancer cells, waste products, trapped proteins, pathogenic bacteria, and viruses, heavy metals, and assorted junk products that the cells need to get rid of.

Your circulatory system (heart, blood vessels, and blood) delivers food and oxygen to your cells, and the products of cell metabolic breakdown must be drained away with its load of waste through the lymph vessels. Now, unlike the artery system, the lymphatic system does not have its own pump. There are only three ways to activate the speed of flow of your lymph away from the tissues it serves and back into the main circulation. Lymphatic flow requires (a) a muscular contraction form of exercise and movement (b) gravitational pressure and (c) internal messages to the one-way valves that are present in the lymph vessels.

Arthur C. Guyton, M.D., professor and chairman of the Dept. of Physiology and Biophysics at the University of Mississippi, School of Medicine, is an international expert on lymphology and the lymphatic system. He states *"The lymphatic group becomes very active during exercise but sluggish under resting conditions. During exercise, the rate of lymph flow can increase to as high as three to fourteen times normal because of increased activity. An increase in tissue fluid protein increases the rate of lymph flow and this washes the proteins out of the tissue spaces, automatically returning the protein concentrate to its normal low level. If it were not for this continual removal of proteins, the dynamics of the capillaries would become so abnormal within only a few hours that life could no longer continue. There is certainly no other function of the lymphatic that can even approach this importance."*

As the lymphatic vessels have one-way valves in them, and the lymph flow only one way (towards the heart) when one jumps up on the Rebounder, the lymph is thrown up and cannot go back down the vessels because of the one way valves. This acts as a suction pump to pull out and suck out the lymph with accumulated toxins between the cells and return it back to the circulation where it is supposed to be.

<u>How to Rebound</u>

Jog on the Rebounder for two minutes, and then jump with both feet on the Rebounder for two minutes and repeat this process over and over for twenty minutes in all. If you get dizzy at first, this is because the toxins are being pulled out of the spaces between your cells too rapidly. You should slow down or stop for a few minutes before continuing if this should happen. If you feel unsteady on the Rebounder, you may want to hook a rope to the ceiling and let it hang down to hold on to or you could screw a little hand-holding hook in the wood door frame and simply hold on to this as you rebound.

8. Drink Water – Live Longer

The average person drinks nearly six times their body weight each year. In our bodies, water is absolutely vital for life. Our health becomes critical if we lose only 10% of our body water and death is certain if we lose 20%. Of our body weight, approximately 70% is water. Even bones contain over 30% water. Our drinking water, beverages, and foods we eat are the sources of water for our bodies. Every cell in our body must have water or it dies. Water bathes the cells in our body and provides the medium or means of transportation for all metabolic elements, which are food nutrients and body chemicals such as hormones, enzymes, vitamins, oxygen and minerals. In these cells, there are literally thousands of chemical reactions taking place at all times to use the food and water we take into our bodies to produce our energy. These processes taking place in the cells are generally referred to as "metabolism." Water is actually produced during these processes. These metabolic elements in the body fluids (primarily water) are constantly flowing in and out of our body cells, and waste products flow out of the body cells into the kidneys for disposal. The heart pumps about 2,000 gallons of this blood plasma through the 70,000 miles of blood vessels in our bodies each day, sometimes at the rate of 40 miles per hour. Actually about a quart of water flows through our kidneys every minute. The kidneys are continually filtering out waste products from the blood, and these products are excreted in the urine.

All body cells have a membrane or sac, which completely surrounds the cells. The body water constantly bathing the cells is vital to maintain a delicate acid-alkali (base) chemical and physical balance between the cells and all body organs. This delicate balance is referred to as homeostasis, and must be maintained or we will die. If we don't have enough water intake, our body metabolism is depressed and when our metabolism slows down, our food has a tendency to turn to fat and we become much more fatigued.

Water is essential to moisten the delicate membranes in our nose, throat, bronchial and breathing tubes, so that oxygen is brought to our blood and carbon dioxide (a waste product) excreted. Water must be available to lubricate our joints, as well as allowing absorption of our food nutrients in our digestive tract. Without adequate water, one will experience constipation, which will produce waste products and toxins that put additional stress on the liver. These accumulated waste products and toxins depress the function of most of our glands. Water is vital in regulating our body temperature. Water is needed for our muscles to function properly and to maintain the right tone. Adequate water prevents wrinkling and sagging of our skin.

It is extremely important that our body maintains a proper equilibrium between the intake and output of body water. This is called water balance. Our water balance comes from the fluids we drink (48%); from the solids we eat (40%), and from the metabolic processes taking place in the body (12%). The output water losses are from the kidneys (56%), skin (20%), lungs (20%), bowels and intestines (4%), and a small amount from tears. Proper water balance must be maintained by having the water intake equal the water output.

The water in the body is distributed in two main compartments. Water outside the cell is called extra cellular water, and the water inside the cells is called intracellular. Intracellular water (about 9 gallons) makes up 50% of our total body weight and extra cellular water makes up (about 4 gallons) 20%. The extra cellular water is further divided into the water around the cells (interstitial, 10-11 quarts) and the blood plasma (intravascular, 3-4 quarts).

When we think about fluid retention, we are primarily concerned with the extra cellular water. This water is stored in the tissue spaces between the cells and the water in the blood plasma. The chemicals sodium and potassium play a very important part in determining whether fluid is retained or not. Various hormones and chemical reactions in the body carefully regulate the concentration of sodium in the blood. When we take in too much inorganic sodium (table salt), the kidneys begin to excrete more sodium in the urine in an effort to bring the delicately balanced sodium concentrate back to normal.

Sodium holds on to water and with excess inorganic sodium in our bodies, we become thirsty. When we drink water, the sodium concentration is diluted and a delicate balance returns. When a person has swelling in the tissues, it generally means they have too much sodium in their body and in order to get rid of this sodium, we must increase the potassium. This is the main way to get rid of fluid retention without the use of drugs.

You may be asking at this point, why not take a diuretic? Diuretics only cause water to leave the body in an abnormal and often dangerous manner. Besides, the water loss is only temporary. The body learns to depend on diuretics like many people are habituated to laxatives. Over a period of time, they have to increase the strength of the laxative for it to be effective.

A Major Problem Today: Most Drinking Water is Polluted

From the above discussion, you can easily understand that water is the key to all bodily functions: digestion, circulation, assimilation, elimination, lubrication, and temperature control. Because of this, we are sure that you can understand that the purity and quality of the water you drink is vital to your body's well being. Another very important point that few people stop to think about is that the earth does not make any new water. In fact, only one percent of the earth's water is suitable for drinking. The other 99% are either ice or unusable salt water. This same 1% is recycled with all the exposure to chemicals, toxins, and poisons.

More and more, everyday throughout our nation and the world, magazines, television, and newspapers warn about the dangers of drinking polluted water. Many of the pollutants in the water are odorless, tasteless, and colorless, but they are dissolved in the water. Unfortunately, for many generations the oceans, rivers, and ground waters have been a catchall for waste products. The main sources of these waste products are agricultural: fertilizers, insecticides, pesticides, herbicides, arsenic, nitrates, industrial (heavy metals, chemicals, solvents, mercury, organic waste, lead, rust, asbestos, dioxin), and man-made (detergents, dissolved solids, sewage, algae, viruses, fungus, parasites, bacteria, hydrocarbons, chlorine). You should easily be able to see the seriousness of the problem when you stop to consider that over 66,000 chemicals are used in the United States and 45,000 pesticides are on the market. We read in a recent issue of Sierra Magazine, an article which reported that of the 1,200 different ingredients found in pesticides that are labeled "inert", only 300 are considered "safe", 100 are known to be dangerous and the risk of the remaining 800 are "unknown'. The seriousness even becomes more apparent when one realizes that there are over 19,000 hazardous waste dumps, 95,000 landfills, tens of thousands of reservoirs that contain liquid waste, and millions of underground storage tanks. There are over three and a half billion gallons of liquid waste created each day, which potentially can pollute our water supply.

It's quite obvious that Big Brother (Government) knows the danger of this polluted water in our society and wants to keep us ignorant of this fact. Would you believe that recent legislative action has made it illegal to claim that any municipally treated water is detrimental to your health? Ralph Nader's (consumer activist) 1988 Report states: "Nationwide, 2,110 organic and inorganic contaminants have been identified in the drinking water at various levels by Federal Land State Survey programs since the Safe Drinking Water Act was passed in 1974. Of these 2,110 contaminants, nearly 2,090 are organic chemicals." This Nader report presents a national portrait of the real drinking water contamination crisis that local, state, and federal officials have been unwilling or unable to manage. The Environmental protection Agency only tests for 33 contaminants and if the standards for these are met, the water is considered safe. What about all the contaminants not tested for? Another factor is that some of the most hazardous contaminants like asbestos and lead usually enter the water after leaving the water treatment plants. Most people do not realize that the majority of the water treatment facilities use aluminum sulfate to precipitate the cloudiness in our drinking water, and according to Colloidal Chemistry Laws, 3 parts per million of this aluminum will cause severe coagulation in our blood. The only way you can protect yourself is to drink distilled water, or reverse osmosis filtered water.

9. The Spiritual Life

We have learned that the best physical health flows from a dynamic relationship with God (The Creator, Allah, Yah, or Jehovah-all the names are beautiful). Nothing counteracts emotional stress more effectively than spiritual insight and its resultant strength. Nearly three thousand years ago, one of the wisest men who ever lived, Prophet Solomon (Peace be upon him), stated the relationship between spiritual and physical health in Proverbs 3: 7-8: "Trust and reverence the Lord and turn your back on evil."

Many people go through their entire life never realizing the tremendous powerful, ever reaching God that can flood out all their negativity. God can cleanse you from top to bottom, inside to outside. In every area of your life, God can show you what is right and what is wrong. This will give us balance in our lives.

The Bible says, "My people perish for lack of knowledge." In the Quran, God says, "Many are caused to sin by appetites void of knowledge." This is so true. Sickness and premature death are commonplace, because we have no knowledge of God's ways. We live entirely differently than the way God intended for us to live. That is one of the reasons there is so much pain and sickness, so many heart attacks, headaches, bad tempers, mental illness, and total lack of joy. We think most of us drift away from God's ways, because of our wishes to satisfy our own desires. We want to gratify our flesh and desire more than we want to serve our God. We are convinced that God has provided a remedy for every disease that might afflict mankind. All disease is caused by some kind of violation of the natural laws of God. We do not obey them, because we do not understand them.

It appears that many of us are simply jaded and have become content to live a life of mediocrity. We have become so perverted that right is wrong (good) and wrong is right (bad). We cannot blame it on others because we all do it. We live in a society that wants to push our children to be super human beings instead of teaching them God's laws and how to live in true freedom and simplicity.

Our physical condition can influence our spiritual lives far more than we realize. If we are disciplined in the care of our physical bodies, we are far more likely to be disciplined in our spiritual lives. Sickness detracts from our relationships and service far more than we understand. God designed our body to be self-repairing and self-healing if we treat it properly. The great majority of Americans today do not have the advantage of learning about good nutrition and the knowledge of God's laws.

In US medical schools today, all students are taught to give out drugs and chemicals to treat symptoms of disease. It is true that some drugs have been developed that have saved millions of lives, but they are certainly used to great excess in our society and all over the world. Over 99% of the drugs and medications given today are cations and can be very harmful to our health if taken over a long period of time.

<u>Mental Attitude and Self Image</u>

With a positive mental attitude, you will look better, feel better, and heal better. God tells us, *"As a man thinketh in his heart, so is he," Proverbs 23:7. Also, Imam Ali, cousin of the Prophet Muhammad (Peace be on both of them) said, "He who knows himself knows his Creator."* We have re-phrased both proverbs to make it easier to understand. "We understand ourselves once we understand the Creator." We have seen these techniques actually change people's lives around 100%, and it has done so for us on several occasions. The truth is that every circumstance of your life can be looked upon from a positive or negative viewpoint.

Another important imaging technique is to always try to feel good about you. Do you basically have positive or negative feelings about the person you see in the mirror? Do you love yourself or hate yourself? Prophet Solomon (Peace be upon him) put it this way; *"A joyful heart is good medicine, but a broken spirit dries up the bones"* (Proverbs 17:22).

Without a positive self-image, you will not properly digest and assimilate the nutrients in your food. If this happens, the food can become toxic within your intestine. Some researchers are convinced that the colon (large intestine) is a holder of the emotions. So much so that a wise doctor in Philadelphia a number of years ago remarked that "the colon is the mirror of the mind and when the mind gets tight, the colon gets tight." The Prophet Muhammad (Peace be upon him) said, "All disease begins in the colon." On the other hand, a positive feeling towards yourself relaxes the intestines, stimulating the proper functioning which will give you the best possible digestion and nutrition.

Most authorities also believe that when you have relationships that are not good, they usually result in a negative self-image. If we do not get along with ourselves, we tend to not get along with others. Other people react to the negative image that we project. Negative relationships affect our bodies just like a negative self-image. For these reasons, we should all strive to develop a good positive mental attitude at all times and to keep a good self-image concerning ourselves. We've seen so many people that live their lives according to what other people may think about them. Frankly, this is a rather stupid attitude, because when the real facts are known, most of the people you meet do not care that much about you. The important thing is for you to be genuine with yourself.

10. Stress and Stress Management

Many human illnesses are directly related to stress, isolation, emotions, pressures from society and the negative effects of the world. Stress, therefore, affects us physically, mentally, and emotionally and influences all our behaviors. Stress may be defined as demand for adaptation. It has been shown, however, that we humans respond to demands not as they actually are, but as we perceive them to be. Stress may be real or imagined.

We constantly face many kinds of stress. These stress factors may be physical (exposures to the extremes of temperature, injuries or accidents), chemical (exposure to pollutants, allergens, poisons, toxins and drugs), microbiological (germs, bacteria, viruses, fungus and other microorganisms), and psychological or extreme emotional states (fear, anger, sadness or sense of loss). Stress affects practically every organ in the body and, if not controlled, can certainly aggravate and complicate most any known disease or illness.

Stress is the response of your mind, emotions, and body to whatever demands are being made on you. So, the important thing is not so much what happens to you, but the way you respond to it. The ideal response is a relaxed, carefree, and positive thinking reaction. Remember there are two kinds of stress: positive and negative. Positive stress is happy, desirable, controllable, and easygoing. Negative stress, however, is maddening, sad, disturbing, uncontrollable and depressing.

Develop a positive attitude about everything you do. The Bible tells us, "As a man thinketh in his heart, so is he." We become what we think. If we constantly think about negative, bad problems, and thoughts, we are going to create more of these bad situations.

a. Tell yourself to totally relax. Simply sit down, close your eyes and take some deep abdominal breaths. Sit in a comfortable chair and tell yourself that you are totally relaxing as you visualize in your mind your feet relaxing first, then your lower legs, then your upper legs, your pelvis, stomach, chest and hands. Then your lower arms, upper arms, neck and head. Visualize yourself, in your "minds eye" as being totally relaxed. A few minutes of this will do wonders to relieve the stress in your entire body.

b. Practice breathing exercises to relax. You should use abdominal breathing to relax. Sit in a very relaxed position in a comfortable chair with your hands on the arms of the chair and your feet on the floor. Breathe in slowly through your nose, as you expand your abdomen, and imagine that you have a balloon inside your abdomen. As you inhale you are slowing inflating the balloon, which will cause your abdominal area to swell. Then, breathe out slowly through your nose. Pull your abdominal muscles in as you press out the air of your lungs. You should take several breaths in this manner, and it will help you relax. Another variation of this type of exercise is to use abdominal breathing as you inhale deeply through your nose.

c. Cultivate a good sense of humor. Laughing always relieves stress. If you know yourself, you know what makes you laugh. If you try to do these things more often, this will help you to relieve stress. Remind yourself to have fun. This may mean going to a comedy show or picking up a book of funny jokes to get you laughing. You might consider keeping a "laugh scrapbook" where you can keep a record of all letters, funny jokes, poems, or anything you have collected that made you laugh. Read these in times of stress.

d. Listen to relaxing music to relieve tension. Listening to your favorite music is an excellent way of relieving stress. Instrumental music performed on the harp, piano, string ensemble or the flute tends to be more soothing than vocal pieces. While you enjoy the music, you will notice that you are breathing more slowly and deeply which means you are more relaxed.

e. Call a relative or friend. When hit with any type of stressful situation, call a close friend or family member and discuss the situation, which can help you get a clearer picture as to how to solve the situation. Do not keep it pent up inside you.

f. Exercise or take a brisk walk to lift your spirits. Any type of exercise and especially brisk walking will result in effective stress reduction. The faster you walk or the harder you exercise, the more your stress will be relieved. This is because certain neurotransmitters are released during the exercise process for about twenty minutes. Try not to think about your problems at this time.

g. Stretch or yawn for better relaxation. Yawning itself is a very effective way to relieve stress. When you yawn try and stretch your muscles as far as you can. If you develop tension in your neck, shoulder, and upper body the simple shoulder shrug will help relax these muscles. Bring your shoulders up to your earlobes for three or four seconds, and then drop your shoulders down and think: shoulders up, shoulders down. Do this three or four times. Another simple exercise is "reaching for the sky. Try to push your arms upwards and slightly backwards, and feel these muscles in your shoulders and upper back stretching. Hold this position for 10-15 seconds as you breathe normally. Stretching any muscles in your body will help you to relax.

h. Take a nature break. If there is any way you can, go to the country, or out to the woods to escape your problems. This can do wonders for a stressful situation. It may be going to the river or just sitting and watching the clouds. Even watching a video or movie about the great outdoors can be very relaxing.

i. Take a vacation or weekender. Getting away from your stressful environment is always relaxing. Try to not feel guilt about not working when you "get away from it all." Relax mentally, physically, and emotionally and learn to let everything go. Tell yourself its okay not to work all of the time. Try to get away for a least a week for the maximum benefits.

j. Get proper rest. Sound sleep each night is a perfect antidote to stress. Stick to a regular sleep schedule and try to begin to relax about an hour before you go to bed. Do not eat a big meal before you go to bed, and be sure that your, sleep in a very comfortable environment. Also, taking a 15-minute nap in the afternoon will be very stress relieving.

k. Prayer will break the anxiety cycle. Praying can strengthen your religious beliefs, and provide you with strength during times of loss or hardship. Praying can teach forgiveness, patience, and understanding. It can relieve some of the negative emotions like anger, bitterness, and hostility. This is an excellent stress reliever.

Of course, there are other stress relieving techniques such as getting a pet (excellent for many), but the important thing is to do something to try to relieve the existing condition.

11. Miscellaneous Nutrition Gems and Pearls

a. Non-herbal tea and coffee. Caffeine is one of a number of biochemical compounds found in non-herbal tea and coffee. Caffeine is also found in chocolate, cola based drinks and a number of medications. An average cup of strong non-herbal tea contains 50 mg of caffeine and coffee 100 mg. Although these can vary from brand to brand the biological qualities of caffeine and related compounds have a number of adverse effects on your health. Caffeine can cause anxiety and nervousness, depression, insomnia, and aggravate any pre-existing psychiatric states. Caffeine can affect your physical body by causing you to pass an excessive amount of urine, diarrhea, bloating, indigestion, tremors, and migraine headaches, rapid and irregular heartbeats. High blood pressure, restless legs at night, and high blood cholesterol are also causes of caffeine consumption. Excessive caffeine can also affect women who have fibrocystic breast disease, as well as PMS. If you drink it at mealtime, the caffeine can decrease the amount of iron absorbed from the vegetables eaten. Caffeine also interferes with zinc absorption. One of the worst things about caffeine is that it stimulates your body to produce excess insulin, and this can aggravate a person's condition that may have hypoglycemia or carbohydrate intolerance. All of us would be wise to eliminate caffeine consumption.

b. Soda Pop and Colas. Soda pop and colas, including diet cola, are some of the worst things that ever happened to the health of America. The great majority of these drinks are loaded with sugar. They act as total cations, because they are sticky and loaded with caffeine. In addition, all sodas, colas, and diet drinks are loaded with other chemicals that are totally cationic in nature and detrimental to your health. A person would be wise to leave out all of these drinks from their diet.

c. Alcohol. Alcohol is probably one of the most socially acceptable "poisons" after non-herbal tea and coffee. Most beers average about 4% alcohol; wine contains 6%, and brandy and whisky about 40%. We should not forget that alcohol is a food and provides calories in the form of carbohydrates. For an overweight person, this can be detrimental. Alcohol has adverse effects on almost every vitamin and mineral. In particular, vitamin B1, B2, B3, B6, folic acid, calcium, magnesium, and zinc are depleted in the bodies of those who consume alcohol. Deficiencies of these nutrients affect one's general health and one's mental health in particular. Alcohol interferes with fatty acid metabolism. The effects of long term consumption of alcohol on the body can be devastating:

liver damage, nervous system imbalance, and brain damage. Certain types of cancer are increased as a result of alcohol consumption, especially cancer of the liver, esophagus, larynx, and mouth. Any woman who drinks alcohol while pregnant is an absolute fool. It is quite common for children who are born of mothers who consume substantial amounts of alcohol during pregnancy to suffer from facial deformities and be mentally retarded.

d. Smoking. Cigarette smoking has a powerful anti-vitamin C effect, and most smokers have a lower than normal level of vitamin C in their blood. Smoking affects the working of the pancreas, which is important in the digestion of our food. Smoking is sure-fire way to get lung cancer.

e. Prescription Drugs and Drug Abuse. The problem with drug addiction and drug abuse seems to be increasing all over our nation. Hundreds of thousands of people take medications to relax them or to sleep every day, drugs such as Valium, Librium, Atrium, Xanax, and Halcyon. It is widely accepted that many people become physically and psychologically addicted to such drugs. They are unable to live without them and their withdrawal from them produces both physical and physiological problems. The medical profession has been slow to recognize and respond to this problem. It is advisable that any person try to abstain from taking any drugs, if at all possible.

OF VITAL IMPORTANCE

a. Totally avoid all hydrogenated oils like margarine and all deep fried foods such as doughnuts, French fries, and potato chips. Read food labels. Our foods are being poisoned today with hydrogenated oils in our boxed foods, mayonnaise, and salad dressings. Use cooking oils with unrefined or non-hydrogenated written on the label. If these terms are missing, the oil is hydrogenated. The best oils to cook with are extra virgin olive oil, coconut oil, and butter.

b. You must increase the proper fatty acids in your diet by eating cold water ocean fish, grass-fed meats, whole grains, raw seeds, fruits, and vegetables. Cold water ocean fish include wild Alaskan salmon, mackerel, herring, orange roughy, and sardines. Fresh fish is the best, but canned fish is okay as they do still have the good oils in them. Eat 3 tsp. of extra virgin olive oil on salads, but keep the oil refrigerated after opening. Walnuts are high in fatty acids and make good snack foods. Eat only breads and cereals that have 100% whole wheat or whole grain written on the label. Most brown breads are not whole grain, but have coloring added. Avoid processed or refined cereals or white flour products such as breads, crackers, macaroni, and spaghetti.

c. With any illness at all, you should follow the above and add the following supplements and follow the directions below.

i. Purchase some cod liver oil capsules or unrefined flaxseed oils from a health food store, and take 4-6 capsules daily. If you can't eat the fish mentioned above, you should take these capsules regularly.

ii. Purchase some unrefined Borage oil and take 1 capsule daily or purchase unrefined Evening Primrose capsules and take 4-6 daily. Eliminate your commercial red meat intake. Since commercial red meat contains antibiotics, growth hormones, and pesticide residues which can aggravate any disease condition.

iii. Avoid all refined sugars, desserts, and all white flour foods.

iv. Get a good hypoallergenic non-yeast whole food multiple vitamin and mineral tablet and take 3-4 tablets daily. Be sure you get at least 1,000 mg of Vitamin C, 50 mg of B3 and B6, 50 mg Zinc, 100 mcg Selenium, and 400 mg of Magnesium in your supplements. The above mentioned vitamins are necessary in the fatty acid chemical reactions.

Super Nutritious Diet Plan

a. **Water.** Drink only distilled water or water from a proven Reverse Osmosis water filtering system. Ideally, one should drink half their weight in ounces. For example, someone weighing 150lbs will drink 75 ounces of water. Drinking this water will help your kidneys get rid of the excess cations you may take in without realizing it. All metabolic processes will function more efficiently by drinking this extra water.

b. **Eliminate Refined Sugar and Refined carbohydrates.** This includes table sugar, splenda, sucrose, white, brown, glucose, refined honey, sorbitol, or any additive that ends in "ose" (maltose, lactose, and fructose). Many foods like cookies, pies, cakes, ice cream, soft drinks, chocolates, puddings, jams, and jellies contain large amounts of sucrose or other refined carbohydrates. Blackstrap molasses, brown rice syrup, and raw unfiltered honey are the exceptions. They are not refined products and carry with them all the nutrients necessary for digestion.

c. **Ensure a Daily Intake of Fresh Green Leafy Vegetables (High Anions).** Such foods are rich in the nutrients that are most commonly found to be lacking in many ill and elderly people. Please keep in mind that ensuring a good intake of raw or wok-cooked vegetables and salads will help protect against some of the more common and more serious diseases in our society.

d. **Eat a Wide Variety of Foods.** Eating the same foods over and over makes it difficult to obtain adequate amounts of all the essential nutrients required for proper nutrition. Also, eating the same foods regularly may make one more susceptible to becoming allergic and addicted to these particular foods, which can add stress to your already overstressed system. Eating a wide variety of foods simply makes good common sense.

e. **Ensure an Adequate Intake of Fiber.** Ideally, our system needs 30-40 grams of fiber daily whereas the average person in our society gets only 8-10 grams of fiber each day. High fiber foods include all beans, salads, fresh fruits, and fresh vegetables. 100% whole grain cereals and breads such as wheat, oats, barley, rye, millet, corn and brown rice (never white). You should not rely too heavily on any one type of fiber such as wheat or bran. One of the best forms of fiber is ground psyllium seed husk. All persons having constipation should add this fiber to their diet daily.

f. **Strive to Eat Only fresh Foods (Foods that spoil).** All additives to foods such as preservatives, coloring agents, emulsifiers, texturizers, flavorings, or chemicals will have adverse effects on your health now and in the future. You will invariably find these additives in most all foods found in cans, bottles, boxes, or cellophane packages. You must read all labels on foods before purchasing. Fresh food without additives or chemicals is greatly preferred.

g. **Strive to Eat High Quality Protein.** Ideally you should eat your protein foods at the afternoon meal. These proteins are found in lean organic grass-fed meats, free range eggs, raw cheeses, nuts, seeds, peas, beans, lentils, sprouted beans, 100% whole grains and wild ocean fish.

h. **Limit Your Intake of Inorganic Salt.** Salt is sodium chloride (NaCl) and sodium is the primary cation found in our blood and all bodily fluids. Excessive intake of inorganic sodium causes fluid retention, high blood pressure, heart strain and numerous other detrimental effects on our body physiology. A wise individual will make every effort to limit and avoid any excess salt intake. Genuine sea salt, Celtic Sea salt, or Himalayan Sea Salt with their high and complete mineral contents, is said to regulate excessive sodium in the blood, raising or lowering it as needed.

i. **Eliminate Alcohol Consumption.** Recent reports conclude that a maximum of two drinks daily is a safe recommendation. However, the Quran says, "avoid alcohol because it keeps you from the remembrance of God and it opens the door for Satan to enter your mind." We prefer to follow God and not scientific reports!

j. **Avoid Becoming Obese by Overeating.** Being significantly overweight reduces life expectancy and aggravates many conditions such as diabetes, hypertension, gout, arthritis, gallstones, and colon cancer. So lose weight, if you are overweight, and try eating high anionic foods. Pure distilled water should be used to decrease the cations and add lemon juice to increase your daily anion intake.

Additional Rules for Healthy Living

a. **Avoid Tobacco Products in All Forms.** Tobacco has many harmful effects whether in smoking or chewing.

b. **Take Prescribed Medical Drugs and Over-the-Counter Drugstore medications Only if Essential** (life threatening). All medications or drugs are 100% cationic (acid) in nature. It is your job to remind your physician to try to decrease or stop any unnecessary medications. Remember that drugs are toxic, and are not essential to health unless there is a defined medical problem. You will never find a person who is deficient in Tylenol or Valium.

c. **Do Not Take Illegal Drugs.** Considerable harm and tragedy is caused by the use of illicit drugs. The danger far outweighs any possible benefits that might result from their use.

d. **Take Regular Physical Exercise.** Regular physical exercise is absolutely necessary to maintain good physical health. We highly recommend the use of a Rebounder or mini-trampoline for at least 20 minutes in the morning; at least 5 days a week. Other forms of exercise such as brisk walking, swimming, cycling, basketball, or any sporting activity are acceptable, but above all, GET YOUR PHYSICAL EXERCISE. Do some form of exercise you enjoy doing.

e. **Take Regular Mental Exercise.** Our mind, like our muscles, needs exercise and with both, if you don't use it, you lose it. The mind affects the body in many known and unknown ways, and good mental health is necessary to enjoy good physical health. Various mental activities like reading, writing, creative arts, and hobbies can be very stimulating to your mind. Turn off the idiot box.

f. **Maintain a Wide Variety of Interests and Activities and Keep Your home and Work Environment Tidy.** A wide variety of interests and activities stimulate your mind and physical body. Working in a clean and tidy environment helps you to be more calm and relaxed. Both of these important areas are stress relieving and foster better health.

g. Follow Definite Goals and Purposes in Your Life. We are all involved in six areas of our lives all 24 hours of each day. These areas are your physical health, mental attitude, business, family, social, and religious life. If you have set your goals in all these areas or if you have agreed to do something for anyone, make sure you act responsibly and complete these vital issues. This will relieve stress and cause an increase in your own self-respect as well as enable you to enjoy a much fuller life. This will place you in a situation where you will be playing a vital part in creating your own future.

h. Take Whole Food Nutritional Supplements. Whole food vitamin and mineral supplements are generally necessary for a healthy individual living a stress-free lifestyle and consuming a natural wholesome diet. Recent studies show that at least 90% of the American people are deficient in one or more nutrients. The only wise course of action is to take supplemental vitamins, minerals, anti-oxidants, trace minerals and fatty acids. This will simply eliminate the possibility of nutritional deficiencies from these vital nutrients.

i. Try to Eliminate Stress from Your Life. Stress aggravates all diseases and can only hamper any healing process. Study the section on stress relief and initiate some of the stress relieving techniques to help attain better health.

j. Study and Learn Good Nutrition and Apply this Knowledge to Your Life. Your future good health or poor health depends upon you and you alone.

k. Get a Pet. Have a pet to love and you can do wonders to help relieve stress in every facet of your life. Recent studies show that pet owners live longer and their quality of life is better.

l. Worship God Everyday. This suggestion is probably the most important of all.

Desirable Practices for Healthy Food Selection and Preparation.

a. Eat only when hungry. Eat only portion sizes you feel you can safely digest. Reason: Over eating taxes your digestion, which results in undigested food.

b. Consume a wide variety of different foods. Reason: A wide variety will provide you body with more adequate types and amounts of vitamins, minerals and other food supplements. This will help prevent food allergies.

c. Avoid eating or drinking the same thing two days in a row. (Exception: pure water) Try to rotate your foods. Reason: variety in food increases potential vitamin and mineral intake and reduces the chance of developing food allergies.

d. Eat slowly and eat only until satisfied. Eat small portions more often and large portions less often. Reason: digestion and assimilation is your key to nutritional health. Your body can digest small amounts eaten frequently more efficiently.

e. Chew food thoroughly. Ideally, chew each mouthful 20-30 times. Reason: digestion begins in the mouth with enzymes in your saliva.

f. Drink liquids between meals, not with meals and preferably 2 hours after and 15 minutes before. Reason: liquids dilute digestive juices.

g. Drink a glass of water upon rising (preferably warm). You may add fresh lemon or apple cider vinegar and a tsp. of raw honey. Reason: this will stimulate regular and normal bowel movements each day.

h. Foods, especially liquids, should not be taken very hot or very cold. Reason: very hot or cold foods create more stress.

i. Drink plenty of distilled or pure water daily, preferably 60-80 ounces. This is especially important with exercise. When perspiring, eating dry foods, and in hot climates.

Reason: water keeps all tissues well hydrated and flushes out impurities that can cause toxic effects. Adequate water also improves elimination. Make sure it is pure water.

j. Raw foods, except meats, should comprise 50% of total food intake and preferably 75%. Reason: raw foods provide more fibers, more vitamins, minerals and food supplements and have more enzymes to give better digestion.

k. At meals, it is best to consume a variety of raw vegetables when you eat cooked foods. Reason: There is greater abundance of enzymes and fiber in vegetables, which will assist digestion, and assimilation of the cooked foods.

l. Avoid overcooking. Reason: vitamins enzymes, proteins and fatty acids are all heat sensitive and can be destroyed or chemically changed by overheating

m. Do not be overly concerned about calories, proteins, fats, carbohydrates, vitamins and minerals while eating wholesome foods. Reason: a normal metabolism is programmed to adjust its selection and absorption of foodstuffs in the presence of a wholesome lifestyle and dietary habits.

n. In a vegetarian meal containing no animal products, some legumes (lentils, beans) should be added when consuming primary grains. Reason: Legumes provide certain proteins needed for balance.

o. For those with compromised or delicate digestion, generally avoid concoctions containing combinations of animal protein (i.e. flesh) and carbohydrates (such as dried fruits, bread, bananas, potatoes, grains) or acid fruits and carbohydrates (such as citrus, tomato, vinegar) or milk and animal proteins all in the same mouthful. Instead, lean more to individual foods consumed separately.

p. Avoid foods to which you are allergic: Reason: allergic foods create a broad spectrum of chronic health problems and upset digestion of other foods eaten at the same time.

q. Eats sweets (including fruits), nuts and seeds alone and in between meals only. Reason: for maximum digestion and assimilation fruit, nuts and seeds are best eaten in moderation and alone. When eaten with a meal or other snack food, they may upset digestion.

r. When emotionally upset, eat less and chew well. Reason: emotional upset changes digestive chemistry and interferes with complete digestion.

s. Avoid distractions while eating such as television, radio, driving or reading. Reason: when attention is fully with a meal and those with whom you share the meal, you can focus on thoroughly chewing and enjoying a relaxed mental state, which assists digestion and assimilation.

t. Read labels and ingredients on boxed, canned and packages food. When dining out, question your server as to ingredients used in the foods you are ordering. Reason: know what is in the food you eat and choose foods that serve your health better.

u. Keep a brief food symptom-feeling journal of everything you eat or drink. Reason: you will learn more about foods and how they affect you by recording them over a period of time and reviewing the records.

v. Be sure to avoid all hydrogenated or partially hydrogenated oils. Reason: hydrogenated oils can block the normal chemical pathways of cholesterol metabolism.

w. Use a product called Willard Water in your distilled or reverse osmosis water for proper hydration of cells.

x. Purchase a shower filter to avoid chlorine exposure.

Heavy Metal Crisis

"Hence gout and some stone afflict the human race; hence lazy jaundice with her saffron face; Palsy, with shaking head and tott'ring knees. And bloated dropsy, the staunch sot's disease; Consumption, pale with keen

but hollow eye, And sharpened feature, showed that death was nigh. The feeble offspring curse their crazy sires, And tainted from his birth, the young expires."
(Description of lead poisoning by an anonymous Roman hermit, Translated by Humelbergius Secundus, 1829)

Lead poisoning is still one of the most overlooked childhood epidemics in America. The media seems to only focus on the common diseases like cancer, heart disease, diabetes, Alzheimer's and so on. Though all of these diseases are extremely important, our children still lack the attention they need regarding this crippling issue.

The history of childhood lead poisoning in cities like St. Louis, Detroit, Chicago and other large and small communities are still a tragic issue. Like other MediSinners of the corporate world, those that produced lead pipes and lead paint were well aware that their product was severely injuring and killing large numbers of young children as far back as the 1920's. Medical journal articles reporting that children were being poisoned by lead paint in their homes began appearing in the U.S. in 1914. After that, repeated articles described how children were lead poisoned from window sills, porch railings, painted surfaces in the home, even play grounds and toys, causing hospitalization from seizures, blindness, stomach cramps, paralysis, and some aggravating deaths.

Lead is a ubiquitous metal that has been used by humans for more than three millennia. It has a long history of creating toxicity within the human body. According to history, the Romans were aware of the health devastations, madness and death. However, they were so intrigued by its diversity that they ignored the consequences at hand. What the Romans did not realize was that their everyday low-level exposure to this metal rendered them vulnerable to chronic lead poisoning. Much like today's modern corporate world of unbridled gluttony and arrogance among the financial elite, the continued thirst for lead manufacturing slowly strangle the great Roman Empire.

Lead poisoning is the most chronic environmental illness affecting modern children in addition to cancer. The efforts are apparently mediocre, at best, due to the serious cases of lead poisoning still being reported in hospital emergency rooms, poison control centers, schools and private physician's offices. In children, virtually no organ system is immune to the effects of lead poisoning. Perhaps the organ of greatest concern is the developing brain. Any disorganizing influence that affects an individual at a critical time in development is likely to have long-lasting effects. Such is the effect of lead on the brain. Lead damages the nervous system, causes headaches, eye spots, metallic waste, inhibits copper enzymes needed for neurotransmitters dopamine, epinephrine and norepinephrine causing hyperactivity, high blood pressure, emotional problems, poor concentration and memory, learning disabilities, sluggish mind to mental retardation, sterility, and personality changes. According to the National Center for Environmental Health, there were about 200 deaths from lead poisoning in the U.S. between 1979 and 1998. Most of the deaths were among males (74%), African-Americans (67%), adults over the age of 45 (76%), and Southerners (70%). According to the agency for Toxic Substances and Disease Registry, there are about one out of every six children in the U.S. with high levels of lead in the blood. Lead poisoning occurs in every group, especially among African-American children in urban area homes. African-Americans and Hispanic children appear to have the greatest risk of developing lead poisoning. Approximately 434,000 U.S. children aged 1-5 years have blood lead levels greater than the CDC recommended level of 10 micrograms of lead per deciliter of blood (this is based on the NHANES (National Health and Nutrition Examination 1999-2000 survey).

The major source of today's lead exposure among U.S. children is lead-based paint and lead-contaminated dust found in deteriorating buildings. Lead-based paints were banned for use in housing in 1978. However, approximately 24 million housing units in the U.S. have deteriorated lead paint and elevated levels of lead contaminated house dust. More than four million of these dwellings are home to one or more young children. The state of Missouri has traditionally been the world's largest producer of lead ore. Ninety-nine percent of the housing stock in the City of St. Louis was built before 1978 when lead-based paints were banned. It is the people that live in these homes that are at high risk, especially children. In 2003, the Health Department of St.

Louis screened 12,011 children for lead poisoning. 1,638 (13.6%) had a blood level of ten micrograms per deciliter or greater, which is the CDC definition of lead poisoning.

Soil Test in Detroit

According to a Free Press investigation, lead-contaminated soil is wide spread throughout metro Detroit, especially in the urban core where many of Michigan's' poisoned children live. This means urban parks and playgrounds still contain this heavy metal! Unfortunately, most of the urban sites will never be cleaned up due to the fact that national strategy for preventing lead poisoning focuses on paint, the main contamination source for children.

There are thousands of growing children that play in toxic dirt in their backyards and neighborhood parks all over the nation that will be innocent victims because they live in the neglected older industrial cities that contain lead. Scientists acknowledge that there needs to be greater focus on the lead in the soil, because it does increase the exposure for children that adds to the lead buildup in their bodies. There are many other sources of lead besides the home. Other sources include: air pollution, ammunition, auto exhaust, contaminated soil, some pottery, and tobacco smoke.

Solutions

One of the first steps to addressing the lead epidemic is dietary modification and detoxification. Since most of the commercial foods and produce contain chemicals it would be best to start with the health food stores. There are many food and herbal based supplements that may remove or prevent further damage from lead toxicity. One such therapy is chelation.

Chelation Therapy

Clinical studies have demonstrated that chelation therapy can bind with heavy metals such as lead and remove them from the body. Chelation is derived from the Greek word "chele" and refers to the claw of a crab or lobster. The primary chelating source, Ethylene Diamine Tetra Acetic Acid (EDTA) which is a synthetic amino acid chelating agent with a particular affinity for toxic metals such as lead, mercury, cadmium (used in chem-trails), and aluminum. When EDTA enters the body it binds with these metals, the material is sequestered, then secreted in bodily wastes.

EDTA Chelation Therapy is a safe and non-painful application and is administered on an outpatient basis. The treatments involve a series of infusions lasting from 90 minutes to 3 hours. Chelation therapy also improves metabolic circulatory function by removing metals.

Chelation procedures were first used in Nazi Germany as a replacement for citric acid. At that time, it was also discovered that radiation poisoning was effectively treated by chelating agents. The chelating agents which remove the heavy metals that emitted radioactivity from the body were the same EDTA used to remove calcium deposits in copper pipes and boilers.

It wasn't until 1948 that EDTA was first used in the treatment of lead poisoning. Since then, chelation therapy has become the premier application in treating lead poisoning, weight normalization, chronic fatigue, memory enhancement, controlling insulin activity, skin, nail and hair improvement and the reversal of impotence.

If you or your children are concerned about lead poisoning or heavy metal detoxification search the web and find a chelation specialist in your area or use Metal Flush by Chi Enterprises (714) 777-1542.

Ten Step Lead and Heavy Metal Detoxification Program:

1. Refrain from foods that contain multiple chemicals which impair maximum detoxification activity.

2. Stop using deodorant that contains aluminum. Replace it with a deodorant that has natural and effective ingredients. Consider a deodorant stone.

3. Fast periodically on a combination of organic vegetable and fruit juices using a combination of sodium alginate, activated charcoal, cayenne, garlic, chlorella, agar powder, bee pollen, stool softener, plenty of distilled and micro-clustered water.

4. Restore depleted nutrients with whole food and herbal based vitamins, minerals, systemic and digestive enzymes.

5. Use an infrared sauna to help remove impurities.

6. Purchase lecithin (non-soy version)

7. Be selective about dinner plates, some products may contain lead.

8. Find a specialist in chelation therapy or a quality supplement of oral chelation.

9. Eat fresh, organically grown greens daily if possible.

10. Make closer observations of yourself and your children.

Other Health Protocols:

Kidney Failure/Disease: Asparagus Extract, Cordyceps, Kidney Chi, and Bathdetox from Chi Enterprise (714) 777-1542
Eye (Glaucoma, Cataracts, Blurred Vision): Bilberry, Eyebright, Alpha-Lipoic Acid, Selenium, Vitamin A, Bates Eye Exercises
Eczema/Psoriasis/Acne: Omega 3 Fatty-Acids, Intestinal Cleansing Formula #1 from Dr. Whitaker (323) 595-8214, Psoracaid from Chi Enterprise (714) 777-1542
Constipation/Irritable Bowel Syndrome/Colitis: Intestinal Cleansing Formula #1 & #2 from Dr. Whitaker (323) 595-8214, Marshmallow, Comfrey, Activated Charcoal
Circulation: Cayenne pepper, Vein-Lite by Chi Enterprise (714) 777-1542
Digestion/Acid Reflux: Apple Cider Vinegar, Food Enzymes, Digestron by Chi Enterprise (714) 777-1542
Fungal Infections/Candida: Pau d Arco, Metal Flush, Olive Leaf Extract
Stress: Whole Food B-Complex, Kava Kava, Minerals, Cod Liver Oil, Cabbage, Brown Rice

Whole Body Tonic for All Ages

The Jurak Classic (JC) Whole Body Tonic draws on the best of the world's vital traditions: emphasizing balance and longevity; counteracting stress; balancing the immune system; improving endurance; increasing physical and mental energy, stamina and circulation and detoxifying and maintaining cellular health.

The individual tonic herbs in the JC Tonic nourish specific cells, tissues, and organs and have been combined to treat the body as a whole. Tonic remedies are well tolerated and have a slow, nourishing effect on the body systems, imparting strength and tone. On a daily basis, one ounce of JC Tonic will detoxify, purify and fortify the body. JC Tonic is a fast and sure way to eliminate internal waste and provide an optimum nutritional environment.

The effectiveness of this 60-year-old formula results from the use of tonic herbs compounded with the ancient method of blending a variety of herbs to enrich the whole range of body systems. It is an idea that had not yet been implemented in Western models of nutritional therapy. If taken on a regular basis, this tonic is a NECESSARY, PREVENTIVE insurance for people of all ages.

I, personally, use the JC Tonic to maintain body balance and a youthful appearance. After months of extensive usage, coupled with fasting, I have experienced rapid hair and nail growth and invigorating energy. I firmly believe that JC Tonic needs to be in the home of anyone who wants to achieve optimum health. When I met the founder of JC Tonic, (Anthony Jurak), I was deeply impressed by his 68 year-old, youthful body. The testimonials I have heard and seen from other JC Tonic users have been astounding. THIS IS A MUST HAVE ITEM IN YOUR HOME. To order your bottle of JC Tonic, please call 866-448-5796 and use customer code #12043.

Dr. Scott Whitaker
July, 2005

37. HERBALIST LIVES 256 YEARS? THE SECRET OF ANCIENT HERBS AND TONICS

Believe it or not in 1933, the world's oldest man died at the incredible age of 256! His name was Dr. Li Chung Yun, a doctor and herbalist, who outlived 23 wives and was living with his 24th, a woman in her 60s at the time of his death. It is recorded that nothing spectacular was in his diet during his first one-hundred years of life. When Dr. Yun reached the second century of his life he went public with some of the herbs and tonics he used to keep his body youthful for all those years.

It was recorded that at the age of 207 he gave 28 lectures at a university in China on health and longevity. According to resources, he lectured for as long as three hours. A professor at Minkuo University claimed to have found records showing that Li was born around 1677-78. On his 150th birthday and 200th birthdays he was honored by the Chinese government. One of the great wisdoms of Dr. Yun was to sit like a tortoise, walk sprightly like a pigeon, and sleep like a dog. Early in his life, somewhere between 1690 and 1750, Li Chung Yun developed a lifestyle of collecting herbs and did so for over a century.

Dr. Li Chung Yung's Protocol for Long Life and Longevity

Though Dr. Li Chung Yung **was not a vegetarian or vegan**, he consumed a limited amount of meat, grains and root vegetables. According to documentation, Li's diet consisted primarily of lightly steamed vegetables, fresh fruit and tonic herbs. The herbs he consumed and recommended most highly for promoting health and longevity were Ginseng, Gotu Kola, Fo-ti,

Polygonum Multi Florum, and Garlic. Dr. Li would often drink two different "elixirs of life," as he would call them, alternating the elixirs every other day, drinking them in the morning and in the evening. This tonic apparently had an impact on his vision, mental clarity, circulation, and spirit. In time he formulated a number of other useful herbal combinations for men and women of all ages. Dr Li Ching Yun's life is an example of how powerful the human body can become and how well Taoist longevity techniques work when it becomes a lifestyle.

Dr. Li was not bedridden in the latter days of his life, like most Americans. He continued to take long hikes in the mountains until the final days of his life. It is also documented that he remained sexually active for at least two centuries, never became senile, and when Dr. Li died, all of his teeth were still intact along with most of his hair. Today, most people lose half their teeth and hair by the age of 35 and all of their teeth and hair by 65. It is truly sad that individuals are dying from diseases like cancer, lupus, diabetes and heart attacks. There is no reason whatsoever that this should be happening. The remedy to premature aging and death is knowledge, wisdom and divine guidance, a lack of either will surely be the foundation of disease, ill-health and premature death, in vain.

Life and Longevity

What does it take for one to become disease free and achieve longevity? Many people die prematurely by common diseases created by dietary neglect, stress and a lack for life. It seems that the human body cannot escape the commercialization of death. The world is constantly promoting terrorism, job exportation, religious confusion, Satanism and environmental calamity.

Longevity is not promised to anyone. It is the law of the universe that we need to follow in order to maneuver our way into long life. You should understand that we have always been surrounded be many forms of evil, devilment and laws of misfortune. An example is the great Tsunami that killed over 150,000 people between Thailand and Africa. Though there might be other possibilities for this devastating tragedy, ranging from earthquake to an underwater nuclear experiment, don't think for a moment that "mankind" was not responsible. We have to constantly be aware of our surroundings, even during our most sedated state. It is very important that we stay close to the vibrations of the universe because whenever evil finds vulnerability there is an open door for catastrophe.

As far as physical health, longevity depends greatly upon our lifestyle, diet and physical constitution. If we continue to feed the body with the essentials, then our body will respond with optimum results. On the other hand, if we thrive on pus saturated milk, commercial tobacco, irradiated foods, synthetic medications, and acidic foods, the end result will be sickness and premature death, in most cases.

We will share with you some of the most effective herbs, supplements, tonics and systems of life that have been used long before allopathic medicine. The effectiveness of these ancient herbal applications is proven to work through primary research and clinical trials not false science. They have supported the human body and its immune system all over the world. So nothing has changed except for the bootlickers and little devils of Satan that give tangible goods and temporary power precedence over their eternal souls. Maybe when they return in the next life, they will come back as gnats and flies.

In order to understand longevity, vitality and internal peace we should understand what the ancient wise men of Taoism called the "Three Treasures." These treasures represent essence, energy and spirit which are called jing, qi, and shen. There are no exact translations for these terms into the English language, but they do translate as essence, vitality and spirit. The main objective of all the ancient healing systems and health-promoting arts is to cultivate, balance and manifest all three treasures. The beauty of this art is that it helps harmonize all aspects of one's wellbeing, helping the patient to achieve these essences of oneness.

The first treasure is jing, the superior ultimate treasure. Though accommodated by a radiant body, the quantity of the treasure is small. According to ancient text, the jing existed before the body. This entity enters our body tissues and becomes the foundation of our body. By retaining the jing within our body we maintain vigor. The jing greatly contributes to longevity without this energy, life is not possible.

Qi (pronounced chee) is the life force which enables the body to think and perform spontaneously. The amount of qi can be measured by power and force. It enables a person to maneuver with vitality. If a person is fatigued, bed ridden, coherent by force, the qi is depleted. The force of qi can be seen in all the elements in the world. It can be seen in water, radiation, animals and all plant life. Our qi circulates through all twelve meridians [the energy channels of the body] to nourish and strengthen the functions of our glands and organs. There are many tonics, supplements and herbal combinations that can build your qi, if you are deficient.

Shen is energy of the mind and spirit. It is a combination of jing and qi energy. When these two treasures are in balance, the mind performs at an optimum level, the spirit become sound, the emotions are under control, the physical body becomes strong, and the immune system becomes more effective and strategic. It is not possible to maintain an optimum life without the balance of jing and qi. Shen will bring a solid peace of mind. When you begin to develop jing you will automatically produce qi. When you generate a large amount of qi, you have developed strong shen. This is the essence of being whole. In order for us to achieve this goal we have to refrain from any MediSins that interrupt the energy flow throughout out our mind, body, and spirit. Here are some examples of MediSins that will destroy our essence of life: alcohol, all refined foods, toxic meats, indoor and out door pollutants, chemical body care products and cosmetics, profanity, negativity, jealousy, envy, hate, denial and feelings of inferiority (destroying another culture or race of people just because you are intimidated and cannot co-exist with humbleness and integrity).

Optimum Health through the Essence of Chinese Tonics

According eastern institutional studies, there are about 247 traditional patent herbal formulas and tonics that are able to pinpoint many health concerns based upon the patient's symptoms. Though very underrated in the United States, these Chinese patent formulas have demonstrated to be quite effective. Its application is often used independently when addressing acute (intense, critical, severe) problems, thus having a very accurate effect, especially with symptoms of the common cold, trauma, fever and pain. When addressing chronic (persisting for a long time) problems of deficiency (qi, blood, yin, yang, etc.), the traditional patent formulas become the therapy of choice.

One of the great things about traditional Chinese medicine is that it looks at the patient as a whole person. Unlike allopathic medicine where it prescribes medicine based upon that isolated symptom using synthetic MediSins that may have to be taken for a long time, maybe years, with no healing results, only side effects, traditional Chinese medicine will base its application on excess or deficiency, which we will discuss later. For example, there may be a case of severe kidney yin with symptoms of night sweating, hot flashes, feverish palms or soles, restless insomnia, and burning sensation over the kidneys. So this appears to be a problem with hormone imbalance or acute menopausal hot flashing. The objective of the Da Bu Yin Wan patent formula 181 is to sedate the deficiency of fire and bring the woman's hormonal structure back to balance. Patients may be given a single application or a proprietary blend (combination of herbs).

Another example, a person experiencing dizziness due to a deficiency of liver blood with accumulation of spleen dampness or stomach phlegm can be treated by combining certain patent formulas like Sho Wu Pian and Er Chen Wan. One formula tonifies chi while the other removes phlegm. Traditional patent formulas are used only as long as the symptoms persist. Once the state of symptoms begins to change, the application of the herbal formula will be assessed or reevaluated to the point of changing or being discontinued. The symptoms are again always based upon excess or deficiency of heat, dampness, cold, the amount of phlegm, stagnation or the exogenous invasions of cold and flu.

The following herbs, roots, flowers and perennials not only protect your body from today's diseases but also help to reverse them: Reishi, Rhodiola, Siberian (eluthero) Ginseng, Tein Chi Ginseng, Imperial Wild Ginseng, Korean Ginseng, Prince Ginseng, Sages Ginseng, Buplerum, Schizandra, Rehmannia,

Dragon Bone, Royal Jelly, Eucommia Bark, Licorice Root, Pearls, Gynostemma, Ginkgo Biloba, Lingustrum, Lo Han Cou, Lyceum Fruit, Polyrachis (whole dried ants), Sea Horse, Sea Dragon, Walnut Kernel, Poria, White Peony Root, White Attractylodes, Cinnamon Bark, Cinnamon Twig, Cordyceps, Asparagus Root, Albizzia Flower and Bark.

These herbal patents are important adjunctive therapy to acupuncture, chiropractry, therapeutic message therapy and reflexology. Though these topical applications are often limited to once a week basis, the daily consumption of the appropriate patent formula will greatly contribute to healing acceleration. Please note some of these herbs are considered super tonics and some supportive herbs.

Understanding the Principles of Yin and Yang

Yin and yang is the foundation of the entire traditional Chinese health care system. It is a phenomenal, natural healing concept that has been exercised for several thousand years stimulating from ancient Africa; the only other healing principle that has withstood the test of time is the system of Ayurveda, also from the ancient east. Yin and Yang is an absolute model of the universal law. Though they are opposite in energy, without the balance of both, the wholeness of life would not exist.

Yin and yang are absolutely interdependent, interacting on a constant cycle so that normality and integrity will maintain, as a whole. In every aspect of physical, spiritual, mental and cosmic life, one force tends to dominate the other, but no total dominance is ever permanent. The same with every kingdom or nation not guided by divine law, it will rise and it will fall at some point. That is divine law. Certain powers of this modern world apparently don't believe in the inevitable.

The Chinese refer to the system of yin and yang as the great principle, which describes the cyclic nature of every living thing or force in the universe. All forms of existence and worldly functions have a cyclic nature and thus are governed by the great principle of yin and yang. Yin and yang are not two different types of energy, but rather two complementary poles of the same basin energy, similar to that of a magnetic field or electric current. Yin and yang are reciprocal states of cyclic change, polar phases in the rhythmic transformation of energy. Take an element like water for example, which would appear to be of yin, but can become yang according to its phase. When heated by the sun to a vaporizing degree it becomes yang, rising upward in a yang direction. When its vapor cools and condenses to form clouds it begins to reach a yin stage transforming back into water falling downward.

In the Western Hemisphere, yin and yang are often associated with the force of male and female energies. The connection between man and woman, both contain aspects of yin and yang. Women are considered yin on the outside, soft and yielding, on the inside they are yang, more firm and resilient. Men are the opposite, yang on the outside, and yin on the inside. Therefore, the yin and yang are measures of polarity and degrees of activity. When anything is too yin or too yang it means that its energy is too weak or too strong, too hot or too cold, too sweet or too bitter.

Your constitution can also determine your system of energy. Men who carry a feminine character have more of a yin constitution. Women who carry a masculine or aggressive energy have a more yang constitution. Because of the various chemical influences in today's world, ranging from xenoestrogens (foreign estrogens) in plastics to estrogen bombarded infant formulas, a greater percentage of men tend to be more yin.

Here are examples of yin and yang constitutions:

Yang Constitution	Yin Constitution
Large Bones and strong frame	Thin bones and weak frame
Aggressive nature	Passive nature
Easily angered, fiery disposition	Not easily angered, passive
Testosterone dominate	Low testosterone or estrogen dominance
Illness tends to be acute	Illness tends to be chronic

The Key to Diagnosis and Healing

When we visit a doctor of allopathic medicine with a complaint of an ailment most of the time he/she isolates the condition. Then without any holistic observation, writes a prescription and sends us home with anywhere from 1 to 15 different medications, all containing side effects. The first step in the ancient healing arts of both Chinese and Ayurvedic medicine is diagnosis. This requires the physician to meet the patient in privacy and apply what the Chinese call the Four Diagnostics (she jen). These four methods of diagnosis are referred to as Interviewing, Observing, Listening and Touching.

First the patient is interviewed in depth and detail about why they are being seen in the first place. There is focus on major symptoms and other factors including habits, and lifestyle. There also needs to be a review of the patient's medical history as well as family history. Then the patient explains very candidly about the initial episodes of the symptoms. From this point there are six topics that are emphasized in order to complete a successful interview so that the patient's healing protocol will be more accurate and effective. For example, chill and fever indicate whether the disease is primarily a yin or a yang condition. A fever with the absence of chills usually indicates an overly yang condition, if the chills are present, it indicates that there is a yang deficiency. Perspiration can determine if a condition is either a yin or yang deficiency and also pinpoint whether the condition is internal or external.

Stool and urine will indicate a cold or hot or a full or empty energy condition depending on whether the patient is experiencing symptoms of constipation or diarrhea. Blood and mucus in the stool are also relevant indications. Dark or scanty urine indicates a condition of excess hot and full energy, while profuse, clear urine is a sign of a cold and empty condition.

Dietary habits and craving for specific foods provide more insight as to what may be the nature or underlying cause of the patient's condition. Aversions to hot fluids and craving cold drinks show that there is a presence of a heat condition in the body. The dominant presence of any particular flavor in the palate can indicate which organ is primarily affected through the flavor's connection with one of the Five Elemental energies and it related organ. A sour taste for example, is connected to the wood energy of the liver.

Excess sleep is an indication of a yang deficiency, where as insomnia is an indication of poor circulation, worry, or a spleen deficiency. A person that normally rises early in the morning indicates an overactive energy of fire within the heart, while aggressive sleep and nightmares are indications of overindulgence in rich foods and drinks combined with dramatic lifestyle and emotional imbalance.

Five Energies

The Five Elemental energies of W**ood, Fire, Earth, Metal and Water** encompass all the myriad phenomena of nature. It is a paradigm that applies equally to humans. The five elemental energies represent the tangible functions of yin and yang energies as they manifest in the cyclic changes of nature which regulates life on earth. Here is an example of how human organs connect with the elements and system of energy:

The heart is a fire-energy yin organ. It is called the king of all organs. This is because its controls the circulation and distribution of blood.

The small intestine is a fire-energy yang organ. This organ is known as the minister of reception because it receives partially digested food and refines and separates the pure from the impure.

The liver is a wood-energy yin organ. It is responsible for filtering, detoxifying, nourishing and storing blood. The liver stores large amounts of sugar in the form of glycogen, which releases into the blood stream as glucose whenever the body requires extra energy.

The gallbladder is a wood-energy yang organ. The organ is responsible for secreting pure bile fluids to help digest and metabolize fats and oils. The energy from the gallbladder supplies muscular strength and vitality. It corresponds with the lymphatic system to clear toxic build up from by-products that are consumed. By doing this it helps eliminate muscular aches and prevents fatigue.

The spleen and the pancreas are energy organs. The spleen is considered the master of digestion because before anything is consumed it must first enter the spleen. The pancreas and spleen both control the extraction and assimilation of nutrients from foods and fluid by producing digestive enzymes and energy required by the stomach and small intestine.

The stomach is known as the sea of nourishment, because it is responsible for providing the entire system with postnatal energy from digestion of food and fluids. In addition to digesting bulk foods and liquids and moving them on to the small intestines for extraction and assimilation of nutrients, the stomach also extracts energy from food and liquids. In coordination with the spleen, it transports this food energy through the meridian system to the lungs, combining air energy from breathing.

These are only examples of how our bodies are connected with the elements of the universe, and why you just can't treat a body with a pill. The diet, lifestyle history, attitudes and symptoms all contribute to the success of helping a person heal.

The Six Motions

There are six motions that can associate with disease and well being:

Joy, though very healthy and pleasing to the body's endorphins cycle, in excess it can be overwhelming to the point of injury. Excessive joy can actually injure the heart and shatter the spirit, because it is extreme. It can slow down and congest the hearts energy, causing the heart to flutter rapidly. Excessive joy is associated with Fire energy, which governs the heart. A person with a weak heart can actually die laughing, a phenomenon well known in western medicine. So those with a weak heart may want to limit their view time with a Chris Rock in concert or a Jay Leno's Tonight show.

Anger is the emotion associated with wood energy and the liver. Extreme anger injures the liver's yin energy, which controls the blood, bile and other fluids. This can also cause the liver's yang energy to flare up (inflammation) creating an out of control condition. Some of the symptoms relating to this condition are headaches, dizziness, blurred vision, mental confusion, bad temper, and liver malfunction. A person that frequently bursts out with anger will eventually damage their liver, so if you are planning to yell at your boss every day remember that your liver is being damaged and it would be wise to look for work elsewhere.

Anxiety is a condition that blocks energy and injures the lungs according to the Internal Medicinal Classic. Anxiety limits your breathing apparatus and suppresses respiration. The lungs govern energy through breathing; therefore the energy circulation becomes impaired by anxiety. Shortness of breath and shallow breathing are indications of intense anxiety. Anxiety can also impair the digestive system; injure the functions of the spleen, pancreas, and stomach, which will eventually lower resistance.

Too much concentration has been found in Asian medicine to injure the spleen, pancreas and stomach also. The term 'concentration' refers to obsessive mental fixation on an isolated problem that constantly preoccupies the mind, including worry. This condition impairs digestion, causes abdominal pain, depletes the immune system and impairs sexual stamina and blood flow.

Grief can injure the heart and lungs and also damage the pericardium (the heart's protective sack) and is linked to the Triple Burner (the combination of three main cavities: thorax, abdomen, and pelvis). Grief will cause the body's storage of vital energy to rapidly dissipate, thus depleting your resistance. It is well known even in western medicine that grief-stricken individuals become highly vulnerable to heart disease, cancer and other forms of physical degeneration.

Fear damages your kidney's energy and causes bladder imbalance. The Internal Medicine Classic states that "if kidney energy is weak, one is prone to chronic fear." Chronic fear and paranoia can easily cause renal failure and permanent kidney damage. When children wet in their beds on a regular basis they are plagued by feelings of fear. This is a result of damaged kidney energy. This is why parents and teachers have to be firm and compassionate with their children. Yelling like a damn fool and talking to them like adults stagnates their kidney energy which can result in other health complications. So if you are not mentally prepared to raise children, don't have any!

THE MERIDIAN CYCLE

The meridian cycle refers to the 24 hours of the day. The word comes from Hours, the falcon god, who flew through the sky in circles. This cycle describes how the energy (qi) flows through the meridians during a 24 hour period. When we arise from our unconscious state (sleep), our nature drives us to defecate. Please note the active time of the large intestine is between 5-7 a.m. Then we break our fast (stomach) between 7-9 a.m. We digest our food (spleen) between 9-11 a.m. The heart is the strongest between 11a.m. – 1 p.m. We eat lunch between 1-3 p.m. (small intestine). Most of the energy is in the bladder meridian between 3-5 p.m., which runs down the back where we do our physical labor. Tea time is 5 p.m. this is the time the kidneys receive nourishment. 7-9 p.m. is the time for the circulation sex meridian called the pericardium or heart governor which is when our day is on the decline, moving toward retirement and connecting with our family. 9-11 p.m. is the time when the circulatory system, digestive system and reproductive system balance each other. It is called the three burning spaces or triple heater meridian. It functions as the immune system and is the time we should be at rest. 11 p.m. – 1 a.m. is the time of the gall bladder which is closely linked to the liver. It is the time when decisions are made consciously and subconsciously.

The liver will go through a self-cleansing and maintenance program between 1-3 a.m. It is also the time when neuro-melanin is secreted which are the building blocks for hormones such as melatonin and serotonin. During this time deep sleep must be acquired in order to produce high quality hormones. This is why most people are very irritated, grumpy and sometimes more violent because of sleep deprivation. The ancient sages used to get up at 3 a.m. in order to meditate. 3- 5 a.m. is the time the lungs are active, they are the reservoir of yang energy and contribute to a great start in the morning. So it's not just the Wheaties that give you that kick start in the morning, as a matter of fact it would be great for the fairly healthy person to start off with five great herbals; Rhodiola, Astragalus, Royal Jelly and American Ginseng, followed by some quality Gynostemma tea.

THE 24 HOUR CIRCULATION OF CHI

Lung Meridian 3 - 5 a.m.
Large Intestine Meridian 5 - 7a.m.
Stomach Meridian 7 - 9 a.m.
Spleen Meridian 9 - 11 a.m.
Heart Meridian 11 a.m. – 1 p.m.
Small Intestines Meridian 1 – 3 p.m.
Bladder Meridian 3 - 5 p.m.
Kidneys Meridian 5 - 7 p.m.
Pericardium Meridian 7 - 9 p.m.
Triple Burner 9 – 11 p.m.
Gall Bladder Meridian 11-1 a.m.
Liver Meridian 1 – 3 a.m.

Note: These are the times that each organ is most active during the course of the day.

American Ginseng considered being a yin tonifying herb Though cooler in nature this ginseng has been shown to be very powerful adaptogenic. Great tonic for both men and women.

Astragalus a potent herb that builds T-cells, very good for the immune system. Very helpful for chronic fatigue

An mein Pian a very effective calming formula, good for insomnia, and anxiety

Chein Chin Tai used for relieving menstrual cramps

Gui Pi Wan Tonifies the blood, the spleen, and nourishes the heart, useful for painful Menses

Ganmaoling a popular cold and flu remedy, used for swollen lymph glands, sore throat, high fever

Sho Wu Chi is a popular liquid tonic preparation for men and women, warms and invigorates blood, nourishes kidneys, liver and benefits the eyes. Has been proven to reverse grey hair, due to its youth enhancing potential

Tan Kwe Gin Builds blood helps regulate menstrual cycle. Good for recovering from an illness or surgery

Tzepao Sanpien Extract The special formula is made from 42 ingredients. It is used in the Asian world to tonify Qi and blood; strengthen kidneys, spleen and lung qi; this tonic can be taken for long periods of time to improves the mind, spirit, strengthen lower back, counteract fatigue, poor memory, insomnia, chronic asthma and weak extremities. Should avoid using with cold and raw foods.

Ten Flavor Tea This formula has been used to tonify the spleen and heart qi, kidney and spleen yang and also nourishes and invigorates blood. It is also used for poor digestion or appetite, fatigue, weak back or legs, anxiety and debility following an illness surgery or even child birth. Should not use if you are experiencing symptoms of heat.

38. THE NATURAL THERAPIES TO CONSIDER

Over the last five years, most of you have heard of some form of holistic medicine. Nearly, if not all forms of media have conducted a story on some so-called new therapy for pain, weight loss, allergies, memory, etc. You now hear stories on aromatherapy, acupuncture, qi gong and other arts of healing. Just to let you know; none of these healing arts are new under the sun. For example, medicinal herbs have been applied to the body since the beginning of human existence.

We have an intricate connection with every element, mineral and cosmic energy source in the universe. As we mentioned throughout the book, the genetic character of all these sources was programmed into our genetic hard drive at the beginning of creation. Unfortunately, the hardheaded, feebleminded, bootlicking western scientists, educators, and doctors wandered astray from this divine law. This is why the human body is made from hundreds of trace elements, minerals, enzymes and other earthly and cosmic particles. In fact, the herbs and plants were here before we were because the Garden of Eden had to be prepared in order for the human journey to begin.

Ancient medicine and its applications are as effective as they were several thousand years ago. For example, acupuncture treatments successfully used to treat certain diseases in China over 3,000 years ago are the same treatments recommended by the World Health Organization (WHO) today. The only thing new is the growing interest and acceptance of this universal therapy.

Here is a look at some of our most popular healing therapies:

ACUPUNCTURE

The purpose of this ancient healing art is to stimulate energetic points on the body with the insertion of a hair like, sterile needle. It remains the only therapy in the world that deals with the human energy system. This system appears to be the most important aspect. Ancient Chinese medicine believes that the imbalance of energy is the foremost cause of disease and direct manipulation of energy is naturally the foremost cure.

Acupuncture was first discovered on the battlefields of ancient China, when the soldiers were wounded by arrows, and the wounds where the arrows penetrated would suddenly disappear from the application of acupuncture. The Chinese physicians found that the body contained an invisible network of energy channels that allows a vital life force called qi to travel back and forth. Twelve major and twelve minor channels were discovered and each channel connected with specific organs and glands. Though these channels are invisible to the eye, they have been sighted by Kirlian photography in the Soviet Union.

Each meridian has designated spots called "vital points" which when stimulated by acupuncture or acupressure cause vital-energy to flow, stop, accelerate, or any other way depending on the physicians application. There are over 800 vital points on the human body, but only several dozen are used in treatment of most conditions. The electrical nature of human energy is the key to the acupuncture's success, because the needles serve as conductors, insulators and accelerators. Many patients of cancer, trauma injury, auto-immune diseases and even AIDS have been successfully treated by acupuncture.

MASSAGE THERAPY

Massage therapy was first applied in ancient Egypt but traditionally recognized in ancient Taoism. The purpose of massage is to relieve fatigue, promote circulation and reestablish equilibrium. One form of massage is acupressure which employs deep muscle to nerve penetration stimulating the vital points along the energy meridians. In traditional Chinese medicine, remedial massage is an art of physical hand pressure and motions called "An-mo and Tuina." Tuina stimulates meridians to release blocked qi and toxins trapped within the body. An-mo creates a more calming effect by using rolling and thrusting motions for relaxation and neutralizing tension and stress.

CHIROPRACTIC MEDICINE

Chiropractic medicine is now the second largest group of primary-care providers in the United States, over forty-five thousand strong. The applications of chiropractic medicine are very effective. Well over thirty percent of the American population receives some form of treatment from chiropractors with 90% stating that the application was effective. Though there are still many people who are ignorant toward the benefits of chiropractic treatment, the healing art is now recognized around the world for its effectiveness.

Chiropractic medicine has been used since the time of Hippo crates to treat back pain. According to the "Chantilly Report", the National Institute of Health recognizes four major principles of chiropractic medicine: (1) the human body has innate self-healing ability and attempts to maintain homeostasis or balance, (2) the nervous system is highly developed in the human system, therefore playing an intricate role between health and disease, (3) the presence of joint dysfunction and misalignment may interrupt the neuro-musculoskeletal system from acting efficiently and may contribute to, or be the actual cause of the disease, and (4) treatment is based on the chiropractic physician's ability to diagnoses and treat existing pathologies and dysfunctions by appropriate manual and physiological procedure.

There are many benefits in the art of chiropractic medicine, which includes correcting poor posture, building muscle tone, cushioning injury and alleviating stress. The main objective of the application of chiropractry is to help the patient's body to return to a normal structure. Not all chiropractors have the same philosophy or the same approach. There are two distinctive schools of thought. These two schools are often described within the chiropractic community as the "straights" (also know as "conservatives") and the "mixers" (also known as "liberals").

The straight chiropractors consider themselves to be technicians of pure chiropractic theory. The straight chiropractors generally limit their practice to manual manipulation of the spine.

"Mixer" chiropractors are noted for using more diagnostic and health care techniques. Their practice is more comprehensive in scope using more holistic principles in their approach to treatment. The mixer is also known to use x-rays to diagnose not only misalignment, but also illnesses.

In addition to spinal manipulation, several different treatments are used by both schools of chiropractry:

Heat Therapy – like a warm bath to soothe tense muscles, chiropractors use a variety of heat sources to relieve pain, promote circulation and healing. Some radiant devices may include ultrasound, microwave, infrared and ultraviolet radiation.

Cold Therapy – similar to icing a muscle injury and sprain, chiropractors mobilize the many healing properties of cold with the application of ice, ice packs or ice massage. This therapy is used to reduce circulation, swelling and pain.

Immobilizing Therapy – This technique uses casts, brace wrapping and splinting.

Traction– stretches the spine and relives strain on a subluxation.

The mixers physiotherapeutic treatment includes:

Hydrotherapy – this is an application of water, which includes underwater exercise, whirlpool, baths, and soaking.

Electrotherapy – is the application of electro-stimulation to improve muscle circulation, and work the lymphatic system and bladder system, which helps to eliminate body fluids.

Ultrasound – transfers electricity into sound waves that send a micro-massage to disperse fluids, reduce swelling, increase circulation, and relieve spasms.

We recommend that you at least become familiar with these natural applications of healthcare. There are many good acupuncturists, chiropractors, and massage therapists across the country and around the world.

QI GONG

Qi Gong (Chee-Gong) is one of greatest physical, mental and spiritual applications in the history of healing arts. Qi Gong is a form of slow moving meditation that stimulates the acupuncture meridians regulating one's breathing technique with precise movement connecting the mind, body and spirit. Qi Gong has been passed down through 14 generations, and it is the most ancient of martial arts.

There are two methods of Qi Gong, static and moving. Meridian Qi Gong is a moving system that encompasses four types of ancient art. The four types of Qi Gong are medical, martial, scholarly, and spiritual. As medical, Qi Gong acts upon the acupuncture meridians and strengthens the internal organs, thus regulating blood pressure, blood sugar and even cholesterol. Qi Gong also stimulates the immune system, strengthens internal organs and tones joints. As scholarly, Qi Gong promotes longevity and self-healing. As spiritual, Qi Gong incorporates the system Taoist yoga and Buddhist Qi Gong. It combines breathing, meditation, self defense, flexibility and strength training. As therapy, it is a way to heal others by emitting electro-magnetic energy, (Qi) from your hands. This Qi emission (therapy) eliminates pain and removes weakness. Clinical studies have shown that Qi Gong helps to reverse osteoporosis, arthritis, heart disease, and diabetes. And, because of its magnificent calming effect internally, Qi Gong has been known to shrink some tumors.

There are several different styles of Qi Gong such as "Blue Dragon" and "Black Dragon" Qi Gong. According to Dr. George Love who is a Licensed Acupuncturist, Doctor of Oriental Medicine and Qi Gong master, one form of Qi Gong is used for health and the other is for longevity. Although, this art appears to be a healing art, it is also a very effective application of self defense. When Qi Gong is performed on a daily basis, it will improve oxygen flow, mental acuity, relaxation and improve digestion. Those that would like to be enlightened should at least participate in this perfected physical and spiritual therapy, it might change your life significantly for the better. To find out more about Qi Gong, contact a Qi Gong instructor in your area or visit www.loveschinesemedicine.com or www.mach1audio.com.

TAI CHI

Tai Chi, also known as Tai Chi Ch'uan, Tai Ji Juan and Taiqi is also a great system of ancient therapy which, originally, was a formidable martial art operating on several levels of awareness. It embodies Taoist philosophy, and according to research it is extremely beneficial to good health and longevity. Tai Chi is a comprehensive series of gentle physical movements, and breathing techniques, with mental and spiritual intent, which enables one to develop a meditative state. It creates a system of serenity and rejuvenation, assisting the mind and body to achieve and maintain balance. It incorporates both inner and outer expressions of the body and mind. This is how we can create the balance of yin and yang's life force energy of qi. By this very method, our system not only develops the ability to balance the "yielding and attacking" aspects in martial art combat, but also injury recovery.

Tai Chi is an ancient, yoga-like Chinese system of ballet-like exercises designed for health, self-defense and spiritual development. The application of Tai Chi supposedly facilitates the flow of qi (chee), "lifes energy" throughout the body by dissolving blockages both within the body and between the body and the environment. Traditional Tai Chi prescribes between 108 and 128 postures, including repetitions. This graceful form of healing and martial art combines mental concentration, coordinated breathing and slow body movements to increase well-being, strength and longevity. Though, there are several different levels, styles and systems of Tai Chi Ch'uan they are all applications of precision, influencing health, spirit and defense.

To become more enlightened with the Tai Chi system of healing, visit a local practitioner in your area or visit www.stltaiji.com or www.traditionaltaichi.com. These educational sites will introduce you to the Yang style and Hu Yuan Chen style of Tai Chi.

There are many good Tai Chi institutions around the world. So it would be a great experience to allow yourself and your children to learn this wonderful system of balance.

MACROBIOTIC APPROACH TO WELLNESS

This treatment modality is thought to promote wellness and optimize overall health. Macrobiotics should be used with, not in place of, standard therapy.

What is macrobiotics? Macrobiotic therapy is a combination of diet, spiritual and social philosophy and a lifestyle of holistic living. The macrobiotic philosophy combines elements of Buddhism with dietary principles based on simplicity and avoidance of "toxic" animal products. Although a relatively new therapy, macrobiotics teaches that it is necessary to maintain balance and harmony between two antagonistic but complementary forces, yin and yang. The diet, originally termed the "Zen macrobiotic diet", was very restrictive and has since been modified by other practitioners in the macrobiotic movement. The diet consists mainly of whole grains (brown rice, millet, quinoa) vegetables and beans with the occasional use of fish and some fruits. Foods that are not allowed in the macrobiotic diet are coffee, diary products, eggs, sugar, meats and processed foods. The macrobiotics diet also requires special methods of food preparation such as using only pots, pans, and utensils made of certain materials such as stainless steel, glass, wood. Absolutely no aluminum or Teflon or microwave ovens should be used for macrobiotic preparation. There is not a single diet for everyone, but rather a dietary "principle" or "law" that considers different climate, age sex, level of activity and changing personal needs.

How does macrobiotics promote wellness and optimize overall health? Traditional Chinese medicine believes that imbalance of yin and yang contributes to illness. Therefore, macrobiotics attempts to rebalance yin and yang and regain health through diet and a change in lifestyle and life philosophy. The macrobiotic diet can reduce fat and plaques and, like other natural fat-reducing diets, may help reduce the risk of certain types of cancers that can be related to high saturated, hydrogenated oil intake such as colon cancer. This lean, holistic diet has been shown to lower blood pressure and reduce the risk of heart disease. Macrobiotics has great stress relieving potential.

Are there any risks involve with the macrobiotic diet? A nutrient, vitamin and calorie restrictive diet can be potentially dangerous for a weak cancer patient. The most serious effects occur when the diet is deficient in calories, vitamin D, vitamin B-12, protein and iron. Increased caloric needs to fight illness and recover from treatment may not be met with the macrobiotic diet, which is high in bulk and low in fat. Some children that are on the macrobiotic diet may have growth and nutrient deficiencies.

GERSON THERAPY

What does the Gerson Therapy involve? Dr. Max Gerson created the Gerson program in 1945 based on his clinical research that cancer patents have a sodium and potassium imbalance in their bodies. The Gerson program is a nutritional approach to cancer treatment and requires that patients comply with a whole food diet that is absent of inorganic sodium bombarded foods, hydrogenated oils, and other dead and refined carbohydrates. The therapy includes high potassium supplementation and large amounts of fruit and vegetables juices. Patients are required to drink 13 glasses of combined organic carrot and apple juice. Frequent coffee enemas are given to detoxify the liver and the body. Previously, patients were required to drink three glass of fresh calf liver daily but this aspect has since been discontinued because several patients experienced toxicity.

The program consists of three central tenets that claim cancer patients do not efficiently metabolize carbohydrates, fats, proteins, vitamins and minerals:

1. Enzymes are critical to support the vitality of intestinal flora
2. The liver and other vital organs must be detoxified and functioning efficiently to support the breakdown of tumors.
3. Potassium and sodium intake must be balanced, usually by sodium restriction and potassium supplementation, to restore metabolism, and health.

Laboratory studies in 1983 and 1985 provided the evidence that upsetting the potassium/sodium balance may play a role in malignancy. The University of Texas M.D. Anderson Caber Center conducted an extensive human studies literature review of the Gerson therapy and found six studies applicable to cancer. several studies indicated higher survival rates and tumor regression in patients treated with the Gerson therapy, especially for patients with melanoma, colorectal and ovarian cancers.

Dr. Gerson wrote a book, the proven success of the metabolic application titled "The Gerson Therapy, A Result of Fifty Cases". This book confirms the success of fifty terminally ill patients. The Gerson application was proven successful in the treatment of tuberculosis, MS, lupus, arthritis and several other degenerative diseases. Though some medical professionals state that the Gerson Therapy is not a decisive cure for any type of cancer, other research and medical professionals see that this therapy creates an optimum foundation for the treatment of degenerative diseases.

How much does the Gerson therapy cost? At the Gerson clinic in Tijuana, Mexico treatment costs about $2,800 per week plus an additional $200 per week for laboratory testing. Some insurance providers reimburse costs associated with treatment.

For additional Information:
Gerson Institute
157 2nd Avenue
San Diego, CA 92101
Telephone (619) 685- 5353
Web site: www.gerson.org

THE FUNDEMENTALS OF AYURVEDA

The treatment modality is thought to promote wellness and optimize overall health. Ayurveda should be with, but not in place of standard cancer therapy.

What is Ayurveda? Ayurveda is a 6000 year old system of ancient traditional medicine, lifestyle and philosophy of India. Ayurveda medicine, similar to traditional Chinese medicine is based on a life force and the pursuit of balance between the body, mind and nature. Illness is believed to be the absence of physical, emotional and spiritual harmony. Its emphasis is on preventing disease and maintaining good health. Ayurveda practitioners use specific diagnostic techniques, such as examinations of the pulse, tongue, face, lips nails, and eyes to pinpoint the disease process. Treatment programs normally include constitutional (individual) diet, body detoxification through the use of fasting and enemas, meditation, yoga, counseling and spiritual therapy.

How effective is Ayurveda? While Ayurveda is not an understood practice by mainstream America or a licensed treatment therapy, increased research is underway to study its effectiveness. According to a report by the National Institutes of Health (NHI), one clinical study showed that in 79% of cases, the health of the patients with various chronic diseases improved measurably after Ayurvedic treatment. Laboratory and clinical studies have suggested that some Ayurvedic herbal preparations may have the potential to prevent and treat certain cancers, including breast, lung and colon. However, randomized clinical trials in humans are needed to make conclusions about the role of Ayurveda in cancer prevention and treatment. The National Cancer Institute (NCI) has added several Ayurveda herbal compounds to its potential anticancer agents and has funded a series of laboratory studies to evaluate two Ayurvedic herbal remedies called (MAK-4 and MAK-5). Their decision was based on preliminary laboratory studies indicating that the two medicines significantly inhibited growth of cancer cells from human and rat tumors. However, until there is documented evidence from carefully controlled studies of the efficacy of Ayurveda herbal remedies, the American Cancer Society urges cancer patients to treat their disease with so-called 'proven' methods of treatments. The Ayurvedic principles of yoga, meditation and counseling can be used in conjunction with conventional cancer treatments.

HOMEOPATHY

This treatment modality is thought to manage the symptoms of cancer, side effects from conventional therapies and/or control pain. Homeopathy should be used with, not in place of standard cancer treatment.

Homeopathy, a highly systematic medical science was developed by a German physician Samuel Hahnemann during the 1800's. Hahnemann was an esteemed physician and chemist who served as a personal physician to the members of the German royalty, his text was one of the most respected in that era of chemistry. Hahnemann studied the records of accidental poisonings from other commonly used medicines of his time, such as mercury, arsenic, belladonna, and silver nitrate, and by testing these poisons on himself and others he discovered that in overdose the "medicines" caused symptoms similar to those of the illness for which they were used. Mercury, used to treat syphilis, could cause syphilis like ulcers. Arsenic and belladonna were known to create certain types of fevers. Silver nitrate, applied for eye inflammation, caused severe irritation and discharge from the eyes. Homeopathic remedies are made from assorted herbs, plants, animals, insects and organic chemicals diluted thousands of times in water or alcohol. In fact, the majority of the homeopathic remedies are so diluted that it is impossible to detect the origin of the active ingredient. Homeopathy should not be confused with herbal medicine. Homeopathic medicine may not always contain herbal ingredients. According to homeopathic practitioners the medicinal solutions contain a "trace" of the original substance.

How do homeopathic applications address the symptoms of degenerative disease and side effects of conventional therapies? Homeopathy is based on Hahnemann's philosophy of "like cures likes;" a substance that causes certain symptoms should also reverse them. Hahnemann tested a huge number of plant, animal and mineral elements on himself in a process called "proving" which involved observing the symptoms they produce and categorizing them as cures for disorders that cause similar problems.

Homeopathy has been practiced in the U.S. for over 170 years. As a matter of fact, it is the preferred medical application by members of the Royal Family in England and homeopathy is widely prescribed by physicians in Europe and Asia.

Homeopathy made its first major debut during the cholera epidemic in Europe during the 1830's. At that time homeopathic doctors had a recovery percentage of 80% compared to conventional doctors 50% recovery rate.

Law of Minimum Dose

The law of minimum dose in homeopathy is using the smallest dose to effect the cure. The magic of "minimum doses" enables the body to heal in the most efficient and least harmful way. The first step in preparing homeopathic remedies is dilution. A common "prime potency" is 6X. The potency is always indicated on the bottles of a remedy.

6X is 1 part raw product-mother tincture-in 1,000,000 parts alcohol/water. Minerals or Cell Salts at this potency can help balance deficiencies in mineral uptake in the body. This is a common problem in America due to the combination of the Standard American Diet (SAD), malnutrition and over toxicity. In potencies 30X and above, none of the original molecules of the mother tincture remains.

The second step in remedy preparation refers to the strength of a remedy. After dilution, the remedy goes through a process of succession. Curative properties are enhanced in this stage. It is the use of potentized and minimum doses that set homeopathy apart. Products in both crude form as herbal mother tincture and homeopathic potentized form are effective.

Hence, you might take St. John's Wort/Hypericum for problems such as depression. You might take Comfrey/Symphytum (herbally or homeopathically) topically for wounds and Eyebright/Euphrasia for tired, sensitive, burning eyes.

Homeopathics prepared from botanicals/herbs, minerals and glands are often for the same indications as their raw counterparts.

Potentization enhances these healing properties and negates the properties that in large doses can cause problems. For instance, using herbal chamomile can in large quantities over a period of time, counteract its calming attributes. Using very large amounts of certain vitamins and herbs can be taxing to the liver. Even properly prescribed medicine kills around 150,000 people annually. Homeopathy is one of several natural applications that offer a safe alternative to home care in first aid and illness.

By 1900, 100 homeopathic hospitals were in operation. The future of homeopathic institutions seemed promising until the AMA began to monopolize the medical industry. Conventional medicine never ceased its aggressive attack on Homeopathy. In the early 1900's Dr. McCormack said "we must admit that we never fought the homeopath on community and got the business." In 1910, the Carnegie Foundation issued a report sanctioning allopathic (conventional) medical schools, while at the same time condemning homeopathic schools. This was based on the premise that homeopath teachers were also practitioners and that courses in pharmacology were taught. With $350 million being gifted to the allopathic institutions homeopathic schools rapidly lost momentum and began to close due to political bias, limited support and money. Though the applications of homeopathy have been proven to be safe and effective the mainstream struggle continues. This is obviously due in part to state laws and the AMA.

Many solutions to today's diseases and various forms of ill-health have been found in homeopathic applications, which can be found in all health food stores, some drug stores and diversified doctors' offices.

EPILOGUE

Since health is a natural state, why is it so hard to achieve? Why does it cost so much to get medical treatments? Why do we remain sick after the treatment? Furthermore, why are natural treatments so rarely used and so difficult to find? And why are those who attempt to provide natural treatments hounded by regulating agencies? In an attempt to answer these questions, we examined the aspects of "health care" which are not about care but disease management.

Drug companies, food processors, advertisers, insurance companies, governments, doctors and citizens are all involved. Their most basic goals, preoccupations, and preconceptions keep truths about health from being sought, discovered, and organized. Our drug-oriented medical system continues to undermine largely our faith in God, natural living, natural healing and our freedom.

Effective natural methods (non-orthodox as they are called by the medical establishment) of health care are difficult to obtain in the United States. For some natural treatments, patients must leave the country, creating further obstacles to achieving health. Citizens always want health, but generally subvert their wishes to the political agenda of the day, even when that agenda results in chaos, war, poverty and other factors that lead to disease.

Past government involvement in so-called health care focused only on the important areas of hygiene, water treatment, sewage disposal and food inspection. Beyond that, involvement has been limited mainly to carrying out the wishes of those who market high-tech disease management and crisis intervention products and services for profit. Vested interests reflect social values. Security, control, status, power and wealth all rate higher than health care in our society, at the present time. This hierarchy will change only when individuals and organizations put health higher on society's agenda.

Business interests that work against clean environment, and therefore against clean food, water, and air include all industries that deplete, exploit, and pollute natural environments in order to make money. The bottom line is business tends to take a heavy toll on nature. **When the economy improves, the environment**

gets polluted; when the environment is treated with respect, the economy suffers. Those who profit from the destruction of nature and of life put us all at peril. We must come to understand and embody the simple fact that, in the long term, life and nature are our only assets. Health results when we respect and align ourselves with both.

Decisions made a generation ago to use artificial fertilizers and intensive farming methods that take more from soils than they give back are coming home to roost. They produce poor soils, poor foods, and poor health. Pesticides meant to decrease crops lost to pests are failing. Crops lost to pests averaged 6% per year after pesticide use. The pesticides eliminated some pests but destroyed their natural predators. The natural balance of nature was altered. Certain predators prey on the insects that destroy crops. When the pesticides were introduced, the predators fed on the insects that had been sprayed and died. When the insects developed their resistance to the pesticides it was business as usual. As a result, there were no more predators to feed on the insects so they eventually destroyed the crops. Concomitantly, crops absorb the chemicals from the pesticides (which are carcinogenic) and are fed to humans for consumption. Sustainable farming methods must fit natural cycles, make use of natural predators for pest control, and maintain fertile, mineral rich soils including soil bacteria and earthworms.

Special interests also mediate against health care more directly. The economic interests of professional disease management (drug, radiation, surgery and high-tech oriented medical practice) are strongly biased against instituting true health care. Accordingly, "disease" seems to yield better profit margins from a business standpoint. Medical doctors get paid for treating, not for curing diseases. If doctors were paid only for keeping people healthier and lost their income when their patients got sick, the entire health care industry would completely change its approach to prevent loss of profits and also loss of its self-respect.

High-tech medicine as presently practiced is not viable for the society that uses it. Treatment costs have increased while levels of health have deteriorated. That's bad investment. For $900 billion each year in expenditures, people should expect and actually receive better positive health care results than they are currently receiving. Giant food processing companies also have vested interests that mediate against health care. Whole foods are relatively cheap. To increase profits, food processors change them into "value added" products, because more can be charged for foods that have been changed by processing technology. Processing has little to do with health, but much to do with convenience and profit. From the point of view of health, processed products have no value since processing removes and / or destroy nutrients and increases toxins. These food-processing companies have played substantial political roles since the early 1900's by blocking evidence about food laws that reflect the findings of science on the requirements of health. Such food laws would expose many processed products as being nutritionally deficient and a destroyer of health.

In private conservations, some researchers claim that the large oil industry conspire to keep negative information about fats, oils, and health from the public in order to profit from the sale of health-destroying products. They claim the industry does not want to make the necessary costly changes in equipment, engineering and methods that would be required to address new information about human health. Health conscious methods would require greater care and would render many of the industry's present methods obsolete. Giant oil, food, drug and medical industries are engaged in the pursuit of money. For them health care seems to be a secondary concern. Consequently, the blindly trusting consumer suffers the effects with compromised health due to the industry's lackadaisical attitude surrounding health care.

In the mid 1970's, President James E. Carter signed a Rockefeller document called the "Global 2000 Report." The basic intent of this report was to reduce the American population to 45% of its current level. This agenda is very much in effect through immune-destroying vaccines, chemtrails (barium spraying from military airplanes on unsuspecting cities throughout America), depleted uranium (radioactive material) from the bombings of Iraq & Afghanistan, and genetically engineered foods. The media feeds us constantly with threats of a WWIII, but they fail to mention that WWIII has already started. People in general are waiting for the big war, but that's not the way it is happening for the moment. This third world war is foremost a quiet war with no classic weapons, but it is no less devastating. This is a war of silent mind control and the implanting of viruses and other lethal diseases upon the population, mostly with the help from vaccines, environmental toxins, and genetically modified foods. Horribly enough, the power elite defense establishment has initiated the genocide of millions of Americans with the contamination of polio viruses that has seeded the entire baby boom generation with cancer viruses. As "age" takes its toll and our immune systems can no longer keep these laboratory-created viruses in check, these "biological time bombs" will begin to activate, with one out of three "boomers" developing cancer.

Indeed, one of the first things President "Slick" Willy Clinton did after the election was to follow the direct orders from David Rockefeller to take over (socialize) 1/5 of the economy - the health care system - that the Rockefeller's oligarchy monopolizes. Deep studies show that 98% of what we call "health care" is in fact disease care.

In the dark ages, we had a society in which "witches" (mostly females) were burnt at the stakes for practicing alternative treatments in the form of herbs and old wisdom. Today the "witches" still exist, but now they call themselves homeopaths, naturopaths and practitioners of alternative medicine. Yet they are still as drastically hunted as they were in the dark ages. Why? It is in these areas that the real cures can be found. If you think like Rockefeller you realize that these "witches" are some of his worst enemies, because they halt the genocide of the world population. By giving poisoned vaccines and vaccines that will compromise our immune system, people get sick and die before their time. When people get sick, they go to the doctor who in return, gives them chemical drugs from the Rockefeller-owned drug companies, which will eventually hammer the last nail into their coffins. With this in mind, one can clearly understand why natural holistic medicine is ridiculed, legislated against and hunted wherever it shows up.

Strange as it may sound, when John D. Rockefeller was actively destroying nature-based medicine in America and setting up Hitler to enforce his I.G Farben cartel agreements throughout Europe, he himself had a naturopathic and homeopathic doctor keeping him alive well into his late 90's. Go figure. People, please wake up and start taking an active role in your own health. The MediSins will be waiting for you, if you do not take heed.

ABOUT the AUTHORS

"The doctor of the future will prescribe no drugs but will interest his patients in the care and nutrition of the human frame and in the cause and prevention of disease."
–Thomas Edison (1847-1931)

Dr. Scott Whitaker, ND

Dr. Scott Whitaker is a Board Certified Naturopathic Doctor & Author with over 15 years experience in herbology, iridology, homeopathy, natural healing, and detoxification. Dr. Whitaker is the Founder/Owner of the Wholistic Health Institute, Inc., a non-profit organization dedicated to the prevention of disease through education. Through preventive natural health protocols and educational workshops, Dr. Whitaker has achieved great success with the individuals he has worked with on a one-to-one basis. His clients have been individuals from all walks of life with health conditions such as alopecia, diabetes, cancer, lymphoma, malnutrition, eczema, heart disease, and AIDS to name a few. The results have been excellent, and the experience unforgettable. Dr. Whitaker has traveled throughout the world learning and applying the healing sciences of China, Asia Minor, North Africa, and Southeast Asia to correct the maladies of our modern time.

Dr. Whitaker received his undergraduate degree from the University of California, Berkeley in Civil Engineering, his Master of Business Administration from the Keller Graduate School of Management in St. Louis, Missouri, and his Doctorate of Naturopathy from the International School of Naturopathy in Los Altos, California. He is also a Certified Natural Health Professional and Iridologist.

Scientific Genius Dies; Saw Work Discredited

By DEL HOOD
The Daily Californian

The scientific genius who built one of the world's most powerful microscopes and invented a machine to treat cancer and other diseases was buried today in Mt. Hope Cemetery.

Royal Raymond Rife, 83, whose Frequency Instrument — a method of electrocuting disease-causing organisms in the body — was the subject of intense debate during the 1950s, died Thursday at Grossmont Hospital of a heart attack.

Alone and virtually penniless, he had been living in an El Cajon rest home since last year.

Acclaimed by the scientific world in the 1930s for his invention of the Universal microscope, a mechanical marvel containing 5,280 parts and a magnifying power 20 times as great as any then in existence, Rife lived to see some of what he considered his most important work discredited by the medical profession.

The Frequency Instruments, used by some doctors across the United States in treating a variety of diseases, were confiscated. Reputations were ruined and one of Rife's associates served three years in prison before winning a reversal of his conviction on grand theft charges.

Though Rife himself was not prosecuted, his reputation was sullied and he clung to the suspicion that organized medicine had conspired against him in his efforts to rid mankind of the scourge of disease.

"Having spent every dime I earned in my research for the benefit of mankind, I have ended up as a pauper, but I achieved the impossible and would do it again," Rife said in an affidavit filed at the time his friend and associate, John Crane, was appealing his conviction.

He accused the American Medical Assn. of rejecting his electronic therapy discoveries and implied the organization had "brainwashed and intimidated" his colleagues as well as "feloniously censored" the publication of his work.

"I certify that the AAA and the Department of Public Health have declared war on Rife's Virus Microscope Institute," said the affidavit signed Feb. 7, 1967.

Rife built his microscope, one of five he invented, so he could actually see disease viruses and observe their activity, a triumph which astounded scientists at the time.

From his observations, Rife developed the theory that every micro-organism has a "mortal oscillatory rate" — a point at which it will shatter or break apart when bombarded by sound waves.

He had conceived the idea of electronic therapy as early as 1922, but it was not until 1934 in the Ellen Scripps home near La Jolla that he was ready to demonstrate "Rife's Ray."

Sixteen patients with incurable diseases were treated by physicians with Rife's Ray in a clinical test of the machine supervised by Dr. Milbank Johnson of Los Angeles.

The claim was made that 14 of the 16 patients were pronounced "clinically cured" by the medical staff within 70 days and the remaining two patients were discharged after three months of treatment.

In the next 20 years, Rife perfected his machine — later to be called the Frequency Instrument — and about 100 of them were in use by physicians in various parts of the world.

Affidavits are on file in the courts from patients who claim they were cured of cancer, butterfly lupus — a skin ailment — and other diseases after treatment with the Frequency Instrument.

Scientists and physicians also claimed success with Rife's invention. One of his closest collaborators was Dr. Arthur Kendall, professor of bacteriology at Northwestern University Medical School, who wrote that he had observed successful treatment of a tumor on a man's cheek.

E. L. Walker of the George Williams Hooper Foundation, an early-day cancer research organization, hailed the device for its effectiveness against typhoid organisms.

"If the ray should prove equally efficient in killing other pathogenic micro-organisms," he wrote to Johnson, "it would be the greatest discovery in the history of therapeutic medicine."

Another devout believer in electronic therapy was Dr. Robert Stafford of Dayton, Ohio, who said the machine had cured some of his patients and relieved others of distress.

But when the State Department of Public Health held its hearing in 1958 to determine if the Frequency Instrument should be approved as a treatment device, all claims in its behalf were rejected.

The hearing board said clinical research "provided no reasonable substantiated evidence of the effectiveness of the Frequency Instrument, consisting primarily of unverified testimonials of physicians and patients . . ."

It concluded that the Frequency Instrument was "a useless device."

Though he held no medical degree, Rife studied optics for seven years in New York and Heidelberg, Germany, and performed more than 50,000 experiments in his research laboratory. He was always referred to in medical journals as "Dr." Rife, believed to be a title conferred by an honorary degree.

His interests extended in many directions. He was a talented musician, an ardent sportsman and at the time of his death still held a speedboat racing title.

Embittered by his treatment from the medical profession, Rife turned to religion after a bout with alcohol and became a member of the Baha'i Faith.

Before his death he offered some of his thoughts to a friend and told her: "The most important thing I ever did was build a microscope."

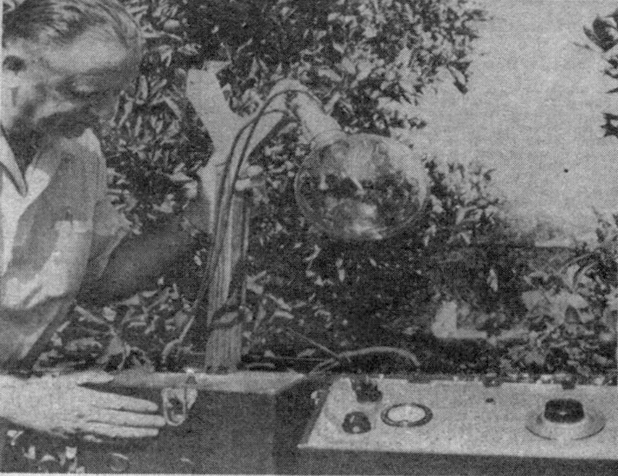

THIS CONTROVERSIAL MACHINE, known as "Rife's Ray" and invented in the 1930s by San Diego scientist Royal Rife, was used to treat a variety of diseases, including cancer, tuberculosis, lupus and leprosy before it was confiscated and declared "useless" by the State Department of Public Health. Some physicians and patients who used the machine, demonstrated in picture by John Crane who was Rife's associate, claimed it cured diseases by electrocuting micro-organisms responsible for the ailments.

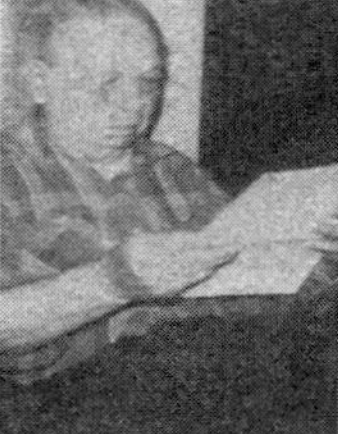

Royal Raymond Rife

Electrical Shock

EL CAJON — Fredrick Gallup, 24, is in serious condition today in El Cajon Valley Hospital where he is being treated for electrical shock sustained while working at a housing project at Granite Hills Drive and Washington Place.

Gallup of 5619 Lindo Paseo, San Diego, was using an electrical saw which apparently developed a short circuit. The fire department said he was unconscious at the scene and fellow workers gave him mouth-to-mouth resuscitation until the ambulance arrived.

Two Aussies Need Homes

EL CAJON — The two Australian exchange students from El Cajon's sister city will be arriving here sooner than expected.

They need places to live.

Joe Cahill, president of Associated Students of Grossmont College, said Susan Walker, 19, and Geoffrey Wilson, 21, are due around Aug. 24.

Originally it was expected they would arrive closer to Sept. 1. They are students at Goulburn Teachers College.

Anyone interested in providing room and board for the Aussies, who will be here for the 1971-72 school year, should contact Harriet Stockwell, 444-1340, or Cahill at 465-1700, Ext. 356.

Both Miss Walker and Wilson will be attending Grossmont College. Two Grossmont College students are in Goulburn preparing to attend Goulburn Teachers College for the next year.

The Dow Jones

NEW YORK (AP) — Dow Jones closing stock averages:

30 Industrials	846.79	+6.79
20 Transportation	209.26	+4.21
15 Utilities	112.38	+0.23
65 Stocks	286.01	+3.03

Sales 11,370,000 shares

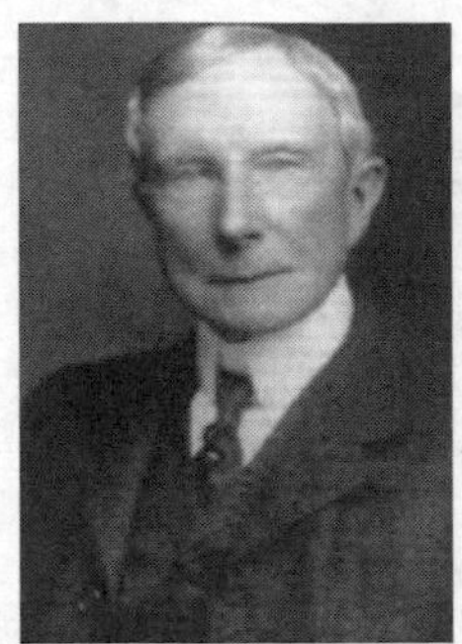

Rockefeller

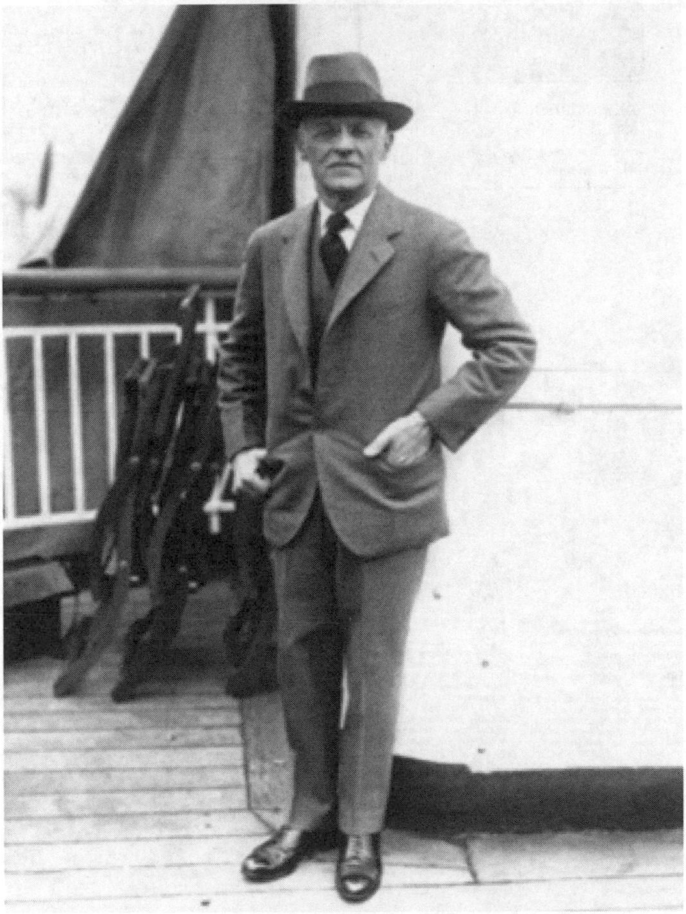

Abraham Flexner

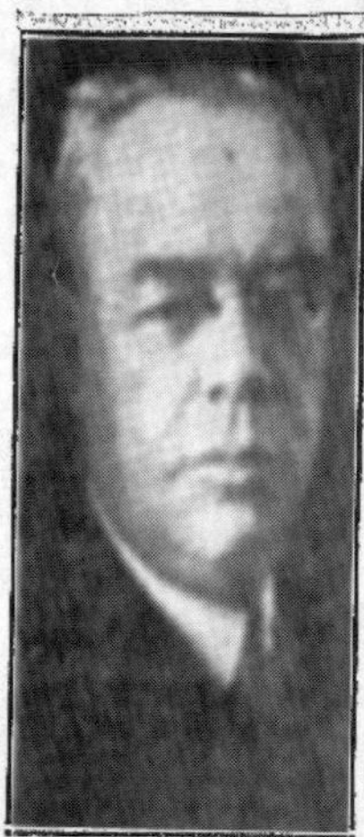

DIES SUDDENLY — Dr. Milbank Johnson, social economist and tax authority, widely mourned here.

DR. JOHNSON DIES AFTER BRIEF ILLNESS

Taxpayers Group Leader Had Varied Southland Career

S.N. 10-3-44

Dr. Milbank Johnson, 73 years of age, nationally-known social economist and chairman of the board of directors of the California Taxpayer's Association since 1926, died early today at the Huntington Memorial Hospital, following a brief illness. Stricken only Saturday, news of his sudden death will come as a great shock to the community. Passing of Dr. Johnson brought to a close a colorful and varied career, marked by a devotion to guiding and counseling young people that their careers, in turn, might be successful.

Those who knew and admired him commented on the fact that Dr. Johnson always was "looking ahead and never was content to live in the past."

Born in Texas

Born in Columbus, Tex., in 1871, Dr. Johnson came to California many years ago, receiving his Bachelor of Science from the University of Southern California in 1890, his LL.D. from the same university in 1917. He also received an LL.D. from Northwestern University in 1920 and his M.D. from that institution. He studied at Johns Hopkins and in European hospitals.

Dr. Johnson practiced in Los Angeles from 1893 to 1901. He was professor of physiology and clinical medicine at U.S.C. from 1897-1901 and from 1901-13 was chief surgeon for the Southern California Edison Company.

From 1913-36 Dr. Johnson was vice-president and director of the Pacific Mutual Life Insurance Company and since his retirement that year has devoted his interest to the California Taxpayers' Association and civic activities.

Many Community Services

Dr. Johnson's community service dates back to 1900 when he was a member of the Los Angeles Board of Health until 1904. He served as president of the Municipal Charities Commission, 1913-17 and as a member of the Board of Freeholders which revised the Los Angeles City Charter in 1910.

During World War I, Dr. Johnson was a member of the executive committee of the California Military Welfare Committee, 1917-19, and from 1920-26 he served as president of the Southwest Museum. During 1925-26 he was president of the California Taxation Improvement Assoiaction. He also was president of the California Conference of Social Agencies, a member of the board of directors of the Pasadena Hospital Association and a member of the executive committee of the National Tax Association. He belonged to the American Medical Association, Southern California Medical Association and Los Angeles County Medical Association, and was one of the founders of the Automobile Club of Southern California. He also was a founder in 1890 of Phi Rho Sigma fraternity, and was a member of Phi Gamma Delta.

A 32nd degree Mason, Dr. Johnson also was a Knight Templar and Shriner.

One of Dr. Johnson's greatest interests, beausce it enabled him to help young people, was the California Educational Aid Foundation of which he was vice-chairman. Its purpose is to provide scholarships for adolescents to secondary schools for training in leadership. Through Dr. Johnson and due to his wise counseling many young people have received a helping hand to outstanding careers.

Surviving Dr. Johnson are his wife, Mrs. Isabel Simeral Johnson and two daughters, Mrs. Louiez Webb and Mrs. Evelyn Bruner.

Funeral arrangements will be announced later.

Star-News
Oct. 3,'44.

GLOSSARY

Adjuvant Therapy: Additional therapy used to assist the primary

Adulteration: The illicit substitution of one substance for another. Example: The use of white sugar instead of natural raw sugar, white bleached flour instead of naturally brown whole flour, white rice instead of brown rice, etc.

Agent Provocateur: A person employed to associate with suspected individuals or groups with the purpose of inciting them to commit an act of trickery, deception or evil for their own personal gain.

Alternative Medicine: Also known as; holistic medicine, natural medicine, Fringe medicine, New Age medicine, non-standard medicine, integrated healthcare. It really should not be look at as alternative because the applications are within the natural laws of health and healing. But due to political and corporate persuasion it is. Alternative therapy treatment is used in place of traditional or mainstream medicine, for example, homeopathy, naturopathy and traditional Chinese medicine. Unlike mainstream medicine, most alternative applications leave no side effects.

Amenorrhea: The absence of the menstrual period.

Amino Acids: The building block of life responsible for the vital production of proteins, hormones, and enzymes. Amino acids are required by all living organisms. Proteins are needed to perform a host of vital functions within the body. There are essential amino acids like arginine, histidine, lysine and non essential like alanine, proline and glycine.

Angina: Angina pectoris is a recurring pain or discomfort in the chest. This happens when some part of the heart does not receive enough blood. Symptoms are burning sensation, fatigue, heaviness, and discomfort in the left arm.

Atherosclerosis: When cholesterol, fat, and calcium deposits (from drinking hard water) or other refined and chemical substances in the blood build up in the walls of the arteries. Eventually, the arteries become narrow, thus reducing the flow of oxygen-rich blood and nutrients to the heart.

Ayurvedic Medicine: Practiced in India for over 5,000 years. The word Ayurvedic means, (science of life). This is a comprehensive system of medicine that combines natural therapies with a highly personalized approach to the treatment of disease. Unlike mainstream western medicine, Ayurvedic medicine places equal emphasis on body, mind and spirit and strives to restore the innate harmony of the individual.

B-cells: White blood cells that are involved in making antibodies

Biological Terrain: Theory discovered by French Physiologist Dr. Claude Benard, that there is intestinal fluid that bathes and nourishes every cell in human body.

Bone Marrow: A soft, spongy tissue inside the bone where red cells, white cells and platelets develop. One on the most important areas of the bodys immune system.

Biopsy: The removal of a small piece of tissue for examination under the microscope to detect or rule out cancer.

Cachexia: A condition caused by chemo-therapy where severe protein loss is caused by loss of appetite. Characterized by weakness and severe muscle wasting.

Cancer: A term for disease in which abnormal cells divide without control. Cancer cells invade nearby tissues and can spread through the bloodstream and lymphatic system to other parts of the body.

Carbotarian: A person who claims to a vegetarian or vegan; however their diets mostly contain processed carbohydrates, unfermented soy, and refined sugar.

Carcinogen: A cancer causing agent., for example, sodium nitrite and sodium nitrate. Though used as preservatives for commercial hotdogs and luncheon meats, excessive consumption can cause cancer.

Carcinoma: The most common type of cancer. It develops in the lining of the lungs, intestines, bladder, breast, uterus, kidneys and prostate.

Chelation Therapy: Defined as "medical therapy" to restore cellular homeostasis through the use of IV metal binding and bioorganic agents such as EDTA.

Congestive Heart Failure (CHF): When the heart is unable to pump enough blood to support the body's needs. CHF occurs when excess body fluids start to leak into the lungs causing breathing complications, fatigue weakness and sleeping problems. The deficiency of CoQ10 and other natural nutrient depleted through malnutrition and certain prescription drugs are directly linked to congestive heart failure.

Coronary Artery Disease (CAD): A heart disease caused by the build up of plaque in the blood vessels feeding the heart. This plaque formation restricts blood flow to the heart muscle.

Deoxyribonucleic A (DNA): the genetic material found in all living cells. This material passes the genetic code from one generation to the next.

Endometriosis: The diseased condition where endometrial tissue develops and grows on the uterus.. Endometriosis can be very painful and cause excessive bleeding. Also called chocolate cyst because sacs are filled with stale blood, this is common. High levels of copper and estrogen are related to cyst formation and birth control pills increases blood copper and estrogen levels.

Endometrium: The inner lining of the uterus that is the surface where the blastocyst/embryo implants during pregnancy. The endometrial tissue that is lost during the menstrual period is the source of tissue for endometriosis formation.

Endorphins: Small molecules secreted by the brain that acts as a natural analgesic. E.g. morphine, does controlling pain.

Enzymes. Enzymes are proteins that cause certain biochemical reactions to occur. In layman terms it is the source which breaks down proteins, carbohydrate, lipids and other material in which food is made.

Fibromyalgia: A chronic, nonarticular rheumatic disease causing chronic fatigue and continuous, frequently severe muscle pain in all four quadrants of the body. Patients can become almost total debilitated and bedridden.

Free Radicals: Toxic chemical species formed from oxygen. Very aggressive and highly active attacks cell walls, membranes, and DNA, causing damage to the cell.

Glucose: A six carbon sugar (therefore a carbohydrate) that is the starting for many metabolic reactions in the body, including the anaerobic energy metabolic pathway, glycosis.

Hemoglobin: An iron containing protein found in red blood cells. Hemoglobin also transports oxygen to body tissues.

Hepatocelluar: Liver cells.

Hepatocytes: Liver cysts.

Iridology: A diagnostic tool based on the assumption that the iris can indicate the general status of internal organs. Iridology is normally used by herbalists and naturopaths.

Kirlian Photography: A process in which an image is obtained by application of a high-frequency electric field to an object so that it radiates a characteristic pattern of luminescence that is recorded on photographic film.

MediSin: Consuming, developing, or even thinking anything unnatural. Any substance that is refined, adulterated to the point of causing decay within the body. Example, white sugar , though used in many commercial food products will cause severe decay in bone tissue and colon area. Prescription drugs that treat but leave toxic side affects. Example, chemotherapy kills some cancer cells but greatly compromises the immune system. Music that is subliminal that interrupts rational thought and behavior.

Medisinner: One who promotes, markets or manufactures medisins.

Metabolic Therapy: Is a natural treatment using natural sources to correct changes in metabolisms that can be caused by disease.

Milieu: A environment or setting.

Nanotransistor: Small transistor

Naturopathic Medicine: A system of medicine that uses natural substances instead of synthetic or chemically derived drugs to treat the patient.

Partial Hysterectomy: A surgery procedure in which the fundus of the uterus is removed, but the cervix is left in place.

Petechial: A minute reddish or purple spot containing blood that appears on the skin.

Phytonutrient: Plant nutrient

Pulse Diagnosis: Considered the most important part of an Ayurvedic examination, the practice performs the diagnosis by placing three fingers on the radial pulse just below the patients wrist.

Premarin: Conjugated estrogen obtained from the urine of pregnant mares, used for HRT.

Quackery: Misleading use of untested, unproven methods to diagnose and/or treat cancer and other medical conditions. This certainly does not mean that natural therapy does not work, most of the more natural and safe applications have not been evaluated by the FDA because of political and corporate influence.

Radical Hysterectomy: Removing of the entire uterus, cervix and some of the vagina.
Sarcoma: A type of cancer that develops in connective or soft tissue, such as cartilage.

Seroconversion: Production of antibodies in response to an antigen.

Thimerosal: Water-soluble, cream-colored crystalline powder. It is 49.6% mercury by weight.

Tongue Diagnosis: The examination of the tongue in the context of its relationships to the internal organs and the eight principles. It includes the detail of tongue's body, color, coating and shape.

Xenoestrogens: Estrogens which are from outside the body and are metabolized into synthetic man-made chemicals. They disrupt hormone profiles. High exposure to these chemicals leads to breast & prostate cancer.

FOOTNOTES

Why is America's health sliding on oil?

1) Bates, C. Essential Fatty Acids and Immunity in Mental Health, Tacoma, WA. Life Science Press, 1987.

2) Brison, G.J. Lipids in Human Nutrition, Inglewood, NJ. Burgess, 1981.

3) Colgan, M Your Personal Vitamin Profile. New York. Quill Books, 1982.

The Carbotarians

1) McArdle, W, Katch, J. Essentials of Exercise Physiology. Lea & Febiger, 1998.

2) Crowe, I. The Quest for Food: Its role in human evolution and migration. Tempus, 2000.

3) L Dunne. The Nutrition Almanac, 3rd Edition (McGraw Hill; New York)

4) L Dunne. The Nutrition Almanac, 31

5) WA Price. Nutrition and Physical Degeneration (Keats Publishing; CT), 1989, 256-281.

6) RL Horst and others. Discrimination in the metabolism of orally dosed ergocalaferol and cholecaliferol by the pig, rat, and chick. Biochem J, 1982, Apr. 20:4:185-9.

7) Krispin Sullivan, CN, Personal Communication on January 3, 2002.

8) H Glerup and others. Commonly recommended daily intake of vitamin D is not sufficient if sunlight exposure is limited. J Int Med, 2000, 247:260-8.

9) K Sullivan. The Miracle of Vitamin D: Wise Traditions, 2000, 3:11-20

10) Sullivan, op cit, In Vivo Threshold for cutanous synthesis of vitamin D3 in skin. Nut Rev, 1989, 47:252-3.

11) Price, op-cit, 256-281.

12) M. Hellebosted and others. Vitamin D deficiency rickets and vitamin B12 deficiency in vegetarian children. Acta Pediatric Scand, 1985, 74:191-5.

13) J Groff and S Gropper, op cit, 317

14) WA Price, op cit

15) RG Munger and others. Prospective study of dietary protein intake and risk of hip fracture in postmenopausal women. Amer J Clin Nutr, 1999, 69:1:147-52.

16) J. Dwyer and others. Diet, indicators of kidney disease, and late mortality among older persons in the NHANES I Epidemiologic follow-up study. Amer J of Pub Health, 1994, 84 :(8):1299-1303.

17) El Wynder and others. J Natl Can Inst, 1975, 54:7

18) MG Enig. Know your fats: The Complete Primer for Understanding the Nutrition of Fats, Oils, and Cholesterol (Bethesda Press; MD), 2000, 84-85.

19) M Gaard and others. Dietary Factors and Risk of Colon Cancer: a prospective study of 50,535 young Norwegian Men and Women. Euro J Cancer Prev, 1996, 5:445-54.

20) E de Stefani and others. Meat Intake, heterocyclic amines, and risk of breast cancer: a case-control study in Uruguay. Cancer Epidemiology Biomarkers Prev, 1997, 6:573-81.

21) S. Francheschi and others. Intake of Macronutrients and Risk of breast cancer. Lancet, 1996, 347: 1351-6.

22) Why not Meat? (Part 2), Down to Earth News, (Honolulu, HI), Dec, Jan, 1998, 1-4.

23) M. Purdy. Are Organophosphate Pesticides Involved in the causation of Bovine Spongiform Encephalopathy (BSE)? J of Nutr Med, 1994, 4:43-82.

24) Ibid

25) D. Brown, BSE does not cause variant CJD: an alternative cause related to post-industrial environmental contamination. Med Hypotheses, 2001, 57:5,

26) K Sullivan. The Lectin Report accessed on January 2, 2002

27) HL Abrams. The Relevance of Paleolithic Diet in Determining Contemporary Nutritional needs. J Appl Nutr, 1979, 1, 2:43-59

Fluoride How America Really Got Brainwashed

1) Dr. John Yiamouyiannis, in interview with Gary Null, 3/10/95. His statement is referenced in the Clinical Toxicology of Commercial Products, Fifth Ed., Williams and Wilkins.

2) Joel Griffiths, "Fluoride: Commie Plot or Capitalist Ploy," Covert Action, Fall 1992, Vol. 42, p.30

3) Ibid. p.27.

4) The Fluoride Story. National Institute of Dental Research.

5) Griffiths, p.28

6) Ibid.

7) Ibid.

8) Ibid.

9) Ibid.

10) Griffiths, op.cit.

11) "H. Trendley Dean." MWWR Weekly. October 22, 1999/48(41); 935

12) The Fluoride Story

Soy: The Meatless Deception

1) P.Golbitz, "Traditional Soyfoods: Processing and Products, "J Nutr 125(1995): 570S-572S.

2) Janel L Christian, Janel L. Greger, Nutrition for Living, 4th ed. (Redwood City, CA: Benjamin Cummings, 1994): A9-A41.

3) Information about Soy and Agriculture can be found in Nutritional Anthropology (Liss, 1987) edited by Francis Johnston.

4) William Shurtleff, Akiko Aoyagi, The History of Soybeans and Soyfoods: Past, Present and Future (unpublished manuscript). Soyfoods Center, Lafayette, CA.

5) William Shurtleff, Chronology of Soymilk Worldwide: Part I: 220 A.D. to 1949, Special Exhibit, Museum of Soy (2001): www.thesoydaily-club.com/mossoymilk/mossoymilk1.asp.

6) R.A. Guy, "The Diets of Nursing Mothers and Young Children in Peiping," Chinese Med J 54, no.1 (1938): 1-30.

7) R.A. Guy, K.S. Yeh, "Roasted Soybean in Infant Feeding," Chinese Med J 54, no.2 (1938): 101-110.

8) R.A. Guy, K.S. Yeh, "Soybean 'Milk' as a Food for Young Infants," Chinese Med J 54, no.1 (1938): 1-30.

9) H.W. Miller, "Survey of Soyfoods in East Asia," Soybean Digest (June 1948):22-23. Summarized in William Shurtleff and Akiko Aoyagi, Bibliography and Sourcebook on Seventh Day Adventist, 1866-1992 (Layfayette, CA: Soyfoods Center):74.

17) David R. Erickson, Ed., Practical Handbook of Soybean Processing and Utilization (Champaign, Il: AOCS Press, 1995).

18) A. Visser, A. Thomas, "Review: Soya Protein Products-Their Processing and Utilization (Champaign, IL: AOCS Press, 1995).

19) Zeki Berk, "Technology of Production of Edible Flours and Protein Products from Soybeans, "Food and Agricultural Organization of the United Nations, Rome, and FAO Bulletin (1992):24.

20) See Note 16: 425-436.

21) Ibid.: 386-388

22) E.W. Lusas, K.C. Rhee, "Soybean Protein Processing and Utilization, in Erickson. See Note 17: 138-146.

29) N.R. Reddy, S.K. Sathe, Eds., Food Phytates (Boca Raton, FL: CRC Press, 2002).

30) R.F. Hurrell et al., "Soy Protein, Phytate and Iron Absorption in Humans, "Am J Clin Nutr 56, No.3 (1992): 573-578.

31) B. Lonnerdal et al., "Effects of Phytate Removal on Zinc Absorption from Soy Formula," Am J Clin Nutr 48, no.5 (1998): 1301-1306

32) L. Davidson et al., "Iron Bioavailability Studied in Infants: The Influence of Phytic Acid and Ascorbic Acid in Infant Formulas Based on Soy Isolate, "Pediatr Res 36, no.6 (1994): 816-822.

33) J.D. Cook et al., "The Inhibitory Effects of Soy Products on Non-Heme Absorption in Man," AM J Clin Nutr 34, no. 12 (1981):2622-2629.

34) N.S. Shaw et al., "A Vegetarian Diet Rich in Soybean Products Compromises Iron Status in Young Students," J Nutr 125 (1995): 212-219.

35) Arpad Pusztai, Plant Lectins (Cambridge University Press, 1991).

36) P. Seeman et al., "Structure of Membrane Holes in Osmotic and Saponin Hemolysis," J Cell Biol 56, no. 2 (1973): 519-527.

37) L.K. Massey et al., "Oxalate Content of Soybean Seeds (Lysine Max: Leguminous), Soyfoods and other edible Legumes, "J Agric Food Chem. 49, no.9 (2001): 4262-4266.

39) F.L. Suarez et al., "Gas Production in Humans Ingesting a Soybean Flour Derived from Beans Naturally Low in Oligosaccharides," Am J Clint Nutr 69, no.1 (1999): 135-139.

40) A. Visor, A. Thomas, "Review: Soya Protein Products, Their Processing, Functionally and Application Aspects," Food Rev Inter 3, nos. 1 & 2 (1987): 1-32.

52) "FAO Food Allergies Report of the Technical Consultation of the food and Agricultural Organization of the United Nations, Rome" (13-14 November 1995).

53) J. Bouquet et al., "Scientific Criteria and Selection of Allergenic Foods for Labeling," Allergy 53, suppl.47 (1998): 3-21.

54) Barbara Keeler, "A Nation of Lab Rats," Sierra Club Magazine (July/August 2001).

55) T. Foulard, I. Malmheden-Yman, "A Study on Severe Food Reactions in Sweden-Is Soy Protein an Underestimated Cause of Food Anaphylaxis," Allergy 53, no. 3 (1999): 261-265.

56) Letter from Ingrid Malmhedn-Ymam, PhD, Senior Chemist, Swediah National Food Administration, Livsmedels Verket to Ministry of Health in New England (30 May 1997): released under Official Information Act.

57) M. Fitzpatrick, "Soy Formulas and the Effects of Isoflavones on the Thyroid, "Inhibition of Thyroid Peroxidase by Dietary Flavonoids on the Thyroid," NZ Med J 113, no. 1103 (2000): 24-26.

58) D.R. Doerge, "Inhibition of Thyroid Peroxidase by Dietary Flavonoids," Chem. Rees Toxically 9 (1996): 16-23

59) R.L. Dive et al., Anti-Thyroid Isoflavones from Soybean," Brioche Pharmacol 54 (1997): 1087-1096.

60) Committee on Toxicology, British Food Standards Agencies (UK), Draft report of the COT Working Group on Phytoestrogens, "4: Sources and Concentrations of Phytoestrogens in Foods and Estimated Dietary Intake."

61) M.A. Jabbar et al., "Abnormal Thyroid Function Test in Infants with Congenital Hypothyroidism: The Influence of Soy-Based Formula," J Am Coll Nutr 16 (1997): 280-282.

62) See Note 57.

63) C.H.G. Irvine et al., "Phytoestrogens in Soy-Based Infant Foods: Concentrations, Daily Intake and Possible Biological Effects," Proc Soc Exp Biol Med 217 (1998): 247-253.

64) C.H.G Irvine et al., "The Potential Adverse Effects of Soybean Phytoestrogens in Infant Feeding," NZ Med J 24 (1995): 318.

65) R.M. Sharpe et al., "Infant feeding with Soy Formula Milk: Effects on the Testis and on Blood Testosterone Levels in Marmoset Monkeys during the Period of Neonatal Testicular Activity," Hum Repro 17, no.7 (2002): 1692-1703.

66) P.L. Whitten et al., "Potential Adverse Effects of Phytoestrogens," J Nutr 125 (1995): 771S-776S.

67) See Note 60. "5: Absorption, Distribution, Metabolism and Excretion of Phytoestrogens."

68) R.B. Clarkson et al., "Estrogen Soybean Isoflavones and Chronic Disease: Risks and Benefits, "Trends, Endocrinal Metab 6 (1995): 11-16.

69) R.S. Kaldas, C.L. Hughes," reproductive and General Metabolic Effects of Phytoestrogens in Mammals," Repr Toxicol 3 (1989): 81-89.

70) See Note 63.

71) R. Santti R et al., "Phytoestrogens: Potential Endocrine Disputers in Males," Toxicol Envir Health 14, nos. 1 & 2 (1998): 223-237.

72) L.S. Frawley, J.D. Neill, "Age-Related Changes in Serum Levels of Gonadotropins and Testosterone in Infantile Male Rhesus Monkeys, "Biol Repro 20 (1979): 1147-1151.

73) D.R. Mann et al., "Blockade of Neonatal Activation of the Pituitary Testicular Axis: Effect on Peripubertal Lutenizing Hormone and Testosterone Secretion and on Testicular Development in Male Monkeys, "J Chin Endocrinal Metab 68 (1989): 600-607.

74) J.S.D. Winter et al., "Pituitary-Gonadal Relations in Infancy: Patterns of Serum Gonadal Steroid Concentrations in Man from Birth to Two Years of Age," J Chin Endocrinal Metab 42 (1976): 679-686.

75) I.L. Sedimeyer, M.R. Palmert, "Delayed Puberty: Analysis of Large Case Series from an Academic Center," J Clin Endocrinal Metab 87, no.4 (2002): 1613-1620.

76) J. Huston, M. Baker, "Hormonal Control of Testicular Descent and the Cause of Cryptorchidism," Repr Fert Dev 6 (1994): 151-156.

77) R. Sharpe, N. Shakkeback, "Are Oestrogens Involved in Falling Sperm Counts and Disorders of the Male Reproductive Tract?" Lancet 341 (1993): 1292-1395.

78) J. Auger et al., "Decline in Semen Quality among Fertile Men in Paris during the Past 20 years," NEJM 332, no.5 (1995): 281-285.

79) Richard Sharpe, MD, as quoted by Aileen Ballantyne in "Why Our Men are Getting Less fertile," London Times (29 August 1995).

80) See Note 64.

81) See Note 74.

82) See Note 73

83) Herman Giddens et al., "Secondary Sexual Characteristics and Menses in Young Girls Seen in Office Practice," Pediatric Research in Office Settings Network 99, no.4 (1997): 505-512.
84) Peter Montague, "The Obscenity of Accelerated Child Development," Ecologist 28, no.3 (1993): 140-142.

85) L. Zacharias, R.J. Wurtman, "Age at Menarche," Nejm 280, no.16 (1969): 868-875.

87) See Note 64.

88) B.L. Strom et al., "Exposure to Soy-Based Formula in Infancy and Endocrinological and Reproductive Outcomes in Young Adulthood," JAMA 286, no.7 (2001): 897-814.

89) L.R. Goldman et al., "Exposure to Soy-Based Formula in Infancy," letter to the editor, JAMA 286, no. 19 (2001):2402-2403.

90) M. Silva, E.C. Reynolds, "Fluoride Content of Infant formula in Australia," Austr Dent J 41, no. 1 (1996): 37-42.

91) S.J. Fomon, J. Ekstrand, "Fluoride Intake by Infants," J Public Health Dent 59, no. 4 (1999): 229-234.

92) R. Weintraub et al., "High Aluminum Content of Content of Infant Milk Formulas." Arch Dis Child 61 (1986): 914-916.

93) W.W.K. Koo et al., "Aluminum contamination of Infant Formulas," J Parenteral Enterol Nutr 12 (1988): 170-173.

94) N.M. Hawkins et al., "Potential Aluminum Toxicity in Infants Fed Special Infant Formula, J Pediatr Gastroenterol Nutr 19, no.4 (1994): 377-381.

95) T.T. Tran et al., "Effect of High Dietary Manganese Intake of Neonatal Rats on Tissue Mineral Accumulation, Stratal Dopamine Levels and Neurodevelopment Status," Neurotoxicol 23 (2002): 635-643.

96) T.T. Trans et al., "Effects of Neonatal Dietary Manganese Exposure on Brian Dopamine Levels and Neurocognitive Function," Neurotoxicol 23 (2002): 645-651.

97) D. Stasny et al., "Manganese Intake and Serum Manganese Concentration of Human Milk-Fed and Formula Fed Infants," Am J Clin Nutr 39, no. 6 (1984): 872-878.

98) P.J. Collipp et al., "Manganese in Infant Formulas and Learning Disability," Ann Nutr Metab 27 (1983): 488-494.

111) D.M. Sheehan, "Isoflavone Content of Breast Milk and Soy Formulas: Benefits and Risks," letter to the editor, Clin Chem 43 (1997): 850.

BIBLIOGRAPHY

Medical Sins I

Bealle, Morris A., The New Drug story, Wash D.C. Columbia Publishing Co., 1958

Braithwaite, John. Corporate Crime in the Pharmaceutical industry, London, Routledge & Kegan

Edward G., World Without Cancer, fourteenth printing, April, 1999.

Mullins, Eustice, Murder by Injection, Third Printing, 1995

Medical Sins II

Carter, James P., M.D., Dr P.H., Racketeering in Medicine

Erasmus, Udo, Fats that Heal Fats that Kill, Alive Books, 1997

Jafari, Annahita, N.D., Lecture, at the Kitchen Physician School of Natural healing, 1996

Kushi, Miichio, with Jack, Alex, the Book of Macrobiotics, Fifth Printing, July 1994.

Love George X. OMD, Lac. Lecture at the "Kitchen Physician of Natural Healing", 1995

Price, Weston A. DDS. Nutrition and physical Degeneration, 6th Edition, 1998.

Robbins, John. Reclaiming Our Health, 1996.

Medical Sins III

Alfie Kohn, "Suffer the Restless Children", Atlantic Monthly, Nov, 1989, p. 98

Amy O'Conner In the news, Vegetarian Times, Oct. 1995, p. 20

Beckham, Nancy, "Why Women Should Not Take HRT", Wellbeing Magazine

Breggin, Peter Toxic Psychiatry (New York: St. Martin's Press, 1991)

Editorial, "Hyperactivity in Childhood", New England Journal of Medicine, 323, Nov.15, 1990.

Ellerbrook, J.M., Lee, J.A.H. "Oral contraceptives and malignant melanoma", Journal of the American Medical Association, 1968.

Gerson, Max, M.D., A Cancer Therapy, 1946.
Goldberg, Burton, The Alternative Medicine Guide, 1992

Goldberg, Burton, Alternative Medicine Guide to Heart Disease, 1997.

Heart Protection Study Collaborative Group. Lancet 2002; 360:7-22.

Kushi, Michio, with Jack Alex, Crime and Diet, Fifth printing, 1997.

Lee, John R., MD What your doctor many not tell you about menopause, Warner Books, New York, 1996

Llaila O. Afrika, African Holistic Health, Fifth Edition, 2004
McCully, K.S. "Homocyteine Theory of Arteriosclerosis: Develop and Current Status" Atherosclerosis Reviews 11 (1983) 157-246.

Moss, Ralph, The Cancer Industry, Revised 1989.

Newman TB, Hulley SB. JAMA 1996; 27:55-60

Passwater, Richard. Supernutrition for Healthy Hearts (New York Dial Press, 1977; Gordon, T., et al. American Journal of Medicine 62.

Rapp, Doris, Is this your child? (New York: William Morrow, 1991

Robbins, John, Reclaiming our Health, 1996.

Sacks FM and others. N Eng J Med 1996; 385; 1001-1009.

Sellman, Sherril, Hormone Heresy, Third Edition 2000.

Whitaker, Julian, M.D., "Heart Surgery Does More Harm than Good." Dr. Julian Whitaker's Health & Healing 7:5 (May 1997) 1-3.

Nutritional Dogma IV

Blaylock, Russell L. MD, Excitotoxins, 1994

Goldberg, Burton, The Alternative Medicine Guide to Weight Loss, 2000.

Kushi, Michio, with Jack Alex, The Book of Microbiotics, 1994.

Kushi, Michio, "Crime and Diet",

Llaila O., Afrika, Afrikan Holistic Health, Fifth Edition, 2004
Malkus, George H., "Why Christians get Sick", Fifteen Printing, 2001.

Nutritional Dogma V

Jensen, Bernard, DC., Tissue Cleansing through Bowel Management, 1981.

Kushi, Michio, Jack, Alex, the Book of Macrobiotics, 1997.

Lee, Lita, Ph.D., Radiation Protection Manual

Malkus, Dr. George H., "Why Christians Get Sick", 2001.

Mullins, Eustice, Murder by Injection, 1995.

Teitel, Martin, Ph.D., Wilson, Kimberly A., Genetic Engineered Foods, 1999.

Vanderhaeghe, Lorna R. and Bouic, Patrick, J.D., Ph.D., "The Immune system Cure", 2000.

Solutions VI

Fratkin, Jake Chinese Herbal Patent Formulas, Eight printing 1995.

Heinerman, John, Ph.D., Health Secrets from the Ancient World, 1991.

Kushi, Michio, and Jack Alex, The Macrobiotic Book, 1997.

Love, George X. OMD., LAC Lecture, 1995.

Morton, Mary, Five Steps to Selecting the best Alternative medicine, 1996.

Reid, Daniel, The Complete Book of Chinese health and healing, 1994.

Reid, Daniel, the Tao of Sex and Longevity, 1989.

Teeguarden, Ron, Master Herbalist, Radiant Health, 1998.